Recent Results in Cancer Research 81

Fortschritte der Krebsforschung
Progrès dans les recherches sur le cancer

H.-P. Lohrmann W. Schreml

Cytotoxic Drugs and the Granulopoietic System

With 6 Figures and 87 Tables

Springer-Verlag
Berlin Heidelberg New York 1982

Priv.-Doz. Dr. Hans-Peter Lohrmann
Priv.-Doz. Dr. Wolfgang Schreml

Universität Ulm, Zentrum für Innere Medizin
Abteilung Innere Medizin III (Hämatologie/Onkologie)
Steinhövelstrasse 9, D-7900 Ulm, Germany

Sponsored by the Swiss League against Cancer

ISBN-13: 978-3-642-81692-5 e-ISBN-13: 978-3-642-81690-1
DOI: 10.1007/978-3-642-81690-1

Library of Congress Cataloging in Publication Data. Lohrmann, H.-P. (Hans-Peter), 1943 – Cytotoxic drugs and the granulopoietic system. (Recent results in cancer research; 81) Bibliography: p. Includes index. 1. Marrow-Effect of drugs on. 2. Antineoplastic agents-Physiological effect. 3. Antineoplastic agents-Toxicology. 4. Granulocytes. I. Schreml, W. (Wolfgang), 1937. II. Title. III. Series: [DNLM: 1. Granulocytes-Drug effects. 2. Antineoplastic agents-Toxicity. 3. Hematopoietic system-Drug effects. W1 RE106P v. 81 / WH 200 L833c] RC261.R35 vol. 81 [RC645.7] 615'.7 81–9316 AACR2

Softcover reprint of the hardcover 1st edition 1982

2125/3140–543210

To our wives and our patients

Contents

1 Introduction

Since cytotoxic drugs were first developed, their damaging effects on bone marrow have attracted considerable interest. We now know that the bone marrow is an organ with rapid cell renewal in which maintenance of the steady-state depends on a high rate of cell production, and that the bone marrow toxicity of cytotoxic agents can be explained by the perturbation of such steady-state conditions. Experimental researchers have analysed in detail the effects of cytotoxic agents upon defined hematopoietic cell populations to define the mechanism of action and the location within the cell cycle at which cytotoxic drugs exert their cytocidal action. From such studies, a classification of cytotoxic agents according to their action upon cells during different phases of the cell cycle has been proposed [80–82]. Others have used the acute perturbation of the hematopoietic systems, caused by application of single high doses of cytotoxic agents, to analyse the patterns of depletion and reconstitution of the various hematopoietic compartments in an effort to shed light on the regulatory mechanisms that are responsible for the delicately balanced cell production of the hematopoietic cell renewal systems. A great deal of information on the structure of the hematopoietic systems has come from such studies, and kinetic parameters of these systems have been defined.

To clinicians, the hematopoietic toxicity of antineoplastic agents has been an undesired though unavoidable side effect of almost all cytotoxic drugs introduced into clinical practice. Although these agents show toxicity to other organs as well, it is the toxicity to the bone marrow which usually limits maximal single doses or determines the minimum time interval between successive treatment courses. Since cytotoxic drug-induced bone marrow failure may be quite severe and life-threatening, dosage adjustments based on peripheral blood counts are an integral part of any study protocol of newly introduced cytotoxic drugs. Careful monitoring of the peripheral blood count has become the routine way to assess bone marrow toxicity of cytotoxic drugs, and to determine the time when recovery allows a new course of treatment to be administered.

The introduction of new and potent anticancer agents and the application of combination chemotherapy, not only to hematologic malignancies but also to solid tumors, has led to a tremendous increase in the use of cytotoxic drugs in clinical practice. More recently, these drugs have been used prophylactically following local treatment modalities, such as surgery and/or radiotherapy of solid tumors ("adjuvant chemotherapy"), in an attempt to eradicate micrometastatic disease. However, this increased use of cytotoxic drugs is not matched by similarly improved understanding of the side effects of such treatment. In this respect, a better understanding of the acute toxicity to the bone marrow with depletion and repletion of the different bone marrow compartments is of obvious importance. Furthermore, clinical phenomena such as the delayed toxicity of some drugs or the occasional occurrence of cumulative toxicity require better understanding. Moreover, in view of ongoing adjuvant chemotherapy studies, the problem of residual marrow damage, persisting after completion of chemotherapy, appears to be of utmost importance. Unfortunately, until recently these problems have attracted little attention, although the methodology to study them is at hand.

Such methodological progress has come from animal studies. Here, an assay has been developed to quantitatively and qualitatively analyse the pluripotent hematopoietic stem cells. Unfortunately, in spite of great efforts, an established assay system for the human pluripotent stem cell is still not realized. However, the in vitro analysis of committed granulopoietic and erythropoietic stem cells has been adopted for the human situation, thus giving us a powerful tool for the study of early, morphologically nonidentifiable hematopoietic cell populations. These techniques have been widely used to approach pathophysiologic questions of human hematologic malignancies, and to better understand the changes accompanying successful treatment of these disorders. Furthermore, hematologic disorders characterized by bone marrow failure, such as aplastic anemia or acute agranulocytosis, have been studied in this way. However, amazingly little work has been done to clarify one of the most frequently encountered forms of human bone marrow failure, namely that following cytotoxic drug exposure.

As Marsh [367] has pointed out, the major difficulty in reviewing the literature on the effects of cytotoxic drugs upon the granulopoietic system is that few, if any data are strictly comparable to other authors' work. When attempts are made to interpret reported results, a great number of variables, such as species, strain, sex, and age, must be considered. The routes of administration vary, as do the doses employed or the time intervals at which drugs are given. With respect to stem cell assays, the source of the cells to be assayed varies: In animals, stem cells within the bone marrow may behave differently than spleen-derived stem cells. The in vitro processing of cells may also affect the data, and the details of the stem cell assays are critical. In dose-survival studies, the exact time interval between application of the cytotoxic drug and the assay of the surviving stem cell fraction is a major cause of varying results. On the other hand, when morphological criteria are used to assess changes in the bone marrow or the peripheral blood, few difficulties should be encountered. Functional assays, such as the measurement of the functional bone marrow granulocyte reserve, again vary with the methodology used.

It is exceedingly difficult to maintain an overview of the vast literature on the effect of cytotoxic agents upon the hematopoietic system, since this work is distributed throughout the experimental and clinical hematologic and oncologic literature. Although much data has been accumulated from both experimental and clinical studies, these data are usually restricted to certain aspects of the effect of cytotoxic drugs on the granulopoietic system, depending on the intentions of the respective studies and on the methodology of the scientists.

Working on the problem of hematopoietic toxicity of cytotoxic drugs in human beings, we felt that a comprehensive review of the known effects of cytotoxic agents upon the granulopoietic system of both experimental animals and human beings would be of value. We decided to provide such a review, thereby allowing others to gain rapid and in-depth insight into the granulopoietic toxicity of cytotoxic agents. It was the aim of our book to collect the data scattered throughout the literature and integrate them into a systematic description of the effects of cytotoxic agents on granulopoiesis. These data are presented for individual cytotoxic agents and the various compartments of the granulopoietic system are discussed separately. The data are presented in tables whenever possible to provide easy access to the information discussed in the text. For some drugs, a rather complete picture of the effect on granulopoiesis can thus be drawn, while, in other cases, only a few aspects have been investigated. Some agents have been used extensively in experimental hematology to induce synchronization or to define the fraction of cells in a specific phase of the cell cycle. At the same time, the clinical application of these drugs may be restricted. On the other hand, some cytotoxic drugs have been tested in preclinical and clinical trials only, and animal data on the effect on the pluripotent or committed stem cells are scarce.

In the second part of this book, we have reviewed the data with respect to more general questions. These subjects are taken from both experimental and clinical hematology: What can be learned of structure, function, and regulation of the granulopoietic system from its response to cytotoxic agents? Are there parameters of predictive value for individual sensitivity to cytotoxic drugs? How can the effect of cytotoxic drugs be ameliorated by nonspecific modulators? What do we know about late bone marrow damage after cytotoxic drug exposure?

The large amount of original material made certain restrictions unavoidable. Toxicity data from clinical studies were selected for review only when detailed results were given. Frequently, only qualitative descriptions of hematopoietic toxicity were reported in the original papers, and these are not analysed here. Similarly, all reports on the hematopoietic toxicity of antineoplastic agents were disregarded when these drugs had been given to recipients pretreated with other cytotoxic drugs or with ionizing radiation. The cytotoxic drug-induced changes of colony-stimulating activity are an interesting problem, but this field of research could not be addressed within the framework of this book.

We hope that this book will provide helpful information for experimental researchers or clinicians using cytotoxic agents, that it may stimulate further research in this field, and that it may contribute to a critical and thoughtful use of these drugs so as to limit the extent of unavoidable toxicity.

2 Structure and Physiology of the Granulopoietic System

The delineation of the structure of the granulopoietic system and the measurement of its normal kinetics have seen major progress in the past two decades. Until not long ago, our knowledge of the granulopoietic system was based almost exclusively on morphological observations: The composition and morphology of the bone marrow cells were studied under normal conditions and in various diseases. Careful studies performed under certain clinical conditions, such as the recovery phase of acute agranulocytosis, have yielded an astonishing amount of information. However, major progress in this field has come from the introduction of techniques using radioisotopes, such as ^{3}H-thymidine or diisopropyl fluorophosphate (DFP^{32}), and the development of stem cell assays. These studies offer detailed information on the structure and physiology of the granulopoietic system. Excellent reviews of this subject have appeared previously [103, 134, 197, 203, 337, 347, 488, 562, 563, 586]. Here, an admittedly superficial outline of current concepts will be given, since an understanding of the structure and physiology of the granulopoietic system is essential for a detailed discussion of the effects of cytotoxic drugs upon this system.

Schematically, the granulopoietic system is composed of a sequential series of cellular compartments whose constituent cells differ from each other by morphological, functional, and/or operational criteria. Most of these compartments are located within the bone marrow (and, in rodents, in the spleen). However, the most mature cells circulate in the peripheral blood (and migrate into the tissues), and a small proportion of stem cells also circulate in the peripheral blood.

The most immature compartment is that of the pluripotent stem cells, which by definition are capable of both replication and differentiation into the granulopoietic, erythropoietic, and megakaryocytic cell lines. This means that, to maintain the pluripotent stem cell pool size, one stem cell must form for each stem cell differentiating into one of the subsequent compartments. Morphologically, these pluripotent stem cells most likely resemble small lymphocytes [59, 252, 644]. Experimentally, pluripotent stem cells are assayed by the spleen colony technique, which has been worked out in rodents (see page 9). Pluripotent stem cells are responsible for bone marrow repopulation after marrow-ablative treatment. Thus, the behavior of pluripotent stem cells is of utmost importance for the overall reaction of the granulopoietic system to cytotoxic drugs. In rodents, pluripotent stem cells are found in bone marrow and spleen, whereas they are restricted to the marrow in higher mammals. In addition, there is evidence that pluripotent stem cells circulate in the peripheral blood in all mammalian species.

Pluripotent stem cells, as defined by the spleen colony assay, do not form a homogenous population. Rather, the pluripotent stem cell pool is composed of a heterogenous group of cells all fulfilling the definition of a pluripotent stem cell, but nevertheless differing in important aspects. Thus, recent work [56, 67, 281] indicates that pluripotent stem cells possess different degrees of "stemness", i.e., they differ with respect to their replicative potential and proliferative activity (see also page 178). Overall, the pluripotent stem cells have a low proliferative activity under steady-state conditions: The proportion of pluripotent stem cells in S-phase of the cell cycle (measured by the ^{3}H-thymidine suicide technique or in vivo by hydroxyurea treatment) has been reported to be less than 20% [23, 44, 620]. However, radiation experiments or transplantation procedures have clearly documented that pluripotent stem cells can rapidly increase their proliferative activity, in response to a pool depletion, so as to normalize their compartment size [133, 155, 227, 420, 421, 466, 628].

It has been suggested that the bone marrow cell production is geared to the cellularity of discrete marrow areas [452]. Later, the same group of workers [366] has postulated that the mechanism for maintenance of a normal pluripotent stem cell compartment size in the bone marrow is mere population size control, where the density (i.e., the mean distance) of stem cells determines stem cell proliferation. Others [420] have postulated that the number of pluripotent stem cells in S-phase of the cell cycle controls the entry of G_0 stem cells into the active cycle. Experimental work has suggested the existence of short-range humoral factors involved in stem cell proliferation control [359, 360].
A minimum size of the pluripotent stem cell compartment appears to be required for differentiation of these cells into the subsequent cellular compartments. If the size of the pluripotent stem cell pool falls below a certain critical value (in mice, values around 10% have been determined experimentally [109]), then self-replication, without simultaneous differentiation of pluripotent stem cells, appears to occur until the threshold compartment size is reestablished. This shift from differentiation to self-replication may be considered a protective mechanism that prevents "burning-out" of the vital pluripotent stem cell pool.
"Committed" stem cells are considered to be the immediate progeny of pluripotent stem cells [379]. By present definition, committed stem cells have only a small capacity for self-replication. The major difference from the pluripotent stem cells is that commitment to one of the hematopoietic cell lines has taken place by mechanisms that are still poorly understood. Following commitment, a committed stem cell can give rise to cells of only one specific pathway of hematopoietic differentiation. For example, a stem cell committed to granulopoiesis can only produce granulocytic cells, but not cells of the erythropoietic or megakaryocytic series. Committed stem cells are assayed by in vitro culture methods: Stem cells committed to granulopoiesis have been defined operationally to be those cells giving rise to granulocytic/macrophage colonies in vitro (see page 10).

Committed stem cells are again located in the bone marrow and spleen of rodents, but are restricted to marrow in higher mammals. Furthermore, committed hematopoietic stem cells are found in the peripheral blood. Committed granulopoietic stem cells still resemble small lymphocytes morphologically, although they can be separated physically from pluripotent stem cells [266, 641]. Committed granulopoietic stem cells proliferate actively. Even under steady-state conditions, the majority of the committed granulocytic cells appear to be in an active cell cycle [298, 378]. Thus, values of 50% for the S-phase fraction of colony-forming units (culture) (CFU-C) have been reported for mice, while in humans, this value has been determined to be around 45% [348]. The difference in proliferative activity between CFU-spleen (CFU-S) and CFU-C is a very important point when cells are exposed to cytotoxic drugs in vivo, since the cytocidal action of these agents is often critically dependent upon the proliferative state of the cells upon which they act (see page 158).

Differentiation of the committed hematopoietic stem cells (and of the ensuing morphologically identifiable proliferating cell compartments) is considered to be primarily humorally controlled by pathway-specific hormonelike substances. In the erythropoietic cell line, this hormone is erythropoietin and, in the granulocytic system, colony-stimulating factor is the prime candidate for such a hormonal regulator (for review, see [337, 379]). In vivo, the regulation of the proliferation of CFU-C may also be controlled by specific inhibitors (more recently it has been suggested that macrophage-derived prostaglandins play such a role [331, 332]). Through differentiation, the progeny of the committed granulopoietic stem cells acquire morphological characteristics making them recognizable as part of the granulocytic system (i.e., the features typical of myeloblasts and promyelocytes). Further maturation leads to the acquisition of neutrophilic granulation and to loss of the early acidophilic granulation.

Among the morphologically identifiable granulocytic cells, an important feature is that only the early forms (myeloblast, promyelocyte, and myelocyte) continue to be capable of cellular division. Once a cell has reached the metamyelocyte stage, it has lost this capacity for division. From this point on, only maturation occurs until the stage of the mature end cell (the neutrophil) is reached. This insight has come from studies using ^{3}H-thymidine (^{3}H-TdR) as a label of newly formed DNA [135] and has led to the division of the morphologically identifiable granulocytic cells of the bone marrow into a proliferating compartment and a maturing, nonproliferating compartment. Kinetic studies indicate the transit time from myeloblast to segmented neutrophil to be 8–10 days in humans. A detailed discussion of granulopoietic system kinetics is beyond the scope of this brief review, particularly since kinetics vary with species. It should be mentioned, however, that the granulocytic system is a rapidly renewing system: To maintain an equilibrium and steady-state, compensating for the high peripheral cell loss, a continuously high rate of cell production is necessary. In man, for example, the total granulocyte turnover rate has been measured to be around 1.7×10^9 cells/kg/day. Since the total peripheral blood granulocyte pool is somewhere around 0.7×10^9/kg, a neutrophil number equivalent to approximately 2.5-times the actual peripheral blood pool size is produced every day to maintain the normal peripheral blood granulocyte concentration. From these considerations, it can be easily understood that any major and long-lasting reduction in granulocyte production will invariably lead to a decrease of the peripheral blood granulocyte concentration, since under these circumstances the cell migration from the blood into tissues will not be matched by sufficient cell production and neutrophil entry from the bone marrow into the blood.

There is one protective mechanism which prevents a minor or short-lived decrease in granulocyte production from immediately affecting the peripheral blood granulocyte concentration. As part of the granulocytic maturation compartment, segmented neutrophils, amounting to as many as 2.5×10^9/kg in man in the steady-state [159, 160], are in the bone marrow awaiting release into the peripheral blood. These marrow segmented neutrophils form the "bone marrow neutrophil storage pool" ("bone marrow granulocyte reserve") upon which the body can draw in a situation of acute neutrophil need. This buffer function between granulocyte production and peripheral granulocyte demand explains why minor short-lived reductions in granulocyte production remain unnoticed when only the peripheral blood granulocyte concentration is monitored. Methods for an estimate of the size of the bone marrow granulocyte storage pool have been developed (see page 12).

Transit through the maturing granulocytic bone marrow compartment appears to proceed in an orderly fashion ("first in, first out"). Egress of mature segmented neutrophils from the bone marrow into peripheral blood appears to be facilitated by an increase in cell surface deformability during maturation to the stage of the segmented neutrophil [345]. However, once a neutrophil has entered the peripheral blood, cell loss by migration into the tissues occurs at random, with a mean intravascular neutrophil half-life ($T_{1/2}$) of 6.7 h (more recently, 25 h has been measured [560]). There appears to be no return of neutrophils from the blood into the marrow, or from the tissues into the blood.

In the peripheral blood, approximately one-half of the neutrophils are marginated to the walls of small blood vessels. There is a continuous rapid exchange between these marginated and the circulating granulocytes. Since the granulocyte count determines the circulating neutrophils only, it underestimates the total number of peripheral blood neutrophils. However, there appears to be no major shift in the relation between marginated and circulating neutrophilic granulocytes in neutropenic states, althoug this question has been insufficiently studied.

From these brief considerations, it is clear that the granulopoietic system is structured as a hierarchy. Within the first three compartments (the pluripotent stem cell compartment, the compartment of committed stem cells, and the proliferating granulocytic pool), proliferation and amplification within each compartment occur. At the same time, differentiation takes place. Once the cells have lost their ability to proliferate, only maturation occurs until the functional end cell, i.e., the segmented neutrophil, is formed. The neutrophil is retained in the bone marrow for 1 or 2 days, than released into the peripheral blood before it migrates into the tissues.

The granulocytic system is regulated such that the formation of new granulocytes meets the peripheral demand for this cell type. For example, under normal steady-state conditions, considerably fewer segmented neutrophils are formed than during an episode of severe bacterial infection. The mechanisms controlling cell formation at any point within the hierarchy of the granulopoietic system are so far only partially understood. From the available evidence, it is clear that humoral factors act at the level of the committed stem cell, thereby increasing or reducing proliferation and amplification within and cell output from this compartment. Colony-stimulating factors, possibly from different sources (such as macrophages or endothelium), appear to be the major stimulating factors acting on committed granulopoietic stem cells. Inhibiting factors, such as prostaglandins, have been described [331, 332], but their regulatory role in vivo is even less well defined than that of colony-stimulating factor(s). As mentioned above, the proliferation within the pluripotent stem cell compartment appears to be mainly locally controlled, i.e., microenvironment-dependent.

Neutropenia of the peripheral blood can be brought about by one of three mechanisms which may be operative in combination: (1) Decreased granulocyte production, so that a new equilibrium between cell influx into the blood and cell efflux from blood into tissues must be established at lower peripheral blood granulocyte concentrations; (2) a shift between marginated and circulating granulocyte pools, the marginated pool growing at the expense of the circulating pool; and (3) increased destruction of neutrophils which cannot be compensated for by a sufficiently increased neutrophil production. With respect to the toxicity of chemotherapeutic agents upon the granulopoietic system, mechanism (1) is the major cause of peripheral blood neutropenia.

A very special problem is posed by the circulation of hematopoietic stem cells in the peripheral blood. The existence of such circulating stem cells has been strongly suggested by observations of bone marrow repopulation by peripheral blood leukocytes [105, 235]. More directly, CFU-S have been demonstrated in the peripheral blood. The circulation of CFU-C and of in vitro erythropoietic burst-forming units (BFU-E) may indicate that pluripotent stem cells are also present in human peripheral blood. Although debated by some authors [383], circulating stem cells may form a link between the various marrow locations, and thus allow the marrow to react uniformly if a local marrow insult should occur.

Although it appears reasonable to assume regulation of peripheral blood stem cells, the relationship between the stem cell pools in the bone marrow and the peripheral blood is only recently being unveiled. There is some evidence that peripheral blood stem cells do not represent the whole spectrum of their bone marrow counterparts. Rather, it appears that the capacity for transit to the peripheral blood is restricted to subpopulations of the bone marrow stem cell compartments. Experimental evidence suggests that the peripheral blood stem cells have a high turnover rate, since they rapidly return to extravascular sites. On the other hand, the peripheral blood stem cell pools appear to mirror, to some extent, the changes in the respective bone marrow compartments: A decrease in the peripheral blood stem cell pool size reflects a reduced bone marrow stem cell compartment size, and the opposite is true for an increase in the peripheral blood stem cell pool size. However, there are reasons to believe that this correlation is not linear [560a].

3 Some Methods Used to Study the Granulopoietic System

In this chapter, a brief survey of the methods used by experimental and clinical researchers is given to facilitate those unfamiliar with the terminology used by hematologists. It is not our intention to give a comprehensive, in-depth description and discussion of the assay methods, or their problems and limitations. Readers interested in the subject are referred to more detailed reviews [379, 563].

3.1 Pluripotent Stem Cell Assay (CFU-S Assay)

Assays for pluripotent hematopoietic stem cells have used the reconstitution of hematopoietic functions following grafting of isologous bone marrow into irradiated recipients (radioprotection assay, erythropoietic repopulation assay, granulopoietic repopulation assay) (for review, see [336]). The shortcoming of these assays is that not only pluripotent stem cells, but also more differentiated cell types with limited proliferation potential (such as committed stem cells) may give – at least abortive – rise to marrow reconstitution. Therefore, these assays do not allow quantification of pluripotent stem cells.

A major breakthroug in experimental hematology has been the development by Till and McCulloch [587] of what is now called the exogenous spleen colony assay. If a suitable number of hemopoietic cells (from bone marrow, spleen, or peripheral blood) is injected i.v. into lethally irradiated isogeneic mice or rats, nodules (colonies) will be found in the spleen of these recipients some 10 days later. A linear relationship exists between the number of cells injected and the number of spleen colonies on day 10. Colonies originate from a single cell (i.e., they are clonal in development) and they contain cells of the erythroid, granulocytic, and megakaryocytic series. Thus, the cells forming spleen colonies are pluripotent; these CFU-S have a high potential for proliferation and differentiation, and they are considered to represent pluripotent hemopoietic stem cells. Of the CFU-S injected, only a certain porportion (expressed as the *f*-fraction) will seed into the spleen and form colonies. However, this proportion can be assayed (10–20%), and the number of CFU-S can therefore be accurately determined in a given sample. Usually, the *f*-factor is assumed to be constant, but it may change following experimental manipulations [212].

Usually, the number of spleen colonies remains constant 8–13 days after transfer of CFU-S into the recipient mice, therefore, spleen colonies are generally enumerated 10 days after injection. However, evidence exists that the kinetics of the development of spleen colonies from normal marrow may be different from those seen after transfer of cytotoxic drug-pretreated marrow [287]. Thus, bone marrow removed following administration of 5-fluorouracil (5-FU) leads to rapidly increasing numbers of spleen colonies 8–13 days after cell inoculation. Furthermore, CFU-S from 5-FU-pretreated bone marrow have been shown to home preferentially in the bone marrow [287]. Although other cytotoxic agents have not been studied in a similar way, the possibility exists that at least some of them may similarly affect the homing and the growth kinetics of CFU-S in bone marrow and spleen, respectively. In these cases, the usual technique of assaying CFU-S (enumeration of colonies on day 10 after cell transfer) will underestimate the true incidence of CFU-S in the cellular inoculum.

3.2 Stem Cells Committed to Granulopoiesis (Granulopoietic Progenitor Cells) (CFU-C)

Using semisolid culture media, such as agar, the in vitro culture of rodent [70, 461] and human [456] hematopoietic tissue has been reported. In this culture system, colonies develop that are composed of granulocytic cells at different stages of maturation, and/or macrophages. A detailed analysis of this culture system has been given recently [379], consequently, a brief summary appears sufficient.
The in vitro development of granulocyte/macrophage colonies is possible from all hemopoietic tissues (such as bone marrow, spleen, or blood). In vitro colony formation is absolutely dependent upon the presence of one or several glycoproteins which are operationally called colony-stimulating factor(s) (CSF). CSF may be obtained from different sources. For human cultures, peripheral blood monocytes [110, 274, 399] and human placenta-conditioned medium [90, 352] have been the major sources of CSF. CSF must be present during the entire culture period, and colony formation is dose-dependent. The formation of granulocyte/macrophage colonies is clonal, i.e., each colony originates from one single cell. Operationally, this cell is called the colony-forming unit (culture) (CFU-C); more recently, the term granulocyte-macrophage colony-forming cell (GM-CFC) has been proposed [379]. CFU-C are considered to be stem cells committed to granulopoiesis. Within the hierarchy of the granulopoietic system, they are positioned between CFU-S and the earliest morphologically identifiable granulocytic cells.

3.3 Agar-Diffusion-Chamber Progenitor Cells

Gordon et al. [241] proposed a modification of the in vitro agar colony assay: Millipore diffusion chambers are filled with a culture medium containing the cells to be assayed plus agar; after the medium has gelled, the Millipore chambers are implanted into the peritoneal cavity of irradiated mice. After 8–9 days, the chambers are removed and the number of granulocyte/macrophage colonies is enumerated. The cells giving rise to these colonies most likely are identical to in vitro CFU-C, although this has not been proven. The major difference of the agar diffusion-chamber technique appears to be that CSF is provided by the host mouse, permitting stable and reproducible culture conditions. However, the major advantage appears to be that human CFU-C can be exposed to cytotoxic agents in vivo, thus allowing studies that cannot be performed in man. Since the method is expensive and time-consuming, meaningful application of the technique appears to be restricted to this experimental question.

3.4 Sensitivity Studies

The sensitivity of pluripotent or committed stem cells can be studied in vivo from the fraction of stem cells surviving administration of a cytotoxic agent. To obtain a dose-survival curve, different doses of the drug are studied. The time interval between drug administration and removal of the target tissue under study (marrow, spleen, blood) for stem cell assay is of critical importance. Dose-survival curves may differ with different time intervals, and they may also vary with different strains and/or species.

For the study of in vitro sensitivity of stem cells to cytotoxic drugs, a suspension of target tissue cells (i.e., a bone marrow or spleen cell suspension) is incubated in vitro at different concentrations of the drug to be tested (this, of course, is not feasible if an agent, such as cyclophosphamide, acquires cytotoxic properties only after in vivo activation). Following in vitro incubation, the cells are washed to remove the cytotoxic agent, whereupon the fraction of stem cells surviving in vitro treatment is determined using the appropriate assay. Sham-incubated cell suspensions usually serve as controls. Duration of exposure and the temperature at which the incubation procedure is performed will influence the results of such in vitro sensitivity studies.

An exponential shape of a dose-survival curve indicates that the cytotoxic agent exerts its cytocidal action upon stem cells regardless of their location within the cell cycle at the time of exposure. However, if the dose-survival curve reaches a plateau beyond a drug concentration, this indicates that the stem cells studied are insensitive to the agent tested in one or more phases of the cell cycle. A "shoulder" at low concentrations of the drug usually is interpreted as an indication of the cells' limited potential to repair the cytotoxic drug-induced damage.

In those cases where cell survival decreases in exponential fashion with increasing drug doses, dose-response curves can be described in mathematical terms. Difficulties in comparing the results of various investigators arise from the different ways to express the data of exponential cell killing. The terms $D_{1/2}$, D_{10}, and D_0 are used, describing the dose of drug to reduce the cell population under study to 50%, 10%, or 37% of control values. In some studies, the exponential line is fitted to the experimental data by mathematical procedures, in others, the curve is drawn by eye. As a rule, the D values are taken from the exponential part of the curve. A shoulder at low doses or an extrapolation number below 100% survival may be present. Thus, when D values are taken directly from the experimental curve, the data are only comparable when the exponential line originates at the 100% survival point.

Despite these restrictions, the exponential character of a dose-response curve offers a more adequate comparison of data: The published data can be transformed and expressed as a uniform parameter, for instance $D_{1/2}$. This transformation can be made from given numbers, extrapolated from graphs, or even estimated from a single dose-survival point, given its position on an exponential curve.

3.5 Recovery Studies

The pattern of depletion and repletion within the different granulopoietic compartments following cytotoxic drug exposure is usually determined as follows: A cytotoxic agent is administered at a given dose-schedule and, at predetermined time intervals thereafter, the hematopoietic target tissue(s) (bone marrow, spleen, blood) are removed for assay. Assay results are expressed per organ (i.e., per spleen, per femur), and normalized according to results of simultaneously assayed sham-treated controls. Using this procedure, the quantitative changes with time following cytotoxic drug exposure may be analysed.

3.6 Proliferative Activity of Stem Cells

For the study of the proliferative activity of hematopoietic pluripotent or committed stem cells, different experimental approaches have been used. All assays are based on the selective kill of DNA-synthesizing cells in S-phase of the cell cycle. Since the fraction of cells in S-phase of the cell cycle reflects the proliferative activity of the particular cell type, determination of this fraction provides a useful estimate of cellular proliferative activity.

In vivo Methods. S-Phase-specific cytocidal agents with a short biologic half-life, such as hydroxyurea (for details see page 121) or cytosine-arabinoside, have been used for selective kill of stem cells in the DNA-doubling phase of the cell cycle. The greater the fraction of cells in S-phase at the time of drug administration, the greater will be the relative reduction of stem cells when the appropriate assay is subsequently performed. As controls, animals pretreated in an identical manner, but not exposed to the S-phase-specific agent are used.

In vitro Methods. Again, the fraction of stem cells killed by in vitro exposure to an S-phase-specific cytotoxic agent is measured. For in vitro incubation, hydroxyurea has been used, and cytosine-arabinoside has been applied. However, the agent most widely used for this purpose is tritiated thymidine (^{3}H-TdR) of high specific activity. It is generally accepted that the loss of colony-forming capacity by CFU-S or CFU-C after pulse-labelling with ^{3}H-TdR of high specific activity is a consequence of the uptake of the label into DNA by cells in S-phase during the exposure period [163, 298]. Obviously, the heavy self-irradiation of the cell nucleus, resulting from incorporation of the label into nuclear material, causes this loss of proliferative capacity or possibly even cell death. The "thymidine suicide" fraction is therefore taken as a measure of the proliferative state of the cell population under study. Increased suicide fractions indicate a shortened cell-cycle length relative to the S-phase length, and/or an increased percentage of the cell under study being in active cell cycle (i.e., a higher growth fraction).

3.7 "Rapidly Proliferating" Stem Cells

The most widely used method for induction of rapid proliferation of pluripotent and committed stem cells is the transplantation of isologous bone marrow into lethally irradiated hosts. In these recipient animals, an exponentially increasing number of stem cells may be found in marrow and spleen after a short period [628]. During this exponential growth phase, the major part (if not all) of the stem cells are in active cell cycle, therefore, this situation allows study of the properties of rapidly proliferating stem cells. Other sources of rapidly proliferating stem cells are the continuously irradiated animal or the animal after endotoxin-treatment.

3.8 Functional Bone Marrow Granulocyte Reserve

Newly formed bone marrow granulocytes are not immediately released into the circulating blood under normal conditions. Rather, they remain in the bone marrow for another 2–3 days during which time surface changes may lead to greater deformability of the cells [345]. The granulocytes thus accumulating within the bone marrow have an important physiologic role: Under conditions of acute peripheral granulocyte demand, they are rapidly released into the circulation ("bone marrow granulocyte reserve"), thus filling the gap between acutely increased demand and delayed increased granulocyte production. Using granulocyte mobilizing agents, an acute peripheral demand for bone marrow granulocytes may be simulated. It appears possible to estimate the size of the bone marrow granulocyte compartment from the maximal increase in circulating granulocytes. The method has been used in man, in whom the marrow granulocyte pool cannot be directly assayed. As mobilizing agents, etiocholanolon [141, 248, 624], endotoxin [140, 198, 276], or hydrocortisone [141] have been used. Although the mechanisms leading to granulocytosis are different with the three agents, results in leukopenic patients are similar [141].

3.9 Bone Marrow Cellularity

The distribution of hematopoietic marrow in the different parts of the skeleton has been studied in mice [75, 543], other mammalian species [189, 190, 431], and in humans [181]. Under normal steady-state conditions, this distribution has been found to be fairly constant [75, 111, 159, 574]; however, it may change following any perturbation, such as the expansion of hematopoietic bone marrow to peripheral bones during tumor-induced neutrophilia [340]. To our knowledge, the effect of single or repeated administration of cytotoxic drugs upon the distribution of hematopoietic bone marrow has not been studied.

Studies in humans have revealed the concentration of bone marrow cells in marrow aspirates to be dependent upon the site [242, 267] and volume [240] of aspiration and on the age of the subject [265a]. Bone marrow differentials, done on aspirated marrow from different sites, gave identical results [242, 267] while the incidence of CFU-C in human marrow obtained from the sternum was reported to be twice that determined in marrow from the iliac crest [242]. In mice, identical relative numbers of CFU-S were found in various parts of the femur and in lumbar vertebrae [570]. Lee et al. [341], determining the CFU-C content in various parts of the skeleton by grinding individual bones, found minor differences in the incidence of CFU-C between different sites in normal animals; in tumor-bearing mice, however, significant changes in the incidence of CFU-C occurred in some parts of the skeleton, while the incidence of granulopoietic precursor cells remained unchanged in others.

The description of the reaction of the hematopoietic systems to cytotoxic drug therapy requires an assessment of the changes of the bone marrow cellularity and of the various hematopoietic compartments as a function of time after administration of the cytotoxic drug(s). However, such quantification presents a major difficulty in larger animals and in human beings. In smaller animals, cellularity of the bone marrow is usually determined by measuring the total nucleated cell count per femur or per humerus; alternatively, the total DNA content of these organs is measured. Relative bone marrow composition data obtained by culture assays (e.g., the number of stem cells per 10^5 marrow cells) or by morphological evaluation (e.g., the percentage of promyelocytes in bone marrow smears) may then be corrected for this cellularity. In this way, exact changes in the size of a given bone marrow compartment as a function of time after administration of a cytotoxic agent can be obtained. Obviously, an equivalent method for direct measurement of bone marrow cellularity is not available for large animals and human beings. Under steady-state conditions, estimates of the bone marrow cellularity have been attempted [451] using indirect parameters such as mitotic indices [317], maturation times and peripheral blood turnover rates. More direct methods for quantification of the bone marrow by ^{59}Fe incorporation into red cell precursors have been developed [151]. However, they are extremely time-consuming, they expose a patient to undesirable ionizing radiation, and they cannot be done repeatedly at short intervals due to the rather long half-life of the isotope. Thus, in larger animals and humans, the problem of exact bone marrow cellularity after chemotherapy is not resolved, and any analysis relies mainly on the relative data obtained by culture methods or by morphological evaluation. However, if the cellularity of the bone marrow changes considerably after chemotherapy (and this is indeed the case, particularly if high doses of drugs are employed) then these relative data can be quite misleading.

In an attempt to arrive at a more quantitative description of the human granulopoietic progenitor cell (CFU-C) compartment, various ways to correct the direct culture data (i.e., CFU-C per 10^5 marrow cells) have been proposed. To correct for the admixture of peripheral blood cells in the marrow aspirate, the number of CFU-C has been related to the number of "early granulocytic cells" (i.e., myeloblast to metamyelocyte) [430]. Other investigators relate the number of CFU-C to that of myelocytes [473] or metamyelocytes [449, 450], considering these ratios as a measure of the amplification within the granulocytic system [449]. This may be of some value in the steady-state. However, such methods are obviously of no value during cytotoxic drug-induced perturbation of the granulocytic system, since these ratios are subject to changes in both compartments which follow different kinetic patterns [41].

In order to better describe the quantitative changes of the human bone marrow CFU-C compartment, the expression of culture data as CFU-C/ml bone marrow aspirate has been recommended [41, 120]. This value is only influenced by admixed peripheral blood CFU-C, whereas it is independent of the admixture of other nucleated peripheral blood cells or of the bone marrow differential count. The admixture of peripheral blood to the marrow aspirate was experimentally shown to be negligible at aspiration volumes below 4 ml [240].

In our studies of cytotoxic drug-induced changes in human granulopoiesis, we have attempted to quantify changes in human bone marrow cellularity using two methods. First, we have used the concentration of nucleated bone marrow cells in standard bone marrow aspirates as an index of the bone marrow cellularity. Second, we have enumerated the number of bone marrow cells per unit bone marrow volume by histomorphometric methods, and used this value as an index of the marrow cellularity following cytotoxic drug therapy (W. Schreml, P. Kubitza, H.-P. Lohrmann, 1980, Attempts at quantification of the changes of the bone marrow cellularity and the hemopoietic marrow compartments in man during cancer chemotherapy, Scand J. Haemat., in press). An example of this method may be found elsewhere (page 32, 33).

4 *Effect of Individual Cytotoxic Agents Upon the Granulopoietic System*

4.1 Nitrogen Mustards

The nitrogen mustards have been the first agents with cytotoxic properties used for the treatment of malignancies. The most completely studied agent of this group of compounds is methyl-*bis*(β-chloroethyl)-amine (mechlorethamine) (HN_2). HN_2 has received the interest of experimental and clinical workers, and both have contributed to a better understanding of the effects of the agent on the granulopoietic system of experimental animals and human beings. In this review, attention will therefore be focussed on studies concerned with the hematopoietic toxicity of HN_2. The effects of other nitrogen mustards, such as ethyl-*bis*(β-chloroethyl)-amine (HN_1) or *tris*(β-chloroethyl)-amine (HN_3), will be mentioned only briefly.
Major differences in the reaction of different strains of mice to HN_2 appear to exist [305] and, furthermore, the route of administration appears to alter its impact on the hematopoietic system [616].

CFU-S Sensitivity Studies. The sensitivity of normal and rapidly proliferating CFU-S (the latter derived from bone marrow or spleen) has been recorded in several studies (Table 1). Usually, exponential survival curves have been obtained, although a few studies described a somewhat greater than exponential reduction of CFU-S survival at low doses of the drug [81, 606, 615, 616]. Identical sensitivity of normal and of rapidly proliferating bone marrow-derived CFU-S was found by one author [167]; however, others [615, 616] described rapidly proliferating CFU-S to be considerably more sensitive to HN_2 than normal CFU-S. There was no difference in the sensitivity of rapidly proliferating marrow- or spleen-derived CFU-S [615]. Following an in vitro incubation of a bone marrow cell suspension with HN_2 (0.05–0.5 μM/l for 60 min at 37° C), identical exponential dose-survival curves were obtained for normal and for regenerating bone marrow CFU-S [435].
Dose-survival studies following in vivo exposure of CFU-S to HN_3 have been performed in mice and rats [166, 167]. Whereas in rats the CFU-S dose-survival curve was almost identical to that determined for HN_2, the murine CFU-S dose-survival curve was suggestive of the formation of a plateau at doses of HN_3 greater than 3 mg/kg. This was true for both normal and rapidly proliferating bone marrow-derived CFU-S. However, spleen-derived rapidly proliferating CFU-S had an exponential dose-survival curve following HN_3.

CFU-S Recovery Studies. There is just one study on the quantitative changes over time of the bone marrow CFU-S compartment following exposure to HN_2 [533]. After 5 mg/kg of the drug, the CFU-S compartment was rapidly depleted; 24 h after drug administration its size reached a nadir of 10% of normal. Thereafter, a gradual reconstitution of the CFU-S compartment was seen, with return to pretreatment size by day 8.

Table 1. Effect of nitrogen mustard on CFU-S: Sensitivity studies in vivo

Species/strain	Time of assay (h)	CFU-S survival (percent of normal) Dose (mg/kg)								Reference
		0	0.5	1	2	5	10	15	20	
Normal CFU-S										
Mouse (C_3H/HeJ)	3	100			15					[277]
Mouse (C_3H/HeJ)	3	100				7	0.5	0.2		[15]
Mouse [(C_{57}Bl/Rij×CBA/Rij)F_1]	16	100		20	5	0.1				[615, 616]
Mouse (AKR/J)	24	100				9	1	0.2	0.06	[81]
Mouse (CBA)	24	100	50	15	2					[167]
Mouse (AKR)	24	100				8	2	0.3	0.06	[606]
Mouse (C_{57}Bl)	24	100		40	8					[172]
Rat (Wilkie)	24	100		80	70					[166]
Rapidly proliferating CFU-S from bone marrow										
Mouse [(C_{57}Bl/Rij×CBA/Rij)F_1]	16	100		2	0.2					[615]
Mouse (CBA)	24	100	50	15	2					[167]
Rat (Wilkie)	24	100	50	25	2.5					[166]
Rapidly proliferating CFU-S from spleen										
Mouse [(C_{57}Bl/Rij×CBA/Rij)F_1]	16	100		2	0.2					[615]

Table 2. Effect of nitrogen mustard on CFU-C: In vivo and in vitro sensitivity studies

	Time of assay (h)	CFU-S survival (percent of controls)					Reference
		Dose of HN_2 (mg/kg)					
		0	5	10	15	20	
In vivo							
Mouse (C_{57}Bl/6N)	24	100	50	0.08	0.007	< 0.001	[78]
	Duration of incubation (h)	Dose of HN_2 (μM/l)					
		0	0.125	0.30	0.6		
In vitro							
Human	1	100	80	60	40		[436]
Mouse (BALB/c)	1	100	60	20	3		[436]
Mouse (BALB/c)							
Normal	1	100	60	20	3		[435]
Rapidly proliferating	1	100	60	20	3		[435]

CFU-C Sensitivity Studies. In several studies, the sensitivity of CFU-C has been investigated following in vivo or in vitro exposure to HN_2 (Table 2). In vivo, mouse CFU-C had an exponential dose-survival curve with a slight shoulder at concentrations below 5 mg/kg drug [78]. In vitro exposure of mouse and human CFU-C to HN_2 similarly reduced the CFU-C survival in an exponential dose-survival correlation [435, 436]. CFU-C from normal and from regenerating bone marrow were equally sensitive to the drug [435]. Human CFU-C were considerably less sensitive than murine CFU-C [436]. The CFU-C kill in vitro was highly temperature-dependent [437].

CFU-C Recovery Studies. Recovery studies of CFU-C following exposure to HN_2 have not been reported.
Following single doses of HN_3 (0.5–1.5 mg/kg), the incidence of CFU-C in dog bone marrow (CFU-C/10^5 marrow cells) declined rapidly; a dose-dependent nadir was reached on day 1. A return to normal values was measured on day 4 following 0.5, 0.75, and 1.0 mg/kg HN_3. When the dogs had been treated with 1.5 mg/kg, the incidence of CFU-C remained near zero on day 4; the animals did not survive longer [1].

Bone Marrow. The studies listed in Table 3 indicate that HN_2 reduces the bone marrow cellularity early, and that the marrow cellularity recovers rapidly. The long-term effect of nitrogen mustard application on the murine bone marrow was studied by Sharp et al. [535], who described a somewhat increased femoral cellularity 40–100 days after HN_2, though between days 8–40 the marrow cellularity was within the normal range.
Studies not listed in Table 3 describe the effect of HN_2 on the marrow cellularity in more general terms. Thus, in the rabbit, a rapid depletion of the myeloid tissue was observed 24–72 h after 2 and 3 mg/kg HN_2, and regeneration of the marrow was

Table 3. Effect of nitrogen mustard on bone marrow cellularity: Recovery studies

	Dose of HN_2 (mg/kg)	Marrow cellularity (percent of controls) Day 0	1	2	3	4	5	6	7	8	Reference
Mouse (CS_1/ASH)	5	100	65			8				80	[533]
Mouse (CS_1/ASH)	5	100	65			8		25	50	80	[534]
Rat	0.9	100	25	8	8	25	25				[265]
Dog (estimated values)	1.0	100			75	20	20	50	75	100	[584]

reported to be completed 1–3 weeks after drug administration [97]. In humans, a reduction of the total nucleated cell count of sternal marrow aspirates from 100,000 cells/μl to 6,400 cells/μl on day 21 was found after two to six daily doses of 0.1 mg/kg HN_2. During week 4 after drug exposure, rapid recovery of the marrow cellularity to 65,000 cells/μl was observed [552]. Spitz [550] described severe marrow hypoplasia and, in some patients, marrow aplasia after total doses of 0.5–2.8 mg/kg HN_2. In mice, the reduction of the bone marrow cellularity was clearly dose-related with an exponential correlation between cellularity and doses of 5–20 mg/kg [78].

Some aspects of the cellular composition of the bone marrow after HN_2 have been described. In rabbits, almost no granulopoiesis was seen during the phase of cellular depletion of the bone marrow (i.e., 2–4 days after HN_2). After day 5, islands of early granulopoiesis reappeared, followed later by more mature granulocytic cells, and normalization of the murine bone marrow composition occurred around day 14 after HN_2 [302]. Other authors reported day 8 murine bone marrow to contain 94% granulocytic cells at various stages of maturation [534]; a phase of relative (but not absolute) bone marrow granulocytopenia was observed 15–30 days after HN_2, whereas normal bone marrow composition was found later [535]. In dogs, the appearance of "hemocytoblasts" preceded the appearance of myeloblasts and promyelocytes, the latter amounting to 40% of all marrow cells on days 7 and 8 after HN_2 [584]. The finding of complete absence of early granulocytic cells from day 4 dog bone marrow smears [53] agrees with these data.

Serial examination of human bone marrow smears revealed a depression of blast forms and promyelocytes during the first week after HN_2, and a moderate increase of these cells during week 2. Myelocytes and metamyelocytes declined during the first 2 weeks after drug administration, and reached peak values in the course of granulocytic regeneration during weeks 3 and 4, respectively [552]. An increase of the proportion of polymorphonuclear cells (PMN) during the initial phase of marrow hypocellularity [22, 552] and its sharp decline during week 3 after treatment [552] reflect the concomitant depletion and repletion of the other cellular compartments of the bone marrow.

In dogs, the functional bone marrow granulocyte reserve was not different from that of controls 2 days after treatment with HN_2 (0.75 mg/kg) [53]. In one study, the functional bone marrow granulocyte reserve of rats was serially determined: The endotoxin-induced increment of peripheral blood granulocytes was reduced to virtually zero from day 2 to day 5 after treatment with 0.4 mg/kg HN_2 [293]. Seven to

Table 4. Effect of nitrogen mustard on peripheral blood white cell (WBC) and granulocyte (PMN) counts

	Dose (mg/kg)	Cell count per µl (percent of controls)												Reference
		Day												
		0	1	2	3	4	5	6	7	8	9	10	12	
WBC														
Dog	0.5	100				50				30			100	[299]
Dog	1.0	100		100	25	15	12	20		60		80	115	[584]
Dog	1.2	100		100		50		12		12		55	100	[342]
Rabbit	1.0	100		80		40	55		100					[245]
Humans	0.2–0.3 × 4	100		60		45		25		25		30		[381]
PMN														
Dog	0.5	100	100		55			45			25		100	[299]
Dog	0.75	100		80		35		8		< 5			50	[53]
Rabbit	1.0	100	90	33	1.5	0	3.5		120					[97]
Rabbit	2.5	100	120	75	10	5	20	50	75	80	100			[631]
Rabbit	3.0	100		80		60		25				100		[302]
Rat	0.2	100			75			100			125		150	[293]
Rat	0.4	100			35			100			175		230	[293]
Rat	0.6	100			10			100			175		230	[293]
Humans	0.1 × 4	100	Nadir 15–22 days after start of treatment											[301]
Humans	0.4 × 4	100	120			80	Nadir during week 3 ~ 20%							[429]
Humans	0.8	100		80			30					20	Recovery to normal day 40	[531]

nine days after treatment, granulocyte mobilization was considerably greater than normal. These data are well in agreement with the cellularity of rat bone marrow reported by Harris et al. [265].

Peripheral Blood Granulocytes. The changes of peripheral blood white cell and granulocyte counts after treatment with HN_2 have been listed in Table 4. With some species variations, the general pattern is a somewhat delayed depression of peripheral blood WBC; in man, lowest values were recorded approximately 21 days after initiation of treatment with HN_2 [142], whereas others [381] observed the WBC nadir to occur around day 14. Dameshek [142] noted the decrease in the leukocyte count to be predominantly a reflection of granulocytopenia. This finding appears to be true for the other species studied (Table 4). The degree of neutropenia is clearly dose-dependent after both HN_2 [97, 293] and HN_3 [1]. In some studies, an increase in peripheral blood granulocytes was noted within the first 24 h after drug administration [97, 429, 631], to be followed by neutropenia; this initial granulocytosis is most likely the expression of the stress (nausea, vomiting) following drug administration. Once peripheral blood granulocytes have recovered to pretreatment values, a rebound may ensue [97, 293, 299], which may occur mainly at higher doses of the drug [293].

4.2 Chlorambucil

Being an aromatic derivative of nitrogen mustard, chlorambucil belongs to the class of alkylating agents. Effective by the oral route of administration, chlorambucil is widely used in the treatment of malignant lymphomas, but has also been used for the treatment of other malignancies, such as testicular tumors or choriocarcinomas. In spite of this, there is little information regarding its effects on the normal hematopoietic systems.

CFU-S. Three groups have investigated the sensitivity of murine CFU-S to chlorambucil. Valeriote et al. [606] studied survival of CFU-S 24 h after doses of 0.2–1.2 mg/mouse (approximately 10–60 mg/kg). There was an exponential survival curve in this dose range ($D_{1/2}$, 16.5 mg/kg), although the existence of a slight shoulder was suggested at doses of less than 20 mg/kg. Tanaka et al. [579] described an exponential survival curve for splenic CFU-S 24 h after chlorambucil, with a $D_{1/2}$ value of approximately 8 mg/kg. Finally, van Putten et al. [615] reported an exponential survival curve for normal bone marrow CFU-S at doses of 0–40 mg/kg chlorambucil given 16 h before assay ($D_{1/2}$, approximately 10 mg/kg). The same authors studied the sensitivity of rapidly proliferating CFU-S from murine spleen; and this survival curve was again exponential, but considerably steeper than that of normal bone marrow CFU-S ($D_{1/2}$, approximately 5 mg/kg).
Recovery studies for CFU-S following chlorambucil have not been reported. There are no reports on the sensitivity or on the recovery of CFU-C following exposure to chlorambucil.

Bone Marrow. A semiquantitative recovery study on the cellularity of rat bone marrow following a dose of 12.5 mg/kg chlorambucil has been reported [185]: The lowest cellularity (approximately 5% of controls) was noted 2 days after drug administration, and complete recovery occurred by day 10 (see also [104]). In the same paper, the proportion of granulocytic bone marrow cells was reported to drop to near zero 2 days after chlorambucil treatment. Thereafter, rapid and overshooting granulocytic regeneration within the bone marrow was noted.

Peripheral Blood. The peripheral blood granulocyte concentration in rats after treatment with 12.5 mg/kg chlorambucil [183–185] showed a slight decrease (nadir on day 3), followed by supranormal granulocyte counts between days 6–14. In drogs, the peripheral blood granulocyte pattern after 5 mg/kg chlorambucil showed the lowest values on day 9 (approximately 50% of pretreatment value), while on day 16, recovery to pretreatment counts was observed [299].

4.3 Aminochlorambucil

Aminchlorambucil has not found clinical application. However, its solubility has made it a convenient drug for experimental workers.

CFU-S Sensitivity Studies. Studies on the sensitivity of CFU-S to aminochlorambucil are listed in Table 5. In the rat, a very shallow exponential dose-survival curve was determined for normal bone marrow CFU-S, though a much greater cytocidal effect on rapidly proliferating marrow CFU-S was noted [166]. A similar study in mice [167] showed normal murine bone marrow CFU-S to be considerably more sensitive to aminochlorambucil than normal rat CFU-S. In contrast to the findings in the rat, rapidly proliferating CFU-S from mouse bone marrow or spleen had exponential survival curves identical to that of normal marrow CFU-S.
Studying the sensitivity of normal murine bone marrow CFU-S to aminochlorambucil, van Putten et al. [616] described an exponential survival curve for doses up to 30 mg/kg. The slope of this curve was considerably less steep than that reported elsewhere by Dunn et al. [167]. The same authors found rapidly proliferating CFU-S from murine spleens to be considerably more sensitive to aminochlorambucil than normal CFU-S.

CFU-S Recovery Studies. A longitudinal study of the depletion and repletion of the femoral CFU-S compartment in rats has reported [174] that following a dose of 2.5 mg/kg aminochlorambucil, an immediate reduction in the size of the CFU-S pool was noted, with lowest values (approximately 60% of pretreatment size) measured 24 h after administration of the drug. Subsequently, rapid recovery took place and pretreatment pool size was reached around day 10. Data determined on day 15 suggest a somewhat excessive expansion of the femoral CFU-S compartment.
Two days after a dose of 2.5 mg/kg aminochlorambucil, normal numbers of rat bone marrow CFU-S were observed [173]. Increase of the dose to 5 mg/kg led to CFU-S values per femur on day 2 that were twice that of controls; however, CFU-S were not measured on day 1 in this study.

Bone Marrow. Changes in the cellularity of rat bone marrow after a dose of 2.5 mg/kg aminochlorambucil were investigated by Dunn et al. [174], and 24 h after drug administration the total nucleated cell count per femur fell to approximately 50% of pretreatment values. Recovery was initially rapid and then more gradual, with return

Table 5. Effect of aminochlorambucil on CFU-S: Sensitivity studies

Species/strain	Time of assay (h)	CFU-S survival (percent of controls)						Reference
		Dose (mg/kg)					$D_{1/2}$ (mg/kg)	
		0	5	10	20	30		
Normal CFU-S								
Rat (−)	24	100	98	95	90		≥ 25	[166]
Mouse (CBA)	24	100	50	10	1		~ 6	[167]
Mouse [(C_{57}Bl/Rij×CBA/Rij)F_1]	16	100	45	25	6	2	~ 5	[616]
Rapidly proliferating CFU-S								
Rat (−)	24	100	60	20	3		~ 6	[166]
Mouse (CAB)	24	100	50	10	1		~ 6	[167]
Mouse [(C_{57}Bl/Rij×CBA/Rij)F_1]	16	100		4	0.2		~ 2.5	[616]

to normal marrow cellularity by day 10. Details on the bone marrow composition after aminochlorambucil have not been reported.

Peripheral Blood. Peripheral blood granulocytes dropped to about 80% of controls 5 days after rats were given 2.5 mg/kg aminochlorambucil [174]. By day 7, the granulocyte level had returned to normal and a considerable rebound of the peripheral blood granulocyte concentration was observed between days 9–15. Studies on the changes of the human granulopoietic system after exposure to aminochlorambucil have not been reported.

4.4 Cyclophosphamide

Cyclophosphamide is probably the most widely used cytotoxic agent. This wide use is paralleled by an enormous amount of experimental work on the drug. Being effective both orally and i.v., cyclophosphamide is metabolized in vivo by liver oxidase enzymes and converted into metabolites with cytotoxic effects [541]. By their chemical structure, these metabolites of cyclophosphamide are alkylating agents. There are excellent reviews on the clinical pharmacology of cyclophosphamide [17, 118]. In clinical practice, the drug is widely used in chemotherapy of both hematologic malignancies and a variety of solid tumors.

CFU-S Sensitivity Studies. The results of dose-response studies of CFU-S to cyclophosphamide, as to other drugs, vary with the mouse strain used, and particularly with the time interval between drug administration and CFU-S assay. Table 6, showing the dose-response of bone marrow CFU-S to cyclophosphamide, clearly demonstrates this variability. In most of the studies listed, an exponential dose-survival curve was determined. However, two groups of workers [154, 278] found a shoulder of the dose-response curve at low concentrations of cyclophosphamide when the assay was performed soon (3 h) after drug administration. One group [614] observed increased sensitivity at doses below 100 mg/kg; at higher doses, an exponential dose-response curve was described.
The sensitivity of rapidly proliferating CFU-S to cyclophosphamide has been studied by several groups. De Wys et al. [155] observed a greater reduction of the femoral CFU-S compartment when cyclophosphamide was given during regeneration from cyclophosphamide-induced perturbation than after the first exposure to the same dose of the drug. Dose-survival studies of rapidly proliferating CFU-S after cyclophosphamide exposure are listed in Table 7. Again, the survival curves are exponential, though a comparison of Tables 6 and 7 clearly indicates that rapidly proliferating CFU-S are considerably more sensitive to the cytocidal action of the drug than normal, mostly resting [23], CFU-S.

CFU-S Recovery Studies. Several groups of investigators have studied changes of the bone marrow CFU-S compartment as a function of time after a single dose of cyclophosphamide. However, since different drug doses, different routes of administration, and different strains have been utilized, the results are not readily comparable. Data are detailed in Table 8. It is clear that cyclophosphamide immediately reduces the size of the bone marrow CFU-S compartment. Usually, lowest values were on day 1 after cyclophosphamide, although in a few studies nadirs

Table 6. Effect of cyclophosphamide on normal murine CFU-S: Sensitivity studies. Where total doses are reported in the original papers, conversions are performed on the basis of an assumed body weight of 20 g per mouse

Mouse strain	Time of assay (h)	$D_{1/2}$ (mg/kg)	Percent CFU-S survival after drug (mg/kg)								Reference
			0	50	100	150	200	250	300	400	
C_3H/HeJ; AKR/J	3	~220	100		85		60		30		[278]
BALB/c	3	~150	100		~70		~25		11		[435]
$(C_{57}Bl/Rij \times CBA/Rij)F_1$	16–20	40	100		18		8		3.8		[614]
$C_{57}Bl$	20	80	100		40		18		7		[391]
RFM/Un or RF/J	24	60	100	55	30	18	9				[579]
$C_{57}Bl$	24	100	100		~35		~10		~2.5		[172]
C_3H/HeJ	24	–	100						~30		[280]
C_3H/HeJ; AKR/J	24	~100	100				25		15	8	[278]
$B_6D_2F_1$	24	50	100	50	25		7				[417]
AKR	24	~100	100	80	50	40	30				[175]
AKR/J	24	50	100		30		6		2		[81, 606]
C_3H/HeJ	24	80	100	55	40		15		6		[66]
$C_{57}Bl/6$	24	150	100	130		~60		~25			[154]
$[C_{57}Bl/6 \times DBA/2]F_1$	24	~100	100		18		10		4.4		[112a]
DBA/2	72	80	100		~30		~10				[6, 7]

Table 7. Effect of cyclophosphamide on rapidly proliferating mouse CFU-S: Sensitivity studies. Methods were marrow cell transfer into irradiated recipients (BMT), in vivo treatment with endotoxin, or daily administration of low doses of total body irradiation (TBI)

Strain (method)	Source of cells	$D_{1/2}$ (mg/kg)	Dose range (mg/kg)	Time of assay (h)	Shape of dose-response curve	Reference
BALB/c (BMT)	Bone marrow	~150	0–200	3	Exponential	[435]
AKR (endotoxin)	Bone marrow	30	0–200	24	Exponential	[175]
C_{57}Bl (TBI)	Bone marrow	50	0–300	20	Exponential	[391]
C_{57}Bl/Rij×CBA/Rij (BMT)	Spleen	40	0–400	16–20	Exponential	[614]

were found on day 2. Nadirs appear to be dose-related, whereas the route of administration does not appear to affect toxicity to the CFU-S compartment [616]. The kinetics of the recovery of the CFU-S pool from the cyclophosphamide-induced damage vary considerably among the different studies. In some reports, particularly when higher doses of cyclophosphamide were used, a transient expansion of the size of the bone marrow CFU-S compartment beyond the normal values was observed during hematopoietic regeneration [154, 155, 445]. In other studies, normalization of the size of the CFU-S bone marrow compartment occurred gradually and sometimes oscillating. In general, the return of the size of the CFU-S compartment to pretreatment values was completed around day 6, although it was delayed in a few studies.

Patterns of depletion and repletion were somewhat different for the splenic CFU-S compartment (Table 9). Again, a dose-dependent nadir was usually observed on days 1 or 2 after cyclophosphamide. However, during regeneration, most investigators reported a considerable transient rebound beyond normal splenic CFU-S pool sizes.

CFU-S circulating in the peripheral blood are also affected by cyclophosphamide treatment. In a paper by De Wys et al. [155], the longitudinal changes of the peripheral blood CFU-S compartment after a single dose of cyclophosphamide (275 mg/kg) are described: By day 1 after drug administration, a reduction of the circulating CFU-S pool size to approximately 4% was measured with subsequent rapid recovery. Pretreatment pool size was reached by day 4, followed by a transient excessive pool size expansion.

CFU-C Sensitivity Studies. Data on the sensitivity of CFU-C to cyclophosphamide are summarized in Table 10. Usually, exponential dose-survival curves have been reported in these studies but, in two papers [78, 417], a slight shoulder of the dose-survival curve was reported at low doses of cyclophosphamide. When tested simultaneously, CFU-C were more drug-sensitive than CFU-S in one study [391]. However, other investigators [435] have reported a nearly identical sensitivity of CFU-S and CFU-C to cyclophosphamide. A comparison of Tables 6 and 10 supports this latter finding. The sensitivity to cyclophosphamide of rapidly proliferating CFU-C was found to be somewhat greater than that of normal CFU-C [391, 435].

Table 8. Effect of cyclophosphamide on mouse bone marrow CFU-S: Recovery studies

Mouse strain	Dose (mg/kg)	Size of CFU-S compartment (percent of day 0)										Reference
		Day										
		0	1	2	3	4	5	6	7	8	10	
RAP	5	100	57		100			97				[382]
$B_6D_2F_1$	100	100	~15	~15		30			~20			[417]
AKR	150	100	25	27	45	60	75	80				[176]
AKR/J	150	100		~30		~60		~80		~80		[609]
–	200	100	32	26	69		257			196		[58, 445]
HSB; $(C_3H \times DBA)F_1$	200	100	~10	~15	~30	~70	~85	~70	~50	~30		[69]
CBA; $C_{57}Bl$	200	100	30		80		30		20			[387]
$C_{57}Bl/6$	240	100	20	~33	~55	100	130		120			[154]
CF_1	250	100			~15				~20		~45	[220]
AKR/J	250	100	5			~15		100				[609]
BALB/c × A	250	100	~8									[219]
CF_1	250	100	9						9		46	[220]
CDF_1	275	100	10	50	~125	~200	~250	~125	~120	100		[155]
$(C_3H \times FW)F_1$	350	100		0.2	6.6	51	42	60		49		[503]

Table 9. Effect of cyclophosphamide on mouse splenic CFU-S: Recovery studies

Mouse strain	Dose (mg/kg)	Size of splenic CFU-S compartment (percent of controls)											Reference
		Day											
		0	1	2	3	4	5	6	7	8	9	10	
RAP	5	100	114		382			338					[382]
AKR/J	150	100		5				100		> 100			[609]
($C_{57}Bl \times C_3H)F_1$	200	100	11	4	46		116			514			[445]
–	200	100	30	10	50		105			500			[58]
AKR/J	250	100		0.2		~ 5		~ 10	700				[609]
CF_1	250	100			< 5				210			~ 300	[219]
$(C_3H \times FW)F_1$	350	100		2.5	10		20	68	926	971			[503]

Table 10. Effect of cyclophosphamide on CFU-C: Sensitivity studies. Where total doses are reported in the original paper, conversions are made on the basis of an assumed body weight of 20 g per mouse

Species (strain)	Time of assay (h)	$D_{1/2}$ (mg/kg)	Percent CFU-C surviving after drug (mg/kg)						Reference
			0	50	100	150	200	300	
Mouse (BALB/c)									
Normal	3	~ 150	100		70		25	11	[435]
Regenerating	3	~ 50	100		10		1		[435]
Mouse ($C_{57}Bl$)	16–20	120	100		50		30	15	[391]
Mouse ($C_{57}Bl$)	18–20	50	100	8	0.5				[237]
Humans	18–20	20	100	50	15	7	2		[237]
Mouse ($C_{57}Bl/6$)	24	80	100	70	35	15		2	[78]
Mouse ($B_6D_2F_1$)	24	100	100	70	45		15		[417]

A special assay technique has been developed by Gordon et al. [237] to test the sensitivity of CFU-C to cytotoxic agents. Using this so-called agar-diffusion chamber technique (for details, see page 10), differences in the sensitivity of human and mouse bone marrow-derived CFU-C have been demonstrated [237].

CFU-C Recovery Studies in Animals and Humans. Most published animal studies have been carried out in mice. Reporting on the incidence of CFU-C in mouse bone marrow (CFU-C per 7.5×10^4 bone marrow cells), Rosenoff et al. [493] observed an initial fall to near-zero values with a subsequent tremendous rebound of bone marrow CFU-C (Table 11). Since the cellularity of the femoral marrow experiences considerable changes during this observation period (see below), such data on the incidence of CFU-C may be quite misleading when the changes of the size of the CFU-C compartment of the bone marrow are considered. On the other hand, the data are analogous to those obtained in humans: They allow for a rough comparison of CFU-C values determined in human beings after cytotoxic drug therapy.

Fortunately, most authors have expressed their results in animal studies as CFU-C per femur (or per humerus), thus referring to the changes of the size of the CFU-C compartment of a distinct part of the bone marrow organ. The data (Table 11) indicate a dose-dependent and immediate depletion of the marrow CFU-C compartment following drug administration. However, recovery is rapid and, in most studies, pretreatment CFU-C compartment size was reached by day 3 or 4. Interestingly, several studies report a second and longer-lasting compartment depletion of moderate degree following this early normalization.

In a few animal studies, the depletion and recovery of the CFU-C compartment of the spleen after cyclophosphamide has been analysed. Data in Table 12 indicate that the reduction of the splenic CFU-C pool, which occurs immediately after chemotherapy, is

Table 11. Effect of cyclophosphamide on mouse bone marrow CFU-C: Recovery studies

Mouse strain	Dose (mg/kg)	Size of marrow CFU-C compartment (percent of control)										Reference
		Day										
		0	1	2	3	4	5	6	7	8	9	
$C_{57}Bl$	84	100	55									[204, 205]
$B_6D_2F_1$	100	100	25	100		80				60		[417]
AKR	150	100	7	~ 30	~ 70	~ 80	~ 90		100		100	[176]
$(C_{57}Bl \times C_3H)F_1$	200	100	11	17	95		55			15		[445]
–	200	100	~ 30	~ 40	~ 100		~ 50			~ 30		[58]
CBA/H[a]	200	100	1	1.5	6	25	40	55	35			[386]
–	200	100	4	19	52	92	560			52		[311]
$C_{57}Bl/6N$	200	100	8	35	65	70	35	27	100	100		[78]
BDF_1	200	100	8			34			28			[602]
$(C_{57}Bl \times DBA)F_1$	200	100	4	20	60	90	> 500		60			[309]
$C_{57}Bl/6$	300	100	< 2	30	60	100	100	100	100			[334]
$(C_{57}Bl \times DBA)F_1$	450	100	0.2			70	260					[309]
BDF_1[b]	200	100	0	270	8,000		170	~ 60		~ 60		[493]

[a] Hypertransfused animals
[b] Values refer to CFU-C/7.5×10^4 marrow cells, not to CFU-C per femur

Table 12. Effect of cyclophosphamide on mouse splenic CFU-C: Recovery studies

Mouse strain	Dose (mg/kg)	Size of splenic CFU-C compartment (percent of control)								Reference
		Day								
		0	1	2	3	4	5	6	7	
BDF_1	200	100	0			0			3,170	[602]
$(C_{57}Bl \times C_3H)F_1$	200	100	10	28	50	280			1,010	[445]
–	200	100	25	40	54	250				[58]
$(C_{57}Bl \times DBA)F_1$	200	100						7,500	32,800	[311]

comparable in degree to that of the bone marrow CFU-C compartment. However, the patterns of recovery of the CFU-C compartment vary in bone marrow and spleen. In none of the studies listed, the splenic CFU-C pool regained pretreatment size before day 4. The major difference between the recovery of the splenic and bone marrow CFU-C pool is the long-lasting expansion of the CFU-C compartment in the spleen after day 4: In the different studies, the number of CFU-C per spleen was 10 to 328-times the normal values during this time period.

In man, data on the behavior of CFU-C after cyclophosphamide treatment are limited, although several reports have appeared more recently. It must be mentioned that in some of these studies, cyclophosphamide was not the only cytotoxic agent given to the patient, but it was combined with another cytotoxic drug.

Senn et al. [528] reported a reduction of the incidence of the CFU-C (i.e., CFU-C per 10^5 marrow cells) to 30% of normal values after 1 g/m^2 cyclophosphamide: This value was maintained for approximately 1 week, whereupon supranormal values (140% of normal) were reached around day 20. Later on, normalization of the relative number of CFU-C was reported.

Using the so-called agar-diffusion chamber technique (see page 10), Gordon [236] studied the incidence of human bone marrow CFU-C following treatment with single

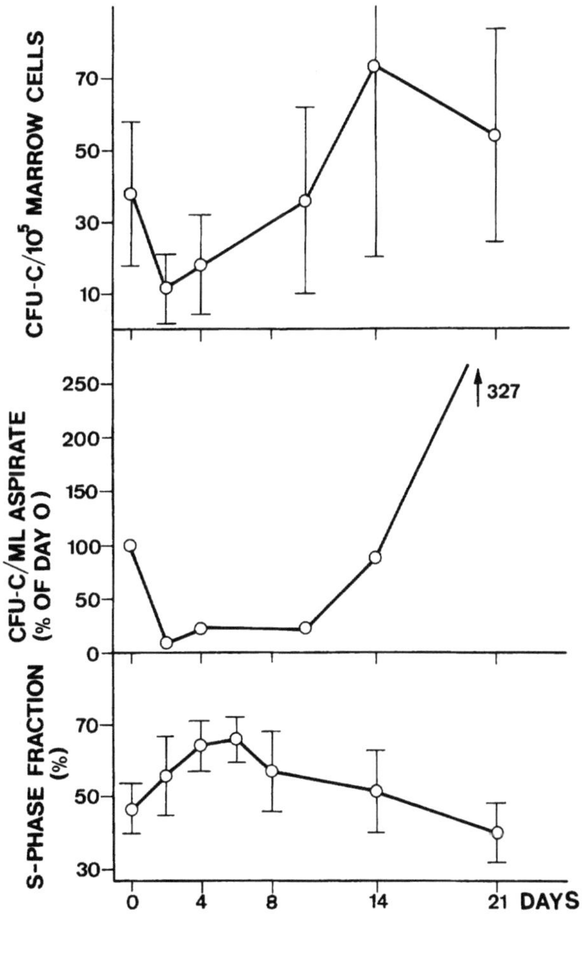

Fig. 1. Changes of the incidence of bone marrow CFU-C (*upper panel*, means ± SD), the concentration of CFU-C in bone marrow aspirates (*middle panel*, median values), and the S-phase fraction of bone marrow CFU-C (*lower panel*, ^{3}H-TdR suicide technique, means ± SD) following high-dose cyclophosphamide therapy (cyclophosphamide, 2,000 mg/m^2 day 0) in humans

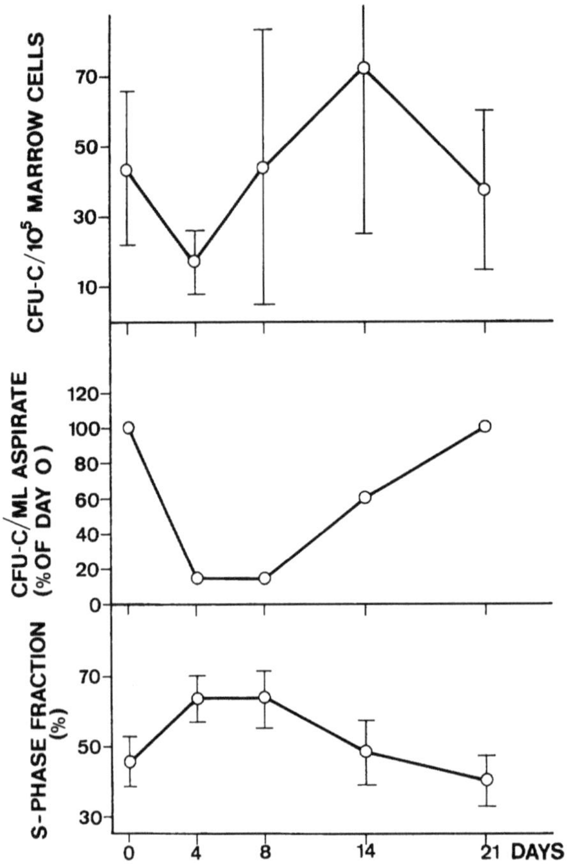

Fig. 2. Changes of the incidence of human bone marrow CFU-C (*upper panel*, means ± SD), the concentration of CFU-C in bone marrow aspirates (*middle panel*, median values), and the S-phase fraction of bone marrow CFU-C (*lower panel*, ^{3}H-TdR suicide technique, means ± SD) following combination therapy with cyclophosphamide (500 mg/m^2) plus adriamycin (50 mg/m^2) given on day 0

high doses of cyclophosphamide. Her data indicate an early and sharp reduction, followed by excessive regeneration approximately 14 days after cyclophosphamide.

Detailed information on the pattern of bone marrow CFU-C in man after single large doses of cyclophosphamide is given in recent reports from our laboratory [352, 353]. Patients were treated with cyclophosphamide (2,000 mg/m^2), in combination with vincristine (1.2 mg/m^2) or adriamycin (20 mg/m^2), and were serially followed-up thereafter. Figure 1 demonstrates the changes in the relative number of bone marrow CFU-C observed in these patients. In another study, we have described the reaction of human bone marrow CFU-C to a combination of "standard" doses of cyclophosphamide (500 mg/m^2) and adriamycin (50 mg/m^2) [353]. The updated results of this study are shown in Fig. 2.

A sequential determination of the incidence of human CFU-C does not take into account that marrow cellularity simultaneously undergoes considerable changes, therefore, these data do not reflect changes in the size of the human CFU-C compartment of the bone marrow. A better quantification of the data is shown in Figs. 1 and 2: Based on the assumption (see page 14) that the cell concentration of standard marrow aspirates can be used as an indicator of marrow cellularity, we calculated the CFU-C concentration (CFU-C per ml aspirate), and considered this value as an approximate measure of the size of the CFU-C bone marrow compartment in man.

Figures 1 and 2 then suggest a considerable reduction in the human CFU-C pool size between days 2–8 to approximately 15% of pretreatment values. After standard doses of cyclophosphamide, return to the pretreatment pool size occurs around day 14, and on day 21, the bone marrow CFU-C compartment is expanded beyond pretreatment size. After high doses of cyclophosphamide, the recovery of the bone marrow CFU-C compartment may be somewhat delayed: The data suggest that pretreatment pool size is only reached by day 21.

Using the histomorphometric evaluation of bone marrow spicule sections as an alternative approach for the assessment of cytotoxic drug-induced (500 mg/m^2 cyclophosphamide plus 50 mg/m^2 adriamycin) changes of human marrow cellularity (see page 14), depletion and regeneration of the different granulopoietic marrow compartments were analysed (Fig. 3). Although the data obtained with the two

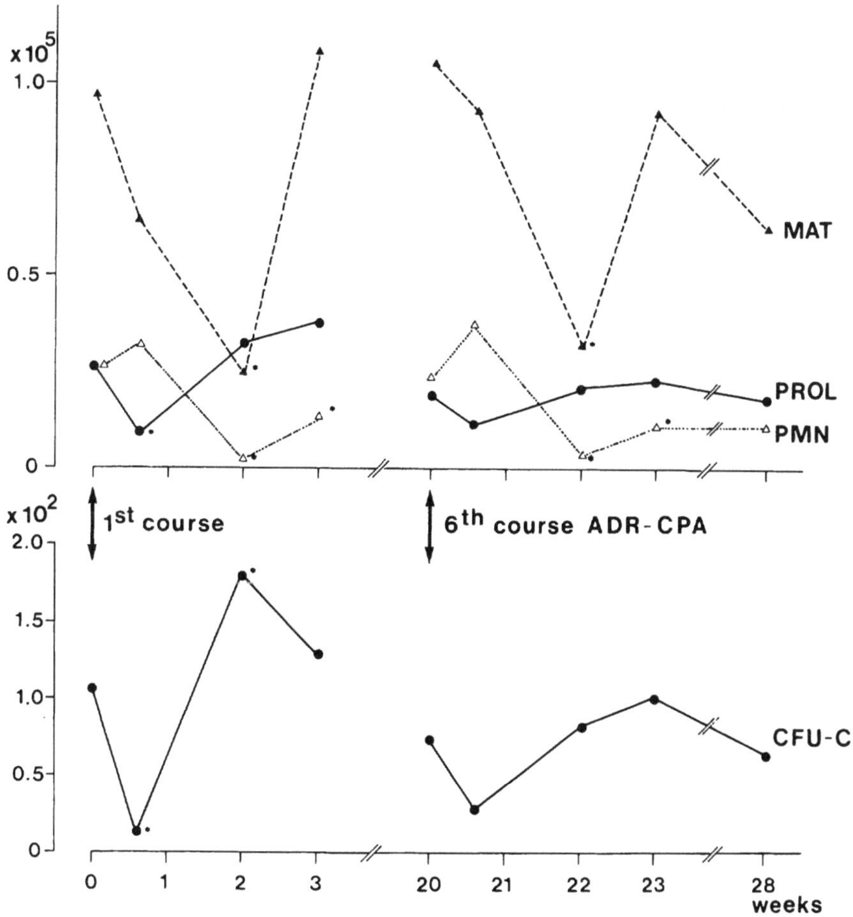

Fig. 3. Changes within the human granulopoietic bone marrow compartments after cyclophosphamide plus adriamycin: CFU-C (*lower panel*); proliferating compartment (PROL, *upper panel*, ●——●); maturing compartment (MAT, ▲— — —▲); bone marrow polymorphonuclear cell pool (PMN, △······△). Median values are given as cell number per mm^3 spicule volume. *: Different from pretreatment values ($p < 0.05$)

Table 13. Effect of cyclophosphamide on bone marrow and spleen cellularity: Recovery studies

Species (strain)	Dose (mg/kg)	Cells per organ[a] (percent of controls) Day 0	1	2	3	4	5	6	7	8	9–10	Reference
Bone marrow												
Rat (−)	50	100		~20		~45		~85		~90		[291]
Mouse (BDF$_1$)	100	100	50	25	18		70				150	[223]
Mouse (AKR)	150	100	50	30	25	40	75	90				[176]
Mouse (ACJ)	150	100						20			80	[355a]
Mouse (CD-1)	200	100		17	23		180			220		[445]
Mouse ([C$_{57}$Bl×DBA]F$_1$)	200	100			Nadir				Return to control			[309]
Mouse (BDF$_1$)	200	100	25			17			100			[602]
Mouse (BDF$_1$)	200	100	40	8	22	60	90	100	100			[494]
Rat (−)	200	100					30		95			[426]
Mouse (C$_{57}$Bl/6)	200	100	28	10		26		70		89		[78]
Mouse (C$_{57}$Bl/6)	240	100	50	20	10	20	50		70			[154]
Mouse (CDF$_1$)	275	100	5	8	30	50	110	100	125	100		[155]
Mouse (C$_{57}$Bl/6J)	300	100			1				100		100	[187]
Rat (−)	325	100					18		30			[426]
Guinea pig	350	100						28				[314]
Spleen												
Mouse (BDF$_1$)	200	100	19			15			38			[602]
Mouse [(C$_{57}$Bl × DBA)F$_1$]	200	100		20		10			60	300		[311]
Rat (−)	200	100					40		68			[426]
Rat (−)	325	100					31		45			[426]

[a] Bone marrow: cells per femur, per tibia, or per humerus

techniques certainly do not reflect compartment changes accurately, they deserve to be further explored.

For some reason, data on the pattern of peripheral blood CFU-C in animals are almost nonexistent. In a short communication, Mueller-Nuebling et al. [411] delineated the changes in the peripheral blood CFU-C pool of dogs after a single high dose of cyclophosphamide (15 mg/kg): Within a few hours after chemotherapy, the peripheral blood was almost devoid of CFU-C. During the following days, rapid repletion of the peripheral blood CFU-C pool was observed, and a rebound to 300–1,000% or more of pretreatment values was recorded between days 8–14.

Several authors described the effect of cyclophosphamide treatment on the human peripheral blood CFU-C compartment. Richman et al. [484], studying mostly untreated patients with ovarian carcinoma before treatment and again on day 21 after chemotherapy with cyclophosphamide (500–700 mg/kg) plus adriamycin (45–70 mg/m^2), frequently observed an increased incidence of peripheral blood CFU-C (i.e., CFU-C per 2×10^5 peripheral blood mononuclear cells) on day 21. Studies were not performed on days 0–21, therefore, this work rather incompletely delineates the longitudinal changes in the peripheral blood CFU-C pool. Although not explicitly stated, one can conclude from the Richman et al. data that the rebound of peripheral blood CFU-C during regeneration was greater after high doses of cyclophosphamide.

Longitudinal changes of the size of the human peripheral blood CFU-C pool after cyclophosphamide were recently reported from this laboratory [351, 353, 354] describing depletion and repletion after standard doses and after high doses of cyclophosphamide. With both regimens, there was an almost immediate and nearly complete exhaustion of the peripheral blood CFU-C pool, with values of 0–10% of pretreatment size on day 2 and/or 4. Following standard doses of cyclophosphamide, the pretreatment pool size was regained by day 14. Few patients had an excessive expansion of the peripheral blood CFU-C pool thereafter. In the majority of the patients, the size of the peripheral blood CFU-C pool remained in the pretreatment range on days 14–21. In contrast to this pattern, an excessive expansion of the peripheral blood CFU-C pool was regularly seen after treatment with high doses of cyclophosphamide, with peak values on days 14–17 after treatment (10 to 50-times pretreatment CFU-C pool size).

Cellularity of the Spleen. Data on the time-course of the cellularity of the spleen after cyclophosphamide are included in Table 13. It appears that the cyclophosphamide-induced reduction of the cellularity of the spleen is longer-lasting than that of the bone marrow (see below): By day 7, the number of cells per spleen was still considerably lower than before cyclophosphamide in all four studies listed.

Bone Marrow: Morphological Studies. In several studies, the cellularity of the bone marrow (usually the femur) after a single administration of cyclophosphamide was followed (Table 13). There appears to be a dose-dependent reduction of cellularity early after drug administration. With doses greater than 200 mg/kg, lowest values (less than 20% of pretreatment values) were usually reported on day 1 or 2. Thereafter, the marrow cellularity began to increase again, and pretreatment values were usually reached at days 5–8. In two of the papers [78, 278], the femoral cellularity was analyzed as a function of the dose of cyclophosphamide. Three hours after 2, 4, or 6 mg cyclophosphamide given i.v. to mice (corresponding to approximately 100, 200, or 300 mg/kg), the femoral cell content was 103, 97, and 90% of controls, respectively.

However, when determined 24 h after the same doses of cyclophosphamide, the femoral cell counts were 34, 36, and 25% of controls [278]. Brown et al. [78], measuring the femoral cellularity 24 h after increasing doses of cyclophosphamide, did not observe any effects of 3 or 30 mg/kg drug. However, when 150 mg/kg cyclophosphamide was given 24 h earlier, the cell content of the femur had dropped to 63% of control values, and it was further reduced to 40% of controls after 300 mg/kg cyclophosphamide.

Unfortunately, the above-mentioned papers do not provide any information on the cytologic changes of the bone marrow following cyclophosphamide. However, this information can be obtained from less current work.

Working with guinea pigs, Kaul et al. [314] described changes of the various granulocytic marrow compartments 6, 9, and 12 days after 350 mg/kg cyclophosphamide. By day 6, these authors observed a striking shift to the left of the morphologically identifiable granulocytic marrow cells, with a drastic reduction of bands and of segmented neutrophils (2.5% of controls). At the same time, myeloblasts and promyelocytes and myelocytes were reduced very little. Nine days after cyclophosphamide, granulocytic regeneration had proceeded through most of the granulocytic compartments, with only the compartment of bands and segmented neutrophils awaiting full repletion (compartment sizes in percent of controls: myeloblasts 128; promyelocytes and myelocytes 265; metamyelocytes 211; bands plus segmented neutrophils 39). By day 12, the proliferating granulocytic compartment was slightly below control size; however, in the more mature granulocytic compartments, a rebound beyond normal values had occurred (metamyelocytes 263% of controls, bands plus segmented neutrophils 239% of controls).

Separating the granulocytic cells of the bone marrow into a proliferating and a nonproliferating group, Host [291] described results of serial compartment size determinations in rats following 50 mg/kg cyclophosphamide. The proliferating compartment was soon depleted (nadir on day 2), returned to pretreatment size by day 4, was somewhat larger than before treatment on days 6 and 8, and final normalization occurred on day 10. The depletion of the nonproliferating granulocytic compartment lasted until day 7, while the subsequent rebound (day 7–14) was greater than that observed in the proliferating granulocytic compartment.

Further information on the cytologic changes of the granulocytic bone marrow in the rat was given by Pliess et al. [460]. Following 150 mg/kg cyclophosphamide, these authors observed an early decrease of the percentages of promyelocytes and myelocytes on day 1 accompanied by a striking increase in the proportion of segmented neutrophils. By days 4 and 5, the latter had almost disappeared from marrow smears and percentages of promyelocytes were increased, followed by an increase of the percentages of myelocytes and later of metamyelocytes, bands, and segmented neutrophils.

A study by Hambsch et al. [256] similarly reported on the composition of rat bone marrow after cyclophosphamide treatment (75 mg/kg). The pattern of changes at the different levels of granulopoiesis is similar to that of the paper just discussed: Promyelocyte percentages were lowest on day 1, were five-times normal by day 5, and were in the normal range by day 6. The nadir of the percentages of myelocytes was reached by day 2 with subsequent rebounding recovery. Percentages of bands and particularly of segmented neutrophils increased during the first 1 and 2 days, respectively. Subsequently, a reduction to near zero occurred before both values returned to pretreatment levels around day 8.

In man, a few studies on the cytologic changes in the granulocytic system of the bone marrow after cyclophosphamide treatment have been reported. Following cyclophosphamide (500 mg/m^2) in combination with adriamycin (50 mg/m^2) [512], we [353] have described a reaction pattern that is qualitatively very similar to that derived from the animal studies discussed above (Table 14). We later added [354] further information on the cytologic changes of the human marrow in response to high doses of cyclophosphamide (2,000 mg/m^2) in combination with vincristine (1.4 mg/m^2) (Table 15). From these data, it is obvious that there is a relative decrease of cells of the proliferating granulocytic compartment shortly after chemotherapy, which is accompanied by a relative increase of the cells of the maturing (nondividing) granulocytic compartment. With granulocytic regeneration, the percentage of proliferating granulocytic cells increases, the proportion of the mature granulocytic cells is, at this stage, considerably reduced, and segmented neutrophils have almost disappeared from the bone marrow. It can be seen from the tables that it takes about 21 days for

Table 14. Changes in human bone marrow differential counts (mean ± SD) after cyclophosphamide (500 mg/m^2) and adriamycin (50 mg/m^2) (data updated from Lohrmann et al. [353])

Day	M/E ratio	Percent of marrow cells		
		Proliferating pool[a]	Maturing pool[b]	PMN[c]
0	1.33	10.6 ± 4.3	36.8 ± 5.8	11.7 ± 7.5
2	4.54	6.9 ± 2.3	52.9 ± 6.1	17.4 ± 5.5
4	4.17	7.0 ± 4.4	50.4 ± 10.6	23.1 ± 9.7
10	0.31	11.2 ± 6.3	21.5 ± 10.2	9.4 ± 5.1
14	0.45	16.0 ± 5.5	12.8 ± 5.4	1.7 ± 1.7
21	1.66	13.0 ± 4.6	43.5 ± 10.4	5.2 ± 3.2

[a] Myeloblast to myelocyte stage
[b] Metamyelocyte to segmented neutrophil (PMN) stage
[c] Polymorphonuclear cells
Abbreviation: M/E, Myeloid to erythroid cell ratio

Table 15. Changes in human bone marrow differential counts (mean ± SD) after high-dose cyclophosphamide therapy (2,000 mg/m^2) (data updated from Lohrmann et al. [354])

Day	M/E ratio	Percent of marrow cells		
		Proliferating pool[a]	Maturing pool[b]	PMN[c]
0	1.27	9.5 ± 3.5	37.3 ± 4.9	8.6 ± 3.3
4	7.69	2.9 ± 1.4	60.1 ± 10.8	28.0 ± 12.6
8	0.09	3.0 ± 3.3	9.6 ± 7.6	4.9 ± 3.6
14	0.80	24.2 ± 6.8	16.0 ± 8.0	0.5 ± 1.6
21	2.08	7.7 ± 4.1	55.4 ± 10.4	6.3 ± 3.4

[a] Myeloblast to myelocyte
[b] Metamyelocyte to polymorphonuclear cells (PMN)
[c] Polymorphonuclear cells

human bone marrow to return to pretreatment composition following cyclophosphamide treatment.

The Proliferative State of Granulopoietic Cells After Cyclophosphamide Treatment. Few papers contain information sufficient to provide a framework for a better understanding of the changes in the proliferative activity of CFU-S or CFU-C in reaction to cyclophosphamide exposure. Three days after a large dose of cyclophosphamide, De Wys et al. [155] reported proliferation of CFU-S with a population-doubling time of 18 h. Attempts to quantify the proportion of CFU-S in S-phase were not made by these authors. Similar conclusions may be derived from other publications listed in Table 8.

Mueller-Nuebling et al. [411] reported an increased ^{3}H-TdR suicidal fraction of bone marrow-derived CFU-C in a dog 2–5 days after treatment with 15 mg/kg cyclophosphamide. In mice, Joyce et al. [309] reported a considerably increased proliferative activity of CFU-C 2, 3, and 4 days after 200 mg/kg cyclophosphamide. Similarly, Ladisch et al. [334] observed increased ^{3}H-TdR suicide fractions 1–6 days after 300 mg/kg cyclophosphamide.

In humans, Gordon [239] utilized the agar-diffusion chamber technique (see page 10) to assay the proliferative state of human CFU-C: By administering the S-phase-specific drug cytosine-arabinoside to chamber-bearing mice shortly after chamber implantation, the fraction of CFU-C in S-phase could be estimated from the fraction of CFU-C surviving this treatment. Exposing human bone marrow-derived CFU-C in vitro to ^{3}H-TdR of high specific activity, Lohrmann et al. [353, 354] investigated the changes in the proliferative activity of human CFU-C after treatment with cyclophosphamide in a similar attempt to obtain information on changes of the proliferative state of these stem cells in reaction to the cytotoxic drug. The data of the two groups are quite similar in spite of the differences in the techniques used: There is an early increase in the proliferative activity of CFU-C, with return to normal at a time (at days 10–14 after cyclophosphamide) when the incidence of bone marrow CFU-C reaches highest values (Figs. 1 and 2).

Szmigielski et al. [573] exposed rabbit bone marrow to ^{3}H-TdR in vitro at different intervals after in vivo administration of cyclophosphamide (50 mg/kg), and determined the percentages of labelled promyelocytes and myelocytes by autoradiography. In rats, the mitotic index of marrow myeloid cells was determined repeatedly after cyclophosphamide (50 mg/kg) [291]. Since different species with different proliferation kinetics of the granulocytic system were used in these studies, the data cannot be put into the appropriate perspective. The interested reader is referred to the original works for details.

Bone Marrow Granulocyte Reserve. An estimate of the granulocyte reserve of rat bone marrow following treatment with a single high dose of cyclophosphamide (50 mg/kg) can be derived from the work of Host [291]. Reporting on the number of "non-dividing myeloid" marrow cells, he provides figures indicating a gradual reduction of these cells with pool size depletion being greatest around day 4, and supranormal values are reached again by day 8. Correlating these changes with those of peripheral blood granulocytes, reported elsewhere by Host [292], one can see that the nadirs of both curves coincide, that both curves show an excessive expansion at the same time (the marrow granulocytes rebounding less than the peripheral blood granulocytes), and that they both return to their pretreatment level at the same time.

In rats, Hambsch et al. [256] determined the percentages of bands and segmented neutrophils in bone marrow smears after cyclophosphamide (75 mg/kg), and compared these values with the extent of the endotoxin-induced mobilization of marrow granulocytes into the peripheral blood. Both values reached nadirs around day 4. Further information on the cyclophosphamide-induced changes of the functional bone marrow granulocyte reserve in rats has been given by Constable et al. [125]: After 80 mg/kg drug, there was no endotoxin-induced increment of peripheral blood granulocytes from day 2–4. Return to control values was reached by day 6, and a considerable rebound of the functional bone marrow granulocyte reserve was noted between days 9 and 12 (more than 300% of control values). An exponential dose-response curve was determined by the same authors when they assessed the functional bone marrow granulocyte reserve on day 4 after variable doses of cyclophosphamide (0–100 mg/kg).
In man, minimal increments of the peripheral blood granulocyte concentrations after mobilization with hydrocortisone were determined 14 days after cyclophosphamide (500 mg/m^2) plus adriamycin (50 mg/m^2), and return to pretreatment values was noted by day 21 [353].

Peripheral Blood Leukocytes. Longitudinal studies of the changes of peripheral blood leukocytes after administration of cyclophosphamide have been performed in several species. In some cases, only peripheral blood white cell counts without further specification are reported (upper part of Table 16). Other workers, however, have specifically listed peripheral blood granulocyte counts, and these data are listed in the lower part of Table 16. From such a tabulation, two points are clearly seen: (1) There is a species-related difference in the kinetics of depletion and repletion of peripheral blood granulocytes, with a more rapid granulocytic regeneration in mice than in rats; (2) there is a close dose-effect correlation: With higher doses of cyclophosphamide, there is a greater and longer-lasting depression of the peripheral blood granulocyte counts, and often there is greater rebound beyond pretreatment values during granulocytic regeneration. The latter point can be most clearly derived from the work of Host [292] in mice and from the extensive work in dogs and monkeys reported by Lee et al. [339] (not included in Table 16, thus, the reader is referred to the original article for details).
Amazingly, references in the literature are scarce when one is looking for a systematic appraisal of cyclophosphamide-induced changes in peripheral blood granulocytes in humans. In the early literature, the drug has often been used in patients pretreated with radio- or chemotherapy, or it has been administered in split doses. These data cannot readily be analysed for our purposes. Again, it appears that the extent and the duration of the drug-induced peripheral blood granulocytopenia depend on the doses used [412, 453]. However, Colvin et al. [121] mentioned that at doses greater than 50 mg/kg, no further prolongation of the peripheral blood granulocyte depression occurred. In the study reported by Nakayama et al. [416], a dose-dependent leukopenia (15–40 mg/kg i.v.) was seen, but the time of the leukocyte nadir (days 11–13) and the duration of leukocyte depression (recovery by day 21) were identical at the different drug doses.
After single high doses of cyclophosphamide, nadirs were usually reached between days 7–12, and a return of peripheral blood granulocyte counts to pretreatment levels was usually completed after 3 weeks [31, 48, 49, 84, 85, 87, 324, 369, 518]. With doses of 800–1,200 mg/m^2 cyclophosphamide, moderate hematologic toxicity was noted

Table 16. Effect of cyclophosphamide on peripheral blood leukocytes and/or granulocytes

Species (strain)	Dose (mg/kg)	Peripheral blood leukocytes (WBC) or granulocytes (PMN) (percent of controls)									Reference
		Day									
		0	1	2	3	4	5	6	7	8	
WBC											
Mouse (Swiss-Webster)	75	100	35		28		40		65		[268]
Dog (–)	100	100	100	90		50	0	All animals dead			[186]
Mouse (Swiss-Webster)	150	100	20		20		30		75		[268]
Mouse (–)	200	100	77	23	19		5			50	[58]
Mouse [(DBA/2 × C_{57}Bl/6)F_1]	200	100		40		35			40		[463]
Mouse (BDF_1)	200	100	50	20	16	11	45	90	110		[494]
Mouse (CD-1)	200	100	23	18	26		56			45	[445]
Mouse (C_{57}Bl/6)	240	100	100	40	70	50	55		80		[154]
Mouse (CF_1)	250	100			35				95		[221]
Mouse (Swiss-Webster)	300	100	25		12		10		40		[268]
Mouse (C_{57}Bl/6)	300	100			12	10	20	55	105		[333]
Mouse [(C_3H/FW)F_1]	350	100	9				7		9	11	[503]

Table 16 (continued)

Species (strain)	Dose (mg/kg)	Peripheral blood leukocytes (WBC) or granulocytes (PMN) (percent of controls)									Reference
		Day									
		0	1	2	3	4	5	6	7	8	
PMN											
Rat (–)	6.25	100	70	50	55	60	80	120	110	100	[292]
Rat (McCollum)	40–45	100	85	75		40		60		200	[637]
Rat (–)	50	100	80	60	40	50	60	100	140	160[a]	[293]
Rat (–)	75	100				10				230	[256]
Rat (–)	100	100	80	50	10	0	0	0	70	80[a]	[292]
Rat (–)	150	100			20	10	20	180		300	[460]
Mouse [(C_{57}Bl × DBA/2)F_1]	200	100		60		5		120	350	500	[309]
Mouse [HSB, (C_3H × DBA)F_1]	200	100	65	40	15	12	75	300	170	~ 350	[69]
Mouse [(C_{57}Bl × DBA/2)F_1]	200	100		62		6	50	106	425	560	[311]
Mouse (CF_1)	200	100		40		10		20		180	[597]
Rat (–)	200	100	60	35	10	0	0	10	40	100	[38]
Mouse (CDF_1)	275	100	70		1.4	0.7	1.8	35	250	240	[155]
Mouse (C_{57}Bl/l)	300	100				< 1	~ 3	~ 30			[333]
Mouse (C_{57}Bl/6J)	300	100			0				130		[187]
Guinea pig	350	100						2		36	[314]

[a] Rebound after day 8

(WBC < 3,000 in 6 of 15 patients and WBC < 2,000 in 1 of 15 patients) [112]. With 30 mg/kg, toxicity was moderate, though increasing the dose to 40 mg/kg led to severe leukopenia in the majority of the patients [519].

A careful analysis of the depression and regeneration of peripheral blood granulocytes in a rather homogeneous group of patients, hematologically normal and without prior radio- or chemotherapy, is included in two recent reports from our laboratory [353, 354]. During the first 4 days after single doses of cyclophosphamide, peripheral blood granulocytes remained within pretreatment range. Thereafter, they steadily declined to a nadir, reached at day 12–14. Between days 14–21, rapid recovery to pretreatment values occurred. Döhle bodies and other morphological aberrations have been observed after cyclophosphamide treatment [300].

Repeated or Chronic Administration of Cyclophosphamide. There is a definite lack of systematic studies on the effect of repeated or chronic administration of cyclophosphamide on the granulopoietic system. Any attempt to draw a comprehensive view of changes in granulopoiesis under such treatment must, therefore, remain fragmentary. This incompleteness is even more astounding, since chronic administration of cyclophosphamide for the purpose of immunosuppression has long been established in clinical practice in treatment of nonhematologic disorders, such as connective tissue diseases.

The changes within the bone marrow stem cell compartment of mice were studied by Pannacciulli et al. [446]. Daily administration of approximately 16 mg/kg cyclophosphamide for 18 weeks initially reduced the femoral CFU-S compartment to less than 50% of pretreatment values. With some oscillations, it returned to its original size by week 6. Thereafter, the CFU-S compartment expanded to twice its normal size before returning to control values by week 18. The initial changes within the femoral CFU-C pool were quite similar, showing a reduction to less than 50% during week 1 followed by a return to supranormal values during week 4. Thereafter, the femoral CFU-C content remained two- to three-times control values throughout week 18.

Changes in bone marrow cellularity during chronic administration of cyclophosphamide have not been recorded systematically. After 3 × 50 mg/kg/day and 5 × 30 mg/kg/day, respectively, a somewhat slower recovery of marrow cellularity was noted than after 1 × 150 mg/kg. However, the degree of depletion of the bone marrow cellularity was similar with the three doses, and maximum marrow hypoplasia was seen on day 6 after initiation of the treatment schedules [355a].

Studying the effect on bone marrow and peripheral blood cells of 200 mg/kg cyclophosphamide given 4 days after an identical first dose, Boyum et al. [69] noted a greater reduction of the femoral CFU-S compartment after the second dose than after the first. Regeneration within the CFU-S pool started earlier and with a shorter doubling time after the second dose; similarly, regeneration of the morphologically identifiable granulocytic cells of the bone marrow started earlier after the second dose of cyclophosphamide. Peripheral blood PMN were more severely depressed following the second dose of cyclophosphamide, but they started to regenerate earlier than after the first drug administration.

Rather extensive studies on the effect of chronic administration of cyclophosphamide on the peripheral blood white cell counts of dogs were performed by Wheeler et al. [637]. Dogs were treated with 3, 4, or 5 mg/kg/day, 5 days per week for 6 weeks. At 3 mg/kg, little toxicity to the peripheral blood PMN count was noted. Toxicity was greater at a daily dose of 4 mg/kg and, at 5 mg/kg/day, moderate to severe neutropenia developed. At doses of 10 and 20 mg/kg/day deaths occurred within 1–2 weeks. An interesting finding was reported by Morley et al. [403]: When dogs were given increasing daily doses of cyclophosphamide, cyclic neutropenia developed at doses of 1.5–3.7 mg/kg/day. From these observations, the authors drew conclusions as to the mechanisms regulating granulopoiesis.

When rats were given three 20 mg/kg doses of cyclophosphamide at 12-day intervals, no change in peripheral blood PMN count was noted [511]. In the guinea pig, daily doses of 15 mg/kg for 10 days caused a disappearance of peripheral blood PMN from day 7–13; thereafter, rapid and excessive regeneration of peripheral blood PMN counts was observed [509]. In these animals, the bone marrow was described to be hypoplastic, being caused mainly by the reduction of the granulocytic bone marrow cells. The regenerative phase after discontinuation of cyclophosphamide treatment was characterized by granulocytic bone marrow hyperplasia [312]. When guinea pigs were given cyclophosphamide (20 mg/kg) every 3 days for a total of six doses, similar changes of the peripheral blood PMN counts occurred [509].

The effect of various dosage schedules on peripheral blood WBC count of rhesus monkeys was investigated by Storb et al. [567]; 2 × 90 mg/kg cyclophosphamide led to severe neutropenia by day 7, with normalization by day 15. Following 4 × 50 mg/kg, the maximal leukocyte depression was again seen by day 7, but regeneration took considerably longer, pretreatment values being reached only by day 30. Animals did not survive doses of 4 × 60 mg/kg.

In rats, 70 mg/kg at 14–18 day intervals led to granulocytopenia at day 3–7; no cumulative toxicity was observed during five treatment courses [636]. Chronic administration (5 mg/kg daily) caused mild granulocytopenia and morphological examination of the bone marrow disclosed a shift to the left of the granulocytic cells [636].

In dogs, 3 mg/kg daily × 28 caused leukopenia, with recovery to normal 7–14 days after cessation of therapy. Doses of 6 mg/kg/day × 28 led to marked leukopenia and granulocytopenia by day 21–28; severe granulocytopenia was observed after 12 mg/kg/day × 11 [638].

In humans, a daily dose of 100 mg led to leukopenia (less than 3,000 WBC/μl) in 17 of 25 patients after more than 2 weeks of treatment [211]. Following discontinuation of drug administration, the WBC count recovered within 1 week. Finkelstein et al. [199] reported leukopenia of less than 1,300/μl to develop after 12 days (range 8–21) of treatment with daily doses of 10 mg/kg cyclophosphamide. Leukopenia occurred earlier in patients with bone marrow tumor involvement. With a dose of 1.5 mg/kg/day, only slight toxicity to the peripheral blood WBC count was noted [536]. In patients with Wegener's granulomatosis, daily doses of 50–150 mg caused a decrease of the peripheral blood granulocyte count and a reduction of the functional bone marrow granulocyte reserve [140]. Interestingly, doses had to be reduced or discontinued in most patients after more than 4 months of therapy because of increasing sensitivity of the granulopoietic system to the drug, indicating cumulative toxicity of cyclophosphamide to the granulopoietic system.

Pegg [453] demonstrated a relationship between daily doses of cyclophosphamide and the extent of peripheral blood leukopenia. Leukopenia of less than 3,000 WBC/μl was regularly noted at doses more than 3 mg/kg/day. Six daily doses of approximately 8 mg/kg caused mild to severe leukopenia [116]. After four daily doses of 15 or 25 mg/kg, severe leukopenia occurred, with nadirs 8–10 days after completion of therapy [412]. After 4 × 30–70 mg/kg cyclophosphamide, granulocyte nadirs (less than 1,000/μl) occurred some 8 days later. A similar degree of neutropenia was noted after $6 \times 30-50$ mg/kg [429].

Clearly, much more systematic work needs to be done to more clearly delineate the reaction of the granulopoietic system to repeated or chronic cyclophosphamide. Of particular importance is confirmation of the work reported by Pannacciulli et al. [446] referred to above that chronic cyclophosphamide causes an expansion of the pluripotent and of the committed granulopoietic stem cell compartments after a short initial depression. If these findings are confirmed[1], the reaction pattern of the hemopoietic system to continuous administration of cyclophosphamide differs basically from that reported after continuous low-dose whole body irradiation: Here, a progressive size reduction of the pluripotent stem cell pool occurs [642] and bone marrow granulopoiesis is considerably reduced [356]. To gain a better insight into the reaction of the granulopoietic system to repeated cytotoxic insults, particularly into the mechanisms by which the system attempts to compensate for the repeated damage, the delineation of possible changes in the proliferative activity of pluripotent and committed stem cells during chronic administration of cyclophosphamide would be of particular interest.

4.5 Melphalan (L-Phenylalanine Mustard)

Chemically, melphalan is a phenylalanine derivative of nitrogen mustard and like the parent compound, it is an alkylating agents. The drug has been extensively used in treatment of multiple myeloma, but it is useful in solid tumors as well, particularly in ovarian carcinoma and breast cancer. The hematopoietic toxicity of melphalan has been extensively studied in experimental animals. In contrast, limited data are available on its effect on the normal human hematopoietic systems.

CFU-S Sensitivity Studies. Dose-survival studies have been performed by a number of investigators to determine the sensitivity of pluripotent stem cells to melphalan (Table 17). Dunn [170] measured the survival of mouse bone marrow CFU-S (normal and rapidly proliferating CFU-S) 4, 16, 24, and 48 h after graded doses of the drug. At 4 and 16 h post-drug, exponential in vivo survival curves showed that rapidly proliferating CFU-S were more sensitive than normal CFU-S, indicating the action of the drug to be proliferation-dependent. However, when the time interval between drug administration and assay for CFU-S survival was extended, the slope of the survival curve for normal CFU-S increased so that the survival curves for normal and for rapidly proliferating CFU-S were similar at 24 and 48 h post-drug. At the same time, the exponential survival curves determined 4 and 16 h post-drug were no longer seen. At 48 h, a curvilinear survival curve was obtained.

In another paper, Dunn [167] described an almost identical sensitivity of normal murine bone marrow CFU-S and of rapidly proliferating marrow-derived CFU-S in the marrow and spleen when assay was performed 24 h after increasing doses of melphalan (1.5–12.0 mg/kg). The shape of the survival curves was curvilinear under these epxerimental conditions.

1 Recently, Schaefer et al. showed that 80 mg/kg cyclophosphamide given to mice at weekly intervals for 41 weeks did not influence the size of the bone marrow CFU-S compartment [505]

Table 17. Effect of melphalan on CFU-S: Sensitivity studies

Species (strain)	Time of assay (h)	CFU-S surviving (percent of controls) Dose (mg/kg) 0	3	6	12	$D_{1/2}$ (mg/kg)	Reference
Normal CFU-S							
Mouse (CBA)	4	100	45	12	2	2.7	[170]
Mouse (CBA)	16	100	40	7	0.7	2.2	
Mouse $[(C_{57}Bl/Rij \times CBA/Rij)F_1]$	16	100	50	25	6	3.0	[615]
Mouse (CBA)	–	100	25		3	3.5	[388]
Mouse (AKR)	24	100	30		6	3	[606]
Rat (–)	24	100	50	20	3	3	[166]
Mouse (CBA)	24	100	8	1	0.1	–	[167]
Mouse (C_3H/HeJ)	24	100	40	18	2	2.5	[66]
Mouse $[(C_{57}Bl/6 \times DBA/2)F_1]$	24	100	30	17	3	2.8	[112a]
Rapidly proliferating CFU-S							
Mouse (CBA)	4	100	10	2.2	0.1	–	[170]
Mouse (CBA)	16	100	20	4	0.1	1.5	
Mouse $[(C_{57}Bl/Rij \times CBA/Rij)F_1]$	16	100	12	2.4		–	[615]
Mouse (CBA)	24	100	8	1	0.1		[167]
Rat (–)	24	100	25	7	0.6	1.5	[166]

Van Putten et al. [615] found normal bone marrow CFU-S to be more sensitive than rapidly proliferating CFU-S from spleen: Both survival curves were exponential. Valeriote et al. [606] reported a sensitivity of normal femoral CFU-S similar to these data (assay at 24 h), whereas a somewhat greater sensitivity of CFU-S to melphalan was reported by Botnick et al. [66] (assay 24 h post-drug).
Ogawa et al. studied the sensitivity of murine CFU-S to melphalan in vitro. When the cells were exposed to the drug for 3 h at 37° C, the sensitivity of normal and regenerating bone marrow CFU-S was identical [435].
Rat bone marrow CFU-S (normal and rapidly proliferating) were studied in vivo for sensitivity to melphalan [166]. Exponential survival curves were determined 24 h after drug administration, and rapidly proliferating CFU-S were more sensitive to the drug than normal CFU-S.

CFU-S Recovery Studies. The response with time of mouse CFU-S after in vivo exposure to melphalan was studied by Dunn [170]. After 6 mg/kg, the femoral content of CFU-S declined almost immediately to 10% of its pretreatment values. Thereafter, a second and more gradual reduction to approximately 1–2% of pretreatment values occurred by day 2. Return of the femoral CFU-S compartment to its normal size was completed by day 7.
Millar et al. [388] observed a decrease of bone marrow CFU-S to less than 1% 24 h after melphalan (15 mg/kg). Thereafter, the marrow CFU-S compartment recovered rapidly and pretreatment values were reached by day 9 without subsequent rebound.
Dunn [170] studied the changes of rapidly proliferating bone marrow CFU-S after in vivo exposure to melphalan. An increased sensitivity of these proliferating CFU-S was documented, with a reduction of the femoral CFU-S compartment to 1% of pretreatment size within 2–4 h post-drug. The number of CFU-S per femur remained at this level until recovery of compartment size commenced approximately 48 h after drug administration.
The changes with time of normal splenic CFU-S after 6 mg/kg melphalan were essentially similar to those of bone marrow CFU-S, although survival of splenic CFU-S was lower than that of marrow CFU-S at all time points [170].
Studying the changes in pool size of CFU-S in the circulating blood (CFU-S/ml blood), Dunn [170] found a decrease to 8% 4 h after drug exposure (6 mg/kg i.v.). A further drop to approximately 2% occurred at 24 and 48 h after melphalan.

CFU-C. The longitudinal changes of the CFU-C compartment have not been delineated following melphalan. In mice, the CFU-C content per femur 24 h after melphalan (2 mg/kg) was reduced to 50% of control values [205].
Several reports described the sensitivity of CFU-C to melphalan, some comparing it directly to that of CFU-S. When the CFU-C content per femur was studied in mice 3 and 24 h after drug, identical exponential curves were determined [434]. The same investigators studied the in vitro sensitivity of CFU-C from normal and from rapidly proliferating bone marrow; exponential survival curves were obtained that were identical not only to each other, but also to those of normal and rapidly proliferating marrow CFU-S. Using somewhat different conditions for incubation of marrow cells with melphalan in vitro, Ogawa et al. [436] found human CFU-C to be more sensitive to the drug than murine CFU-C, though both cell types displayed exponential survival curves.

Bone Marrow. The changes in murine bone marrow cellularity after a single dose of melphalan (6 mg/kg) were measured by Dunn [170], and a reduction of the femoral cell content to 40% at 24 h and to 9% at 48 h was seen. At 96 h, regeneration of the femoral cellularity (17%) was beginning. Simpson et al. [540] determined a linear correlation between dose of melphalan and marrow cellularity measured 4 days later, but they also observed an impressive circadian variation of the effect of melphalan on the reduction of the marrow cellularity, in that greatest toxicity was seen when the drug was given during the dark period.

Peripheral Blood. The recovery of peripheral blood WBC in humans following single high doses of melphalan (60–125 mg/m^2) was reported by Hedley et al. [271] who showed a minor reduction in WBC count during the first 6 days, followed by a rapid drop (to less than 500 WBC/µl) from day 10–14. Recovery was incomplete 35 days after drug administration. In another paper [376], the same group of investigators reported the changes of peripheral blood neutrophilic granulocytes after 60–125 mg/kg melphalan, and granulocytes were absent from the peripheral blood from day 12–20, but they recovered to near normal levels by day 32. There are indications of cumulative toxicity to the granulopoietic system after repeated melphalan treatments [549].

4.6 Busulfan

Busulfan, an alkylating agent with the chemical structure of an alkyl sulfonate [171], is effective by the oral route. Its pharmacokinetics have been described [622]. In early studies the cytocidal action of busulfan was found to be similar to that of radiation [30]. The drug has been used almost exclusively in myeloproliferative disorders, particularly in chronic myelogenous leukemia [224]. Its use requires experience, since frequently its effects upon the granulocyte and platelet counts are delayed, making determination of the dosage difficult. On the other hand, overdosage may lead to irreversible bone marrow failure.

CFU-S Sensitivity Studies. Several groups have studied the sensitivity of normal and rapidly proliferating CFU-S to busulfan (Table 18). With normal CFU-S, the dose-survival curve usually was exponential, though in one paper [42] a slightly curvilinear survival curve was described, and another group [387] reported no increased toxicity of busulfan at doses greater than 30 mg/kg (the time of assay after administration of busulfan was not stated). When rapidly proliferating CFU-S (after bone marrow transplantation or continuous irradiation) were studied for their sensitivity, one group of authors [42] described a curvilinear survival curve which was not different from that of normal CFU-S. In contrast, others [616] described an exponential survival curve for rapidly proliferating CFU-S which was somewhat steeper than that for normal CFU-S.
In vitro, the sensitivity of CFU-S to 20 µg/ml busulfan (2 h, 37° C) was measured [146] and a reduction to 2.7% of controls was found.

CFU-S Recovery Studies. The recovery of the bone marrow CFU-S compartment after a single dose of busulfan has been studied in mice and rats (Table 19). Rapid reduction

Table 18. Effect of busulfan on normal and rapidly proliferating bone marrow CFU-S: Sensitivity studies

Mouse strain	Time of assay (h)	$D_{1/2}$ (mg/kg)	CFU-S surviving (percent of controls)						Exponential dose-survival curve	Reference
			Dose (mg/kg)							
			0	10	20	40	60	80		
Normal CFU-S										
CBA or $C_{57}Bl$	–	~ 8	100		15	4	4		+ (plateau at > 30 mg/kg)	[387]
RFM/Un	24	35	100		60	45	25	16	+	[579]
C_3H/HeJ	24	8.5	100	30		5				[67]
–	24	20	100	60		5			– (Curvilinear)	[42]
$(C_{57}Bl/Rij \times CBA/Rij)F_1$	16	~ 15	100		40	15	5		+	[616]
Rapidly proliferating CFU-S										
$(C_{57}Bl/Rij \times CBA/Rij)F_1$	16	~ 15	100		40	9	1.5		+ (Shoulder at low doses?)	[616]
–	24	20	100	60		5			– (Curvilinear)	[42]

Table 19. Effect of busulfan on bone marrow CFU-S: Recovery studies

Species (strain)	Dose (mg/kg)	Bone marrow CFU-S (percent of controls) Day 0	1–3	4–6	7–9	10–12	13–15	16–18	19–21	22–24	25–27		Reference
Mouse [(CBA × C_{57}Bl/6)F_1]	10	100	60	40	40		50		80				[145]
Rat (Wilkie)	10	100	10				37		54			Day 35: 80	[168]
Rat (–)	10	100	20	20	30		80		90				[174]
Mouse [(CBA × C_{57}Bl/6)F_1]	20	100	15	20	40		20		40				[145]
Mouse (C_{57}Bl/6)	25	100				61[a]							[34]
Mouse (CBA; C_{57}Bl)	30	100	5	10	5								[387]
Mouse (NMRI; DBA/2)	30	100					7	3			14		[524]
Mouse [(CBA × C_{57}Bl/6)F_1]	40	100	1	1	2		4		20		60		[145]
Mouse [(BALBc × A)F_1]	40–50	100	10									Day 42: 45	[221]
Mouse (C_{57}Bl)	40	100	3										[553]
Mouse (–)	40	100		3		3			6			Day 30: 20 Day 40: 80	[43]
Mouse (–)	40	100	3	< 1	< 1	< 1	< 1	8	15	40			[599]
Mouse [(C_{57}Bl × DBA/2)F_1]	40	100			~ 1								[635]
Mouse (CF_1)	44	100	2	2	2	2	3						[480]
Mouse (CF_1)	44	100	4.5	< 1	< 1	< 1	2.1	~ 5	16.9	15.9	35		[481]
Mouse (CF_1)	44	100	< 1	< 1	< 1	< 2	< 3						[598]
Mouse [(C_3H/Hg-Mg)]	44	100		< 0.2	< 0.2								[213]
Mouse (DBA/2)	60	100		<10									[418]
Mouse [(C_3H × DBA)F_1]	60	100	0.1	0.03	0.1	1			2			Day 55: 30	[308]
Mouse (MF_1)	60	100	< 1	< 1	< 1	< 1	< 1	< 1		4			[479]
Mouse ($B_6D_2F_1$)	60	100	0.5	2	3	3–4	3–4		30			Day 35: 35	[57]

[a] Expressed as CFU-S/10^5 cells, and not CFU-S/femur as the other values in the table

Table 20. Effect of busulfan on splenic CFU-S: Recovery studies

Species (strain)	Dose (mg/kg)	Splenic CFU-S (percent of controls)								Reference
		Day								
		0	1–3	4–6	7–9	10–12	13–15	16–18	19–21	
Mouse (NMRI; DBA/2)	30	100					< 4	< 0.2		[524]
Mouse [(C_{57}bl × DBA/2)F_1]	40	100			~ 1					[635]
Mouse (–)	40	100	0.5						100	[43]
Mouse [(CBA × C_{57}Bl/6)F_1]	40	100	0.4	0.4	0.3			[145]		
Mouse [(C_3H/Hg-Mg)]	44	100		< 0.1	< 0.1					[606]

in the size of the bone marrow CFU-S compartment regularly occurs and the data document dose-dependency of this toxicity. Subsequent to the initial rapid depletion, a long-lasting depletion of the bone marrow CFU-S compartment was regularly observed. Regeneration of the CFU-S compartment occurs only very gradually. From the data published, it can be concluded that it takes more than 14 days in both species (in most studies, this time is considerably longer) before the CFU-S compartment of the bone marrow returns to pretreatment size.

Studies on the recovery of the splenic CFU-S compartment following busulfan treatments are listed in Table 20. When measured simultaneously, the effect of the drug was greater on the splenic than the bone marrow CFU-S compartment [43]. However, reconstitution of the splenic CFU-S pool proceeded more rapidly than that of the bone marrow compartment.

The proliferative activity of CFU-S in the spleen was found to be increased on day 14 (no earlier measurements performed) and had returned to control values 26 and 42 days after busulfan [43]. The proliferative activity of bone marrow-derived CFU-S following busulfan treatment was studied by several groups. Blackett and Millard [43] observed an increased kill of marrow CFU-S by cytosine arabinoside 5 and 14 days after busulfan. On days 26 and 42 after the drug, the proliferative activity of CFU-S had returned to the control level. Dunn [168] used the ^{3}H-TdR suicide technique to determine the proliferative activity of rat bone marrow CFU-S. Two days after a dose of 10 mg/kg busulfan, there was no difference in the proliferative activity between the treated animals and controls. However, 13 days after busulfan, the fraction of CFU-S surviving in vitro exposure to ^{3}H-TdR was significantly reduced (to about 0.40, compared to controls of about 0.85), indicating an increase in the proliferative activity of the busulfan-exposed CFU-S at this time. Twenty-one days after busulfan, the proliferative activity of CFU-S had returned to the normal range.

CFU-C Sensitivity Studies. Blackett et al. [42] measured the sensitivity of murine marrow CFU-C following in vivo administration of busulfan (assay performed 24 h post drug). There was a somewhat curvilinear dose-survival curve, suggesting a shoulder at lower doses and an exponential curve at higher doses of the drug. Survival of CFU-C was greater than that of CFU-S assayed simultaneously, which agrees with data reported by others [145, 146, 389].

Delmonte et al. [146] determined a reduction of mouse femoral CFU-C to 12% of controls 24 h after 40 mg/kg busulfan. He also described the preferential killing of lighter density CFU-C by the drug [147]. Exposure of CFU-C in vitro to the drug (2 h, 37° C; 20 µg/ml busulfan) resulted in a decrease of CFU-C to 22.9%.

Gordon et al. [239] assayed normal human stem cells identical with or closely related to CFU-C for their sensitivity to busulfan (agar-diffusion chamber method). Again, a survival curve can be constructed composed of a shoulder at low doses and an exponential part at high doses of busulfan.

CFU-C Recovery Studies. Little work has been published on the pattern of depletion and repletion of the CFU-C compartment in animals following busulfan treatment (Table 21). In mice, a reduction of the size of the femoral CFU-C compartment to 23% was described 24 h after 40 mg/kg busulfan [553]. Others [43] observed a reduction of the murine marrow CFU-C compartment to about 25% of pretreatment size during the first 1 or 2 days after a single dose of 40 mg/kg busulfan. However, a further decrease of the size of the CFU-C compartment ensued, with nadirs of 1–2% of pretreatment

Table 21. Effect of busulfan on bone marrow and spleen CFU-C: Recovery studies

Species (strain)	Dose (mg/kg)	CFU-C (percent of controls) Day 0	1	2	4	6	8	10	14	18	22	26	30	34	Reference
Bone Marrow															
Mouse ($C_{57}Bl$)	40	100	23												[553]
Mouse ($C_{57}Bl$)	40	100	25	25	1–2				5		10		60		[43]
Mouse (DBA/2)	30	100							9	9		13			[524]
Mouse [(CBA × $C_{57}Bl/6)F_1$]	10	100			50		100		60		55				[145]
	20	100			10		50		20		60				[145]
	40	100			5		1		3		20			100	[145]
Mouse ($B_6D_2F_1$)	60	100		20	6	2	5	1.5	5		25		90	85	[57]
Dog (beagle)	10	100[b]					70		70		100	200			[2]
	20	100[b]					7		30		20	70			[2]
	30	100[b]					< 1		5		10	10		Day 56: 15	[2]
	40	100[b]					< 1		NA[a]						[2]
Spleen															
Mouse (NMRI or DBA/2)	30	100							16	5.5					[524]
Mouse [(CBA × $C_{57}Bl/6)F_1$]	40	100	2		3		3								[145]
Mouse ($C_{57}Bl$)	40	100		2						100		400		100	[43]

[a] All animals dead, no analysis possible
[b] Values expressed as CFU-C/ml marrow aspirate

size reached around day 5. Thereafter, CFU-C showed the same slow recovery as the CFU-S assayed in parallel.

Seidel et al. [524] studied the effect of a single dose of 30 mg/kg busulfan on the CFU-C pool in bone marrow and spleen. In the bone marrow, the number of CFU-C per femur was 9% of controls on day 13, 9% on day 18, and 13% on day 26. The number of CFU-C per spleen was 16% of controls on day 13, 5.5% on day 18 (day 26 was not reported).

The most detailed study on the changes with time of the femoral CFU-C compartment after busulfan has been reported by Delmonte et al. [145]. With three different doses (10, 20, and 40 mg/kg, respectively), the incidence of femoral CFU-C was decreased time- and dose-dependently. By 2–5 days, maximal depression to 21%, 9.3%, and 1.5% of control values was measured in the three dosage groups, respectively. Incipient repopulation of the femoral CFU-C compartment was observed 5–6 days after treatment. Normalization of the bone marrow CFU-C compartment size was noted by day 21 in the 10 and 20 mg/kg dosage groups though, in the 40 mg/kg group, total repletion of the femoral CFU-C pool required 35 days.

Very recently, Boggs et al. [57] reported a recovery study for bone marrow CFU-C in $B_6D_2F_1$ mice. Following 60 mg/kg busulfan, CFU-C gradually declined. With some abortive rises, the minimum size of the bone marrow CFU-C compartment (2% of controls) was reached by day 9. The subsequent recovery led to near normal values after day 30.

In dogs, the number of CFU-C per ml bone marrow aspirate following busulfan doses (10–40 mg/kg) was measured [2]. A dose-dependent reduction of CFU-C was determined. With a dose of 20 mg/kg, the nadir was observed on day 7 and recovery to control values took 28 days to be completed. With 30 mg/kg busulfan, there were almost no CFU-C detectable on day 7 and on day 56 the recovery was incomplete, the value for CFU-C per ml aspirate being in the range of 15% of controls.

In mouse spleen, CFU-C were reduced to 2% of control values by day 2 after 40 mg/kg busulfan, with a more rapid recovery than in the bone marrow leading to a normalization of the splenic CFU-C compartment size by day 20. On day 25, an excessive expansion of the splenic CFU-C compartment was noted, but normal values were again recorded on days 35 and 42 [43].

The splenic CFU-C compartment was similarly studied by Delmonte et al. [145]. During the first 7 days after treatment with 40 mg/kg busulfan, the number of CFU-C per spleen was decreased to a degree (2.2% of control values) comparable to that of the femoral CFU-C.

The proliferative activity of murine CFU-C following busulfan administration was derived from the fraction of stem cells surviving repeated cytosine arabinoside injections. Bone marrow CFU-C showed increased proliferative activity 5 and 14 days after busulfan, with return to a normal proliferative activity on day 42. In the spleen, CFU-C were intensively proliferating on day 14 after busulfan (day 5 not tested), with return to their normal proliferative activity at 26 and 42 days [43].

Data on the recovery pattern of normal human CFU-C following busulfan are not available, most likely because this drug has been almost exclusively used in the treatment of myeloproliferative disorders, whereas it is not part of any treatment protocol of human solid tumors.

Studies of the reaction pattern of normal peripheral blood CFU-C to busulfan have not been reported in experimental animals or in humans.

Of some interest are calculations of the ratio of femoral CFU-S to femoral CFU-C following treatment with busulfan [146]. The drug depressed the number of CFU-S more profoundly than the number of CFU-C, and this depression was time- and dose-dependent: In both the 10 and 20 mg/kg groups, the CFU-S : CFU-C ratio reached its nadir (43% and 30% of control values, respectively) by day 7. Normalization of the CFU-S : CFU-C ratio by day 28 was seen in the 10 mg/kg group but not in the 20 mg/kg group. In animals treated with 40 mg/kg busulfan, the nadir of the CFU-S : CFU-C ratio occurred as early as 2 days after treatment and normal values were recorded by day 21.

The splenic CFU-S : CFU-C ratio showed a depression to 2–9% of control values during the first 7 days after 40 mg/kg busulfan (measurements beyond this time point were not made).

Bone Marrow Cellularity. Busulfan depletes the cellularity of the bone marrow for a prolonged period of time. This impact appears to be dose-related with respect to both severity of marrow hypoplasia and the duration of time to normalization (Table 22). Minimum marrow cellularity has been reported to occur at days 4–10 in these studies in both rats and mice. As long as 3 weeks after exposure to the drug, the cellularity of the marrow was still subnormal in all studies. Longer observation periods have not been reported.

Cytologic Changes of the Bone Marrow. Following 60 mg/kg busulfan, the number of murine granulocytic bone marrow cells decreased to a nadir of less than 10% on day 5. A transient recovery to 60% of normal by day 10 was followed by a decline to a second nadir of approximately 30% of normal on day 14. By day 35, granulocytic bone marrow cells had not returned to the pretreatment level [57]. In mice, the number of proliferating granulocytic cells of the bone marrow fell to a first nadir (10% of pretreatment numbers) around day 4 after busulfan (60 mg/kg), rose to approximately 60% by day 7, and then fell again to approximately 20% for a prolonged period of time (up to day 20) [308]. Thirty-five and 55 days after busulfan, the number of proliferating granulocytic cells in the marrow was in the pretreatment range. The nonproliferative granulocytic marrow cells followed a similar pattern, but they lagged approximately 24 h behind the decline and regeneration of the proliferating granulocytic marrow cells.

The number of blast cells per femur was studied after treatment of mice with 40 mg/kg busulfan [145]. Blast cell levels were severely depressed 1–3 days after drug exposure, evidence of beginning blast cell regeneration was noted by day 4, and return to low normal blast cell levels was recorded by day 7.

Finley et al. [200] described the changes in the composition of murine granulocytic marrow 2–10 days after busulfan. On day 2, no changes were detectable. However, on day 6 the early granulocytic cells were absent, whereas an increase in the proportion of myeloblasts and myelocytes was seen on day 10.

Niskanen [427, 428] reported detailed results of the changes of the bone marrow cytology following 12 mg/kg busulfan in white rats. The proliferating granulocytic cells reached lowest values (about 30% of controls) on day 4, followed by a gradual return towards normal (28 days after busulfan, the proliferating granulocytic cells had still reached only about 80% of normal). The nonproliferating (nonmitotic) granulocytic marrow cells showed a very similar pattern of depletion and repletion, althoug there was a lag period between the changes of proliferating cells and the respective changes of the nonproliferating granulocytic cells.

Table 22. Effect of busulfan on bone marrow cellularity: Recovery studies

Species (strain)	Dose (mg/kg)	Cellularity (percent of controls)												Reference
		Day												
		0	2	4	6	8	10	12	14	16	18	22	26	
Mouse [(CBA × $C_{57}Bl/6)F_1$]	10	No changes of marrow cellularity												[145]
Rat (–)	10	100	80	30		80		60	60			90		[174]
Rat (Sprague/Dawley)	12	100	70	40		40	40			50		60		[427]
Rat (–)	15	100	50[a]	75	50	50			30			50		[183]
Mouse [(CBA × $C_{57}Bl/6)F_1$]	20	100		70	100									[145]
Mouse (DBA/2; NMRI)	30	100						66			76		92	[524]
Mouse [(CBA × $C_{57}Bl/6)F_1$]	40	100	50	40	70	80			50				80	[145]
Mouse (–)	40	Little depression (to 70–80%) through day 26												[43]
Mouse (–)	40	100			21	71								[599]
Mouse (Rf/Up)	50–60	Semiquantitative analysis, hypoplasia days 4–24												[14]
Mouse (MF_1)	60	100	11		11	18	13		36		32	57		[479]
Mouse ($B_6D_2F_1$)	60	100	40 50	20	3	10	2		10			55	Day 35: 90	[57]
Rat (–)	No experimental data given in detail ("gradual fall and recovery of marrow cellularity")													[136]

[a] Estimates

Elson et al. [183] did not separate the changes of the proliferating and of the nonproliferating rat marrow compartment. Rather, they reported on the overall changes of the granulocytic marrow cells. Between days 2–6 after busulfan (15 mg/kg), a steep reduction was observed. Between days 6–15, the granulocytic cells continued to be less than 20% of normal. The gradual recovery observed later failed to return the granulocytic cell count of the marrow to normal by day 26.
Reissmann [479] studied the bone marrow content of myelocytes and segmented neutrophils after 60 mg/kg busulfan. Myelocytes gradually decreased to low values (less than 20% of normal) by day 16. During the same time, segmented neutrophils almost completely disappeared from the bone marrow.
Changes within the myeloblast compartment resulting from a single dose of 40 mg/kg busulfan were studied by Udupa et al. [599]. There was a rapid drop of the percentage of myeloblasts, with a nadir of 25% reached on day 4. Myeloblast counts increased transiently to 60% of normal on day 6 and dropped again to around 20% of normal on days 12–16. Early after busulfan, there was a considerable reduction of the percentage of labeled myeloblasts after in vivo exposure to ^{3}H-TdR. However, the percentage of labeled myeloblasts returned to normal by day 4 and thereafter remained normal for the observation period. The myelocyte to metamyelocyte transition rate, as determined from the percentage of metamyelocytes labeled 16 h after injection of ^{3}H-TdR into previously busulfan-treated mice, dropped to less than 10% of normal by day 3, remained at that level through day 5, and then rose to 60% of normal by day 8. Thereafter, a second long-lasting reduction of the myelocyte to metamyelocyte transition rate was determined with values of less than 10% between day 12–16 after busulfan. The changes of the myeloblast counts preceded the respective changes of the myelocyte to metamyelocyte transition rate by approximately 2 days during the phase of the transient recovery and of the second long-lasting depletion.
Studies of the cytologic changes of a normal, i.e., a nonleukemic, human bone marrow after busulfan exposure are not reported in the literature. The bone marrow granulocyte reserve has not been studied following busulfan exposure.

Peripheral Blood Granulocytes. In a variety of mammalian species, the longitudinal changes of peripheral blood granulocytes after busulfan exposure have been studied. From the tabulation of these data (Table 23), the long duration of the busulfan-induced depression of the granulocytic bone marrow compartments (see above) is reflected in the peripheral blood by a dose-dependent long-lasting neutropenia. In mice, peripheral blood neutrophils have by far not returned to pretreatment concentrations as long as 2 months after single high doses of busulfan [308]. Comparing the busulfan-induced neutropenia to that after other cytotoxic drugs, such as cyclophosphamide, it becomes obvious that granulocytopenia after busulfan develops more slowly. Although no findings on the effect of busulfan on a normal (i.e., nonleukemic) granulocytopoiesis have been published in man, the more gradual development of granulocytopenia in experimental animals resembles the delayed reduction of granulocyte counts that occurs in patients with chronic myelogenous leukemia after initiation of busulfan treatment.

Granulopiesis After Repeated Exposure to Busulfan. The data discussed above indicate that the complete recovery to pretreatment size of the different granulopoietic compartments after a single exposure to busulfan takes considerable time. Thus, it is conceivable that repeated administration of busulfan at intervals shorter than that

Table 23. Effect of busulfan on peripheral blood granulocytes: Recovery studies

Species (strain)	Dose (mg/kg)	Blood granulocyte count (percent of controls)											Reference
		Day											
		0	1–3	4–6	7–9	10–12	13–15	16–18	19–21	22–24	25–27	28–30	
Mouse [(CBA × C_{57}Bl/6)F_1]	10	100	35						100				[145]
Rat (–)	10	100	90	50	< 10	< 10	15	~ 15	20	~ 50	80		[174]
Rat (–)	10–15	100				10–20					100		[183]
Dog (beagle)	10–40						—Nadir—						[2]
Rat (Sprague/Dawley)	12	100	50	35	25	15	22	30	40	50			[427]
Rat (–)	15	100	110	60	20	< 5	~ 5	15	35	40			[184, 185]
Dog (mongrel)	15–20	100		~ 90	~ 25	~ 20	~ 15						[299]
Mouse (Swiss)	16.3	100	155	65		25							[200]
Mouse [(DBA × C_{57}Bl/6)F_1]	20	100		23					100				[145]
Rat (Sprague/Dawley)	35	100	53	24	0	0	†						[500]
Mouse (–)	40	100	85	18	35	45	20	10					[599]
Mouse (–)	40				70–80% of normal through day 26								[43]
Mouse [(DBA × C_{57}Bl/6)F_1]	40	100		3					30			< 100	[145]
Mouse (CF_1)	44	100	66	20	28	20	16	20	32	75		90	[597]
Mouse (MF_1)	60	100	100	60	30	20		2	2				[479]
Mouse [(C_3H × DBA)F_1]	60	100	50	20	45	40			8			Day 55: ~ 50%	[308]

required for normalization of compartment sizes may lead to cumulative toxicity, i.e., to progressive shrinking of compartment sizes. However, even with full quantitative normalization of compartment sizes, animal studies indicate the possibility of a permanent qualitative defect of the pluripotent stem cell population following short-term busulfan treatment.

Morley et al. [401] studied the effect of busulfan, given repeatedly at short intervals for a limited period of time, on the hematopoietic system of mice. The animals developed marrow aplasia with resulting peripheral blood pancytopenia several months after completion of busulfan therapy. Further studies revealed that this phase of overt marrow aplasia was preceded by a phase of "latent aplasia". During this latter phase, peripheral blood counts and the marrow cellularity were normal, but the size of the pluripotent and of the committed stem cell pools was progressively shrinking [402]. Busulfan-induced damage to the hemopoietic microenvironment as a major cause of this hematopoietic failure could be ruled out [404]. Thus, a primary busulfan-induced stem cell failure appeared to be the most likely cause of the ensuing hemopoietic failure [406]. Although others observed no overt marrow aplasia after similar busulfan treatment, the reduction in size of stem cell compartments was confirmed [65, 66, 68, 202]. Concomitant with the reduction of the size of the CFU-S pool, an increased proliferative activity of the CFU-S was demonstrated as long as 56 and 104 weeks after completion of busulfan treatment [281].

The following studies shed light on the nature of the delayed stem cell and hematopoietic failure after short-term busulfan treatment. Measuring the extent of CFU-S self-replication within individual spleen colonies, Schofield [512] demonstrated diminished capacity for self-maintenance of CFU-S after busulfan treatment. In a series of experiments, Botnick and Hellman and their coworkers extended and supported these findings. Using the number of possible serial transfers of bone marrow as a measure for the self-replicative capacity of pluripotent stem cells, these authors demonstrated a considerable loss of the potential for proliferation and self-replication of stem cells following repeated exposure to busulfan [65, 66]. More directly, the same group later demonstrated a busulfan-induced loss of CFU-S self-replication within the femoral cavity of supralethally irradiated mice [67, 281].

From these data, a hypothesis of the nature of the busulfan-induced damage to the hematopoietic system has been put forth [275]. It appears that the more differentiated compartments are little affected in a direct manner by busulfan. The damage to these differentiated hematopoietic compartments appears to be indirect, as a result of damage to earlier compartments. The long duration of the recovery period allows the conclusion that the capacity for regeneration is severely impaired following busulfan treatment. An explanation for these observations may come from the suggestion [67] that busulfan treatment preferentially and irreversibly destroys the most immature cells among pluripotent stem cells. For a discussion of this hypothesis, the reader is referred to the chapter on residual bone marrow damage following cytotoxic drug exposure (page 177).

4.7 Dimethyl Myleran (DMM)

DMM, a dimethylated homologue of busulfan (Myleran), has attracted some interest from experimental and clinical researchers. However, the available data do not allow a comprehensive view of its action upon the granulocytic system.

CFU-S Sensitivity Studies. The sensitivity of murine CFU-S to DMM was investigated by van Putten [616]. Both normal and rapidly proliferating CFU-S gave exponential dose-survival curves at doses of 5–35 mg/kg DMM (assayed 16 h post-drug), although the sensitivity of rapidly proliferating CFU-S to DMM was somewhat greater than that of normal CFU-S.

CFU-S Recovery Studies. A longitudinal study of the effect of DMM on the pluripotent stem cell pool has not been published. In mice, a reduction in size of the femoral CFU-S compartment to approximately 35% has been observed 13 days after a dose of 3.5 mg/kg DMM. At this time, the proliferative activity of the CFU-S was increased (^{3}H-TdR suicide technique) [170].
The "granulocytic repopulating ability" (a measure for the bone marrow content of a poorly defined population of granulopoietic stem cells) was depressed for a prolonged period after treatment with 2 mg/kg DMM [126]. Return to normal values was not observed within a follow-up period of 25 days.

CFU-C; Bone Marrow. Studies of CFU-C have not been performed following administration of DMM.
A dose of 10 mg/kg DMM reduced the marrow cellularity of mice to 20% of controls by day 3 [566].
An analysis of changes in bone marrow cytology following DMM is not reported in the literature.
Taking the endotoxin-induced increment in peripheral granulocytes as a measure of the functional bone marrow granulocyte reserve, Constable et al. [125] found a decrease of this value to 50% on day 3 and to 15–20% from day 4–9; 50% values were again reached by day 11 and pretreatment values were seen on day 13 with no subsequent excessive values.

Peripheral Blood. Some toxicological studies on the effect of graded doses of DMM on the peripheral blood white cell and neutrophil counts have been performed, mainly in the context of autologous marrow transplantation utilized as a rescue procedure from severe cytotoxic drug-induced marrow failure. Lethal doses of DMM were reported to be 7.5 mg/kg in rats [575] and dogs [322], 10.0 mg/kg in rhesus monkeys [86], and 15 mg/kg in mice [203a]. Death resulted mainly from severe hematopoietic toxicity in these studies. In rhesus monkeys, severe dose-dependent peripheral blood granulocytopenia occurred from days 11–25 at higher concentrations of the drug, and recovery from granulocytopenia was gradual [86]. Similarly, in dogs a dose-dependent granulocytopenia and a slow recovery of peripheral blood granulocyte counts was noted. Between days 7–15, granulocytes were absent from the peripheral blood at doses greater than 5 mg/kg DMM [322]. In rats, a single dose of 8 mg/kg led to a rapid reduction of peripheral blood granulocytes, while between days 4–6 near zero levels were recorded. Thereafter, a somewhat oscillatory gradual rise of the peripheral blood PMN count occurred and, on day 13 after DMM, the count had returned to approximately 30% of pretreatment values [595].
In man, preferential toxicity of DMM to the granulopoietic system was noted by Bierman et al. [39] in a few patients treated for advanced solid tumours with this drug. However, the authors did not provide detailed information on extent or duration of granulocytopenia, or on the kinetics of granulocyte recovery. From data reported by Clifford et al. [113], a considerable reduction of the peripheral blood leukocyte

concentration is apparent at DMM doses of 2.0–3.5 mg/kg (given as three split doses at 2-day intervals). However, no information on the time course of the decline and the subsequent recovery of peripheral blood granulocyte counts can be derived from the paper.

4.8 Methotrexate (MTX)

The antimetabolite MTX is a typical S-phase-specific cytotoxic agent. Its very complex effects on malignant and normal cells, including granulopoietic cells, are a consequence of its pharmacologic characteristics. Inhibition of dihydrofolate reductase leads to depletion of 1-carbon-carrying tetrahydrofolates, and thus to a block of thymidilate and purine nucleotide synthesis. In various systems, including normal and leukemic hematopoietic cells, the threshold level for blocking DNA synthesis has been established [458, 568]. In vivo and in vitro, the availability of exogenous nucleosides and the ability of cells to utilize these resources determine whether MTX will cause the cessation of nucleic acid synthesis [458]. A complex mechanism for blocking cells in the cell cycle has been described in L cells [63]. In this model, cell kill resulted from the inhibition of thymidilate synthesis, while the concurrent inhibition of purine synthesis appeared to prevent efficient killing. "Purineless death" is discussed as a link between growth rate and cytotoxicity of MTX [295].
Since the killing effect of MTX is limited to cells in S-phase, the dose-survival curves show a characteristic plateau produced by the resistance of cells in other phases of the cell cycle.
Goldin et al. [233] first explored ways to modify MTX toxicity by "rescue techniques". By circumventing the MTX-induced metabolic block with citrovorum factor (leucovorin) or by substituting precursors of nucleic acid synthesis like thymidine or hypoxanthine, the therapeutic index of MTX could be improved (reviewed in Bertino [36]).
In view of these very complex interactions, it is not surprising that a complete picture of MTX influence on granulopoiesis is not available to date.

CFU-S Sensitivity Studies. The dose-survival of pluripotent bone marrow stem cells has been assessed after single doses of MTX and during continuous application (Table 24).
Due to their low proliferative activity, normal CFU-S are little sensitive to MTX. In the mouse, most authors found no significant decrease of bone marrow CFU-S 16–24 h after a wide range of MTX doses (Table 24) [370, 420, 617]), although Dunn and Constable [172] reported a depletion of the CFU-S pool to about 50–60% with a plateau at doses greater than 50 mg/kg (Table 24). In two papers from the same group, evaluating combinations of various cytotoxic agents, an unusually low CFU-S survival was reported with a plateau at 30% with 50–150 mg/kg MTX [178, 612] (Table 24).
In the study of Nečas and Neuwirt [420] (Table 24), the proliferative activity of murine CFU-S, after a single dose of 5 mg/kg MTX, was reported to increase slightly, from 20 to 30% of CFU-S in S-phase (^{3}H-TdR suicide technique), with a time lag of approximately 24 h and a maximum at 30 h. This time course was interpreted to be the result of partial synchronization of CFU-S. Similarly, rat CFU-S showed little response to MTX in vivo when bone marrow or spleen cells were assayed 4 h after exposure in

Table 24. Effect of MTX on CFU-S: Sensitivity studies

Species (strain)	Source of CFU-S, experimental conditions	Time of assay after MTX (h)	CFU-S survival (percent of controls) Dose (mg/kg)																	Reference
			3.75	5	7.5	15	20	25	30	50	60	75/80	100	150	200	250	300	400	1500	
Mouse (NMRI)	Bone marrow	24		100																[420]
Mouse (Swiss)	Bone marrow	24									100									[370, 371]
Mouse (C_{57}Bl × CBA)	Bone marrow	16									100	100								[617]
Mouse (C_{57}Bl)	Bone marrow	24								51			47		58					[172]
Mouse (C_3H × DBA/2J)	Bone marrow	24								30				30						[178, 612]
Mouse (C_{57}Bl × DBA)	Endogenous CFU-S, MTX immediately after irradiation	9 days after irradiation								100				75		< 10		0		[56]
Mouse (C_{57}Bl × DBA/2)	Posttransplant spleen, MTX 48 h after transplantation	120	80		65	55	65		60			10								[530, 531]

Table 24 (continued)

Species (strain)	Source of CFU-S, experimental conditions	Time of assay after MTX (h)	CFU-S survival (percent of controls)																	Reference
			Dose (mg/kg)																	
			3.75	5	7.5	15	20	25	30	50	60	75/ 80	100	150	200	250	300	400	1500	
Rat (Wilkie hooded)	Bone marrow derived CFU-S, recovered in control animals[a]																			
	Bone marrow	4								90		90	90							[169]
	Spleen									90		90	90							
	During exponential phase[b]																			
	Bone marrow									12		12	12							
	Spleen									12		12	12							
Mouse (AKR/J)	Bone marrow, "continuous" MTX administration	24						30		30			30	30					30	[82]
Mouse (C_{57}Bl/6N)	Bone marrow, continuous infusion														37					[458]

[a] 36 days after transplantation of bone marrow
[b] 4 days after transplantation of bone marrow

animals that had received a bone marrow transplant 36 days previously [169] (Table 24).
When MTX was given to mice by repeated injections, thus establishing a continuous drug exposure for 24–48 h, a plateau at approximately 30% CFU-S survival is observed [82] (Table 24). A similar depression of CFU-S is observed at the end of a 24-h continuous infusion with a cumulative dose of approximately 200 mg/kg [458] (Table 24). In these experiments, the serum level was kept constant at $0.5–2.0 \times 10^{-5}$ *M*.
Endogenous CFU-S were studied in mice injected with MTX immediately after sublethal irradiation. A dose of 50 mg/kg did not decrease the number of endogenous CFU-S, though at higher doses a progressive cell kill was observed [56] (Table 24). The dose-survival curve of rapidly proliferating bone marrow-derived CFU-S exposed to MTX 48 h after marrow transplantation showed a plateau at approximately 60% CFU-S survival up to doses of 30 mg/kg; 10% CFU-S survival was determined after 80 mg/kg [530, 531] (Table 24). In this set of data, the spleen colonies were counted 7 days after transplantation, i.e., 5 days after MTX. When 15–30 mg/kg MTX was given on day 5 after transplantation, all visible colony growth was abolished on day 7. However, on day 12 after transplantation, CFU-S counts did not differ from control animals. The authors concluded that the small number of surviving stem cells was able to restore a normal number of spleen colonies when sufficient time was given for recovery.

CFU-S Recovery Studies. Since single doses of MTX have shown no or little cytotoxic effect on the CFU-S pool, recovery experiments are not meaningful.
Few studies on the changes of CFU-S have been performed during continuous MTX administration (Table 25). Bruce et al. [82] gave 50 and 150 mg/kg per day in three or six divided doses for 24 or 48 h and observed an exponential decline of CFU-S during the first 12 h, followed by a plateau at 30% CFU-S survival up to 72 h. Pinedo et al. [457] kept the serum level of MTX constant at $0.5–2.0 \times 10^{-5}$ *M* by an implanted delivery system. They observed a decline to 37% CFU-S survival at 24 h and a further decrease to 12% at 48 h. This further decrease of the CFU-S pool at low MTX levels has been interpreted as an efflux from the CFU-S pool in the process of CFU-C "recruitment" at the same time [459] (see also page 68).

Table 25. Effect of MTX on murine CFU-S: Percent survival during continuous drug administration

Strain	Dose (level) of MTX	CFU-S survival (percent of controls)				Reference
		Time of exposure (h)[a]				
		0–12	24	48	72	
AKR/7	50 or 150 mg/24 h by repeated injections	Exponential decline	30	30	30	[82]
C_{57}Bl/6N	Constant level at $0.5–2.0 \times 10^{-5}$ *M* (approximately 200 mg/24 h)		37	12		[457, 459]

[a] CFU-S measured at the end of exposure period

Table 26. Effect of single doses of MTX on murine CFU-C: Sensitivity studies

Strain	Source of CFU-C, experimental conditions	Time of assay after MTX (h)	Survival of CFU-C (percent of controls)													Reference
			Dose (mg/kg)													
			2	5	15	30	50	60	100	120	200	250	300	400	500	
$C_{57}Bl$	Bone marrow	18–20							75–80		75–80		75–80			[237]
$C_{57}Bl/6N$	Bone marrow	24		95			65					55			50	[78]
BDF_1	Bone marrow	24							66							[602]
	Spleen	24							154							
$C_{57}Bl$	Bone marrow	24			85		88							115		[204, 206]
	Bone marrow, *C. parvum* (−24 h)	24			82		78							75		
$C_{57}Bl$	Bone marrow	24						102		58						[626, 627]

Table 27. Effect of repeated/continuous MTX administration on murine CFU-C: Sensitivity studies

Strain	Source of CFU-S	Dose schedule	Time of assay (h)	CFU-C survival (percent of controls)						Reference
				Cumulative dose (mg/kg/24 h)						
				2	15	50	100	120	200	
				Serum level (m*M*)[a]						
				4.5×10^{-8}	1.8×10^{-7}	1.2×10^{-6}		7×10^{-6}		
BDF_1	Bone marrow	Three divided doses every 6 h	6[b]				78			[602]
	Spleen	Three divided doses every 6 h	150[b]				742			
$C_{57}Bl/6N$	Bone marrow	Continuous infusion	24[c]	64	64	46		43		[457]
			48[c]	78	55	56		67		

[a] From reference [457]
[b] After last MTX dose
[c] Duration of continuous infusion

CFU-C in Vivo Sensitivity Studies. Experiments on the in vivo dose-response of CFU-C after single doses of MTX are listed in Table 26. The dose-survival curves regularly show a plateau. Although the level of this plateau varies somewhat, a remarkable resistance of CFU-C to single MTX doses is evident.

When the bone marrow CFU-C of C_{57}Bl mice were stimulated to a higher proliferative state by *Corynebacterium parvum* (*C. parvum*), MTX reduced the CFU-C content per femur to approximately two-thirds of the value observed after MTX alone [204, 206] (Table 26).

Uyeki [602] (Table 26) reports a difference in survival between bone marrow and spleen CFU-C. The behavior of the bone marrow and spleen CFU-C pool will be further discussed with the recovery studies.

Repeated [602] or continuous [457] administration of MTX caused somewhat greater CFU-C kill than single doses (Table 27).

Few data are available on the in vivo sensitivity of human CFU-C. In our laboratory, we have studied granulopoietic precursor cells in bone marrow after high-dose MTX (200 mg/kg over 6 h) followed by citrovorum factor rescue over 72 h [516]. Forty-eight hours after beginning MTX administration the incidence of bone marrow CFU-C decreased to 60% of control values, while the circulating CFU-C pool decreased to 10% of pretreatment size. In these experiments, the proliferative activity of bone marrow CFU-C was measured, using the ^{3}H-TdR suicide technique. A small increase of the proliferative state of bone marrow CFU-C was observed on day 7 (53% kill by ^{3}H-TdR versus 42% on day 0, $P < 0.05$).

CFU-C in Vitro Sensitivity Studies. Pinedo et al. [458] (Table 28) determined the CFU-C survival at various MTX concentrations, present in the cultures during the entire culture period. When undialysed serum was used, no CFU-C kill occurred even at very high MTX concentrations. When dialysed serum was used, a progressive cell kill occurred without formation of a plateau. This system clearly demonstrates that the cytotoxic action of MTX can be reversed by metabolites present in undialysed serum. The in vitro MTX exposure of CFU-C was used by the authors [457, 458] to elucidate several aspects of the pharmacology of MTX. The fact that CFU-C, preexposed in vivo to MTX, showed the same in vitro sensitivity as nonexposed CFU-C indicates no selection of a MTX-resistant CFU-C subpopulation, which would explain the resumption of DNA synthesis during continuous in vivo MTX exposure. This model has also been used to study the reversal of MTX cytotoxicity to mouse bone marrow cells by leukovorin and nucleosides [458]. At low concentrations of MTX, equimolar concentrations of leukovorin led to a complete rescue, while at higher concentrations of MTX, the concentration of leukovorin had to exceed that of MTX. While leukovorin reversed the MTX toxicity to CFU-C competitively, rescue by nucleosides was noncompetitive.

Recent data [321] on the in vitro sensitivity of human CFU-C (Table 28) show that a plateau at around 30% survival is achieved with concentrations 10^{-5} *M* or more when the drug is present during the entire culture period. Two-hour drug exposure before plating did not reduce CFU-C survival even at 10^{-3} *M* MTX concentration, while 6- and 24-h exposures were effective only at this highest dose level.

CFU-C Sensitivity in Diffusion Chambers. Utilizing the agar-diffusion chamber system, murine and human CFU-C were exposed to various doses of MTX given as single injection to the primary host and transferred to a secondary host 20 h later [237]

Table 28. Effect of MTX on bone marrow CFU-C in vitro (upper part) and in diffusion chambers (lower part): Sensitivity studies

Species (strain)	Experimental conditions	CFU-C survival (percent of controls)							Reference
		Concentration (*M*)							
		10^{-9}	10^{-8}	10^{-7}	10^{-6}	10^{-5}	10^{-4}	10^{-3}	
Mouse (C_{57}Bl/6N)	Incubation in vitro, continuous exposure								
	Undialysed medium	100	100	100	100	80	40		[458]
	Dialysed medium	100	50	0					
Mouse (C_{57}Bl/6N) preexposed to MTX in vivo	Dialysed medium		50						[457]
Human	Continuous exposure	105	93	62	44	33	30	26	[321]
	2-h exposure					100	100	108	
	6-h exposure					146	120	25	
	24-h exposure			91	117	77	82	4	
		Dose (mg/kg)[a]							
				100	200	300			
Mouse (C_{57}Bl)	Exposure in diffusion chambers for 18–20 h			40	10	4			[237]
Human	Exposure in diffusion chambers for 18–20 h			40	10	4			

[a] Exposure to MTX in diffusion chambers in primary hosts

(Table 28, lower part). Identical exponential dose-survival curves were found for both murine and human CFU-C with a $D_{1/2}$ of around 70 mg/kg.
These experiments also illustrate the importance of the experimental conditions. When agar was omitted from the diffusion chambers during MTX exposure, no exponential CFU-C kill was observed, but the CFU-C survival curve showed a plateau at approximately 50%. The authors discuss two possibilities for this difference: The presence of agar in the diffusion chamber could cause prolonged MTX availability or the state of CFU-C proliferation may vary due to experimental conditions.

CFU-C Recovery Studies. In view of the minor effects of single doses of MTX on the CFU-C compartment, it is not surprising that time-course experiments reveal no major changes in this situation (Table 29). In the experiments of Vogler et al. [626] (Table 29), a second dose of MTX caused slight to moderate reduction of CFU-C survival followed by excessive recovery. Both CFU-C depression and "overshoot" were dependent on dose and the time interval between the two doses. In the experiments of Uyeki [602] (Table 29), few changes were observed in the bone marrow CFU-C compartment, while the splenic CFU-C pool was greatly expanded.
When a constant serum level of MTX was maintained ($0.5-2.0 \times 10^{-5}$ *M*), CFU-C decreased to approximately 40% by 24 h and recovered to 60–65% by 48 h [459] (Table 29). This increase of CFU-C during continuous MTX administration together with a decrease of CFU-S during this time period [457, 459] (Table 25) was taken as evidence of CFU-C recruitment [459].
In man, we have studied the time course of bone marrow and circulating CFU-C after high-dose MTX with citrovorum factor rescue [516] (Table 29). While bone marrow CFU-C showed little response to high-dose MTX-citrovorum factor rescue (HDM-CFR), the peripheral blood CFU-C pool decreased to 10% on day 2.

Bone Marrow Cellularity. Data on dose-response and time course of bone marrow cellularity after MTX are summarized in Table 30. When assayed 24 h after MTX, the bone marrow cellularity decreases to a plateau at 60–70% of normal over a wide range of single MTX doses. The nadir of bone marrow cellularity is reached 2–4 days after MTX.
Under continuous administration of different MTX doses a plateau of cellularity is found at around 30% of normal. However, this value is reached more rapidly at higher continuous MTX levels [457] (Table 30).

Cytologic Changes of Bone Marrow. Some data on cytologic changes of bone marrow during and after MTX are given in early work on the folate antagonists. Ferguson [195] reported on the hematotoxicity of single and repeated doses of MTX in mice, rats, and dogs. The data are most extensive on the changes in rat bone marrow. After single injections of 50 mg/kg, the erythroid:granulopoietic cell ratio (E:G ratio) decreased from 0.4 to 0.08 during the 72 h following the drug, indicating a substantial loss of erythropoietic precursors. A similar preferential sensitivity of erythropoietic cells has been described in man [161]. Vogler et al. [626] reported on the absolute size of the proliferating and nonproliferating granulocytic compartment in mice after single doses of 60 mg/kg, and after two doses given 3 or 6 days apart. After the single dose, a nadir was reached on day 2 for the proliferating (43%) and nonproliferating granulocytic (55%) cells. The proliferating compartment showed a rebound (150%) by day 6 and a rebound of similar degree was reached in the nonproliferating compartment on day 11.

Table 29. Effect of MTX on CFU-C: Recovery studies

Species (strain)	Dose of MTX (mg/kg), experimental conditions	Survival of CFU-C (percent of controls)																Reference
		Time after MTX																
		Hours		Days														
		1	3	1	2	3	4	5	6	7	8	9	10	11	12	13	14	
Mouse ($C_{57}Bl$)	Bone marrow																	[626]
	60 mg/kg, day 0			102	88	190	148	112	174	97	132	73	91	55	104			
	2 × 60 mg/kg, day 0 + 3						86	66	44	136	207	105	97	96	69			
	2 × 60 mg/kg, day 0 + 6									74	88	198	221	91	163			
	120 mg/kg, day 0			51	50	111	82	121	89									
	120 mg/kg, day 0 and 60 mg/kg, day 3						15	180		190		465						
Mouse (BDF_1)	100 mg/kg																	[602]
	Bone marrow	68	89	66/75			80			118								
	Spleen			154			747			427								
Mouse ($C_{57}Bl/6N$)	Continuous infusion																	
	$0.5-2.0 \times 10^{-5}$ *M* (~ 200 mg/kg per 24 h)			38	60													[459]
	7×10^{-6} *M*			45	65													[457]
Human	200 mg/kg in 6 h followed by citrovorum factor rescue																	[516]
	Bone marrow (incidence)				62					81							102	
	Peripheral blood				10					110							100	

Table 30. Effect of MTX on bone marrow cellularity: Sensitivity and recovery studies

Species (strain)	Dose of MTX (mg/kg)	Bone marrow cellularity (percent of controls)																Reference
		Time after MTX																
		Hours				Days												
		1	3	12	18	1	2	3	4	5	6	7	8	9	10	11	12	
Mouse ($C_{57}Bl$)	60					61.8	46.4	51.5	63.5	103.9	99.3	117.1	112.2	90.8	139	121	102	[627]
	120					69.5	44.7	52.7	48.9	91.7	87.6							[626]
Mouse (BDF_1)	100	105	115			77 92[a]		68				88						[602]
Mouse (NMRI)	5, 10, 20					80												[420]
Mouse ($C_{57}Bl/6N$)	5					76												[78]
	50					81												
	250					62												
	500					60												
Mouse ($C_{57}Bl$)	Continuous infusion at serum level																	[457, 459]
	1×10^{-5} *M*			30														
	2×10^{-6} *M*				40	30												
	2×10^{-7} *M*					50	30											
	5×10^{-8} *M*					60	40											
Rats	3×0.8 every 12 h					90	60	55	40	45	80	70	65	80	90	110	120	[263]

[a] From different set of data

A second dose, given on day 3, was followed by a further decrease of proliferating and nonproliferating cells 2 days later. When the second dose was delayed until day 6, the granulocytic compartments were depressed to 30–35% four days later.
In guinea pigs, 4 mg/kg MTX, repeated every other day for 14 days, led to a severe reduction of erythropoietic cells (E:G ratio before treatment 0.17, after treatment 0.02), though no change occurred in the ratio of proliferating to maturing granulocytic cells [312].
In humans, the data of Rizzoli [487] show a relative decrease of the proliferative granulopoietic cells in the bone marrow differential during and immediately after high-dose MTX with normalization during leukovorin rescue. In our experiments with high-dose MTX and citrovorum factor rescue [516], the E:G ratio decreased significantly on day 2. On the same day, there was a preferential reduction of the proliferating granulopoietic compartment as compared to the maturing granulocytic cells.
Megaloblastic changes, more prominent in erythropoiesis than in granulopoiesis, are a common finding after MTX exposure [161, 338, 458, 582].

Bone Marrow Granulocyte Reserve. A systematic study on MTX-induced changes of the bone marrow granulocyte reserve, using an endotoxin stimulus, was reported by Constable and Blackett [125] in rats. An exponential dose-effect curve was found with a $D_{1/2}$ of 1.0 mg/kg MTX (extrapolated from the graph), when measured 4 days after drug. This exponential dose-response curve could be explained by the fact that the proliferating granulocytic cells are all in cell cycle, and no effective block prevents the entry of these cells into the sensitive S-phase during the time of effective MTX levels. A time-response curve after 5 mg/kg MTX showed a rapid decline to zero values for mobilizable granulocytes on day 4, with rapid recovery to excessive values on day 9. Few data on the functional bone marrow granulocyte reserve after high-dose MTX with citrovorum factor rescue in man are contained in our report [516]: No significant difference was found on days 7 and 14 after therapy.

Peripheral Blood Leukocytes. It is of interest that most systematic studies on peripheral blood leukocytes have been performed in rats (Table 31). Single high MTX doses led to a rapid fall of PMN counts within 1–3 days [194]. Lower MTX doses, as used by Harding [262], i.e., 0.5–1.0 mg/kg × 3 within 24 h, induced a similar degree of granulocytopenia, but the nadir was not reached before day 7. In these experiments, an experimentally produced pyogenic infection caused earlier and more severe granulocytopenia. Several studies are concerned with the effect of two doses applied at various time intervals. Harding [263] administered a second MTX course at intervals between 1–21 days. At moderate doses (0.05 mg/kg × 3 every 12 h per course), maximum PMN depression, to less than 5% of pretreatment values, occurred with an interval of 6 days between the two courses. Doubling MTX doses resulted in maximum granulocytopenia when the time interval was 3 days. Continuous administration of low daily doses (0.1–0.4 mg/kg) to rats reduced the PMN count to 50% within 5 weeks and to 10% of normal by 7 weeks [194].
In mice, the rather high dose of 60 mg/kg MTX caused a depression of WBC, but no significant change of neutrophils [626]. MTX (60 mg/kg), given 3 days after an identical first dose, did similarly not affect blood neutrophils. However, when the interval between the first and second dose was extended to 6 days, severe neutropenia (15% of normal) was observed on day 8.

Table 31. Effect of MTX on peripheral blood PMN and WBC (animal data)

Species (strain)	MTX dose, schedule	Result	Reference
Rat (Wistar)	50 mg/kg, acute	Progressive decrease of granulocytes to 16% of control within 72 h	[194]
	0.1–0.4 mg/kg/day, chronic	Reduction to 50% by 5 weeks, to 10% at 7 weeks	
Rat (Angus × PVG/c)	0.5–1.0 mg/kg × 3 within 24 h	Reduction to 30%, nadir around day 7	[263]
	Two courses et various time intervals	Lowest granulocyte level (5%) on day 1, with MTX on days 0 and 6	
	After ligation of ureter	Earlier and more severe leukopenia during pyogenic infection	[262]
Mouse (C_{57}Bl)	60 mg/kg, single dose	WBC, 50% day 1, overshoot day 6	[626]
	Repeated day 3	No additional change of neutrophils	
	Repeated day 6	Drop of neutrophils to 15% on day 2 after second dose	
Guinea pig	5 mg/kg every 2–3 days until day 12	Undulating pattern; reduction to 50% on day 17	[509]
Rat (–)	30 mg/kg	Reduction of WBC, 30% day 2; overshoot, 150% days 8–12	[444]

In guinea pigs, MTX (5 mg/kg) given every 2–3 days until day 12 caused a reduction of circulating neutrophils to 50% by day 17 [509].
Taken together, these animal experiments suggest that the time schedule of application is more important than the dose given: When MTX is given repeatedly, the degree of granulocytopenia is a function of the time interval between successive doses.
In man, the variety of doses and time schedules, with and without leukovorin rescue or other rescue techniques, does not permit a systematic description of peripheral granulocytopenia after MTX.
Hansen et al. [260] tested the tolerance by escalating doses in widely spaced intervals in 34 patients. Hematotoxicity was defined as a fall of WBC below 5,000/mm^3. Using this rather low limit of toxicity, there was a wide variation of sensitivity between patients from doses as low as 50 mg/m^2 to as high as 900 mg/m^2 MTX.
Douglas and Price [161] collected hematotoxicity data from the literature. In seven studies covering a wide range of doses, less than 20% of treated cases were reported to have experienced hematotoxicity when the interval between injections was 1 week or longer. In contrast, a toxic effect on granulopoiesis was observed in 30–100% of patients in the nine studies that had used shorter intervals or repeated daily applications.
In a widely quoted paper on MTX toxicity, Goldie et al. [232] gave data on eight courses of HDM-CFR with doses of 100–20,000 mg total dose given over 12–48 h. The authors concluded that toxicity was dose-independent, but was a function of the duration of infusion. The same data were more thoroughly presented by Douglas et al. [161]: In 14 courses of HDM-CFR given within less than 24 h, the decline in total leukocyte count was $-8.3 \pm 23.3\%$ (with several cases showing an increase in WBC count), while in ten courses given over 30–48 h, the decline was $-30.5 \pm 26.6\%$.
The data of Stoller et al. [565] on 395 HDM-CFR courses given to 78 patients clearly show that hematotoxicity occurs only if a high serum MTX level persists for more than 48 h. Continuing their work, Stoller et al. [566] adjusted the dose of leukovorin to the projected 36-h MTX serum concentration derived from the serum concentrations at 18 and 24 h. Three of 110 courses with normal MTX pharmacokinetics induced myelosuppression. When MTX clearance was delayed, additional leukovorin was given and only one of five courses showed hematotoxicity.
In 349 HDM-CFR courses given to 43 pediatric patients with osteosarcoma, only 1.5% of courses led to depression of WBC counts below 2,000/mm^3 [454]. Levitt et al. [344] compared various dose ranges of MTX with and without leukovorin rescue with respect to myelosuppression. In 14 of 15 patients, doses of 80–230 mg/m^2 induced granulopenia below 2,500/mm^3. With citrovorum factor, granulopenia was seen in one of eight courses with 300–480 mg/m^2, and in 7 of 17 courses with 500–1080 mg/m^2.
In general, there is remarkably little toxicity of HDM-CFR on granulopoiesis when the MTX plasma level does not remain above a "safe" threshold for a prolonged period of time. By utilizing a modified infusion scheme in keeping with this postulation, Salasoo and Freedman [497] administered 85 courses of HDM-CFR with a mean low WBC count of $3,300 \pm 1,200/mm^3$.
In five patients treated with HDM-CFR, we have thoroughly evaluated the changes of granulopoiesis [516]. A slight, statistically not significant decrease of the peripheral blood granulocytes was observed. In one additional patient, four consecutive courses

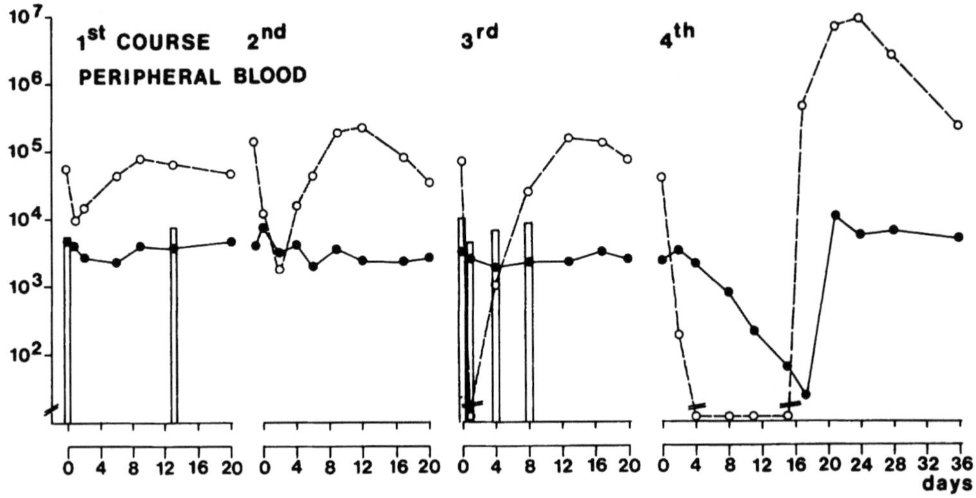

Fig. 4. Collected data on peripheral blood during four courses of HDM-CFR in one patient with osteosarcoma. Between individual courses, cyclophosphamide and adriamycin were given: ● PMN/μl; ○ CFU-C/l; bars indicate functional bone marrow PMN reserve. (From reference [516] with permission of the publisher)

were studied, three of which did not induce granulocytopenia while the fourth led to the disappearance of circulating CFU-C after day 4 and to progressive granulocytopenia with agranulocytosis on day 16 (Fig. 4). The severe toxicity of this last course could not be predicted from parameters of granulopoiesis seen before the beginning of the last HDM-CFR course. These parameters had recovered to normal values from the interspersed courses of cyclophosphamide and adriamycin, and there was no impairment of renal function. However, widespread metastases had occurred by the time of the fourth HDM-CFR course involving the lungs and skeleton. It has been observed during the early experience with MTX that unexpectedly high toxicity may be observed in individuals with a slight degree of bone marrow insufficiency due to replacement by tumor or previous exposure to radiation therapy or alkylating agents [122].

4.9 5-Fluorouracil (5-FU)

5-FU, a fluorinated pyrimidine base, was introduced in 1957 by Heidelberger et al. [273]. The major effect of 5-FU is inhibition of DNA synthesis [64], though effects on RNA metabolism have also been described [118, 261, 272, 589]. Due to the long half-lives of its metabolites, the action of 5-FU in vivo is prolonged [98, 346]. As derived from its dose-response characteristics in vitro and in vivo, described for the granulopoietic system in this chapter, 5-FU is considered to be a cytotoxic agent active on proliferating cells but independent of the cycle phase.

CFU-S Sensitivity Studies. In vivo dose-response studies have been performed on various strains of mice. Relevant data from these studies are summarized in Table 32. Where dose-response curves have been reported, an exponential cell kill has regularly been observed, and the values for $D_{1/2}$ agree when the CFU-S assay was performed

Table 32. Effect of 5-FU on murine CFU-S: Sensitivity studies in vivo. Source of CFU-S was bone marrow, except for transitional and rapidly proliferating CFU-S which were derived from spleens after bone marrow transplantation. *CPA*, cyclophosphamide

Strain, schedule, proliferative state of CFU-S	Time of assay (h)	$D_{1/2}$ (mg/kg)	Shoulder (mg/kg)	CFU-S survival (percent of controls) Dose (mg/kg)								Reference
				20–25	40–50	75–80	100	125–135	150	180–200	275–300	
AKR/J, given in six divided doses every 4 h	24 after first dose	27	15		70			5		2	0.1	[81]
AKR Normal	1	60	10		70		40			10	3	[80]
Transitional		60	10		70		40			15	4	
Rapidly proliferating		11	0		15		< 0.1					
AKR Normal	24	26	50		100	68	32	17	9			[175]
Endotoxin (−24 h)		15	11	100	13	3	< 1					
ARK Normal	6							50				[176]
Endotoxin (−24 h)								2				
150 mg CPA (−36 h)								2.5				
Irradiation (−36 h)								2				
(C_{57}Bl × CBA) Normal	16	35	[a]		20		10			1–2		[616]
Rapidly proliferating		8.6	25		10		0.2					
C_{57}Bl, i.v.	24				19	9	6					[172]
MF_1	24								1.3			[482]
CBA/H, given in six divided doses every 24 h	24 after last dose							26				[294]
BALB/c × C_{57}Bl	24								0.1			[287]
BALB/c × C_{57}Bl	96								4.4			[306a]

[a] Extrapolation number 0.7

16–24 h after 5-FU. CFU-S assay at 1 h resulted in a higher $D_{1/2}$ of about 60 mg/kg [80] (Table 32). Some apparent differences in the studies presented in table 32 result from the existence and extent of a shoulder at low doses of the drug.

When 5-FU was given in six divided doses every 4 h, the slope of the survival curve is not different from that seen after a single injection of the drug [81] (Table 32). This may be explained by the prolonged half-lives of cytotoxic metabolites of 5-FU [98, 346].

The effect of 5-FU on normal, transitional, and rapidly proliferating cells has been compared [80] (Table 32). CFU-S in their normal low proliferative state and transitional CFU-S showed virtually identical sensitivity to 5-FU, but rapidly proliferating CFU-S were much more sensitive. Pretreatment with cyclophosphamide or with total body irradiation (TBI) 36 h before administration of 5-FU also rendered the CFU-S more sensitive [176] (Table 32).

In a similar way, Van Putten [616] compared normal CFU-S to spleen-derived rapidly proliferating CFU-S on day 7 after bone marrow transplantation (Table 32). The differences in sensitivity of these CFU-S populations are well in agreement with the data of others reported in Table 32.

In one study [80], the dose-response curve was also established for CFU-S exposed to 5-FU in vitro for 1 h at 37° C. An exponential survival curve without a shoulder was observed, with a $D_{1/2}$ at a concentration of 50 μM [80] (Table 35).

The effect of endotoxin on the cytotoxic action of 5-FU on granulopoiesis has been extensively investigated. These data will be considered separatly (see page 165).

When the CFU-S from 5-FU-treated donors were determined at 8 to 14 days in the recipient spleen, a steep linear increase of the colony count was observed (if the 10-day count is taken as 100%, CFU-S count on day 8 was 24% and, on day 12, 230%). Thus, estimates of the CFU-S count of 5-FU-pretreated marrow suspensions may be misleading when the number of spleen colonies is counted 10 days after cell transfer, since with normal hemopoietic tissue the number of spleen colonies has reached a plateau 10 days after cell transfer (see page 9). Furthermore, the same authors obtained evidence that stem cells from 5-FU-pretreated animals preferentially home to the bone marrow of irradiated recipients [287].

CFU-S Recovery Studies. Few systematic studies have been performed on the changes of the pluripotent stem cell pool after single doses of 5-FU. During the early phase after 100–125 mg/kg, a rapid decline of CFU-S appears to exist, reaching a minimum after 24 h [80, 172, 175, 176, 616] (Table 33).

The effect of endotoxin [482] (Table 33) on the pattern of depletion and regeneration of the CFU-S pool is described elsewhere in more detail (see page 165).

Administration of erythropoietin on day 1 after 5-FU did not change the pattern of regeneration in the CFU-S bone marrow compartment [487] (Table 33).

CFU-C Sensitivity Studies in vivo. As for the CFU-S compartment, data on the in vivo sensitivity of the granulopoietic progenitor cell (CFU-C) compartment are restricted to the mouse model (Table 34). Exponential dose-survival curves have been reported in three studies, with some variations in $D_{1/2}$ values and the presence and extent of a shoulder.

Comparing the $D_{1/2}$ values for CFU-C (Table 34) with those for CFU-S (Table 32), it appears that normal CFU-C are somewhat more sensitive than normal CFU-S and that their sensitivity is similar to that of proliferating CFU-S.

Table 33. Effect of 5-FU on murine bone marrow CFU-S: Recovery studies

Strain and pretreatment	Dose (mg/kg)	CFU-S survival (percent of controls)															Reference
		Time after 5-FU															
		Hours							Days								
		1	4	6	8	12	16	20	1	2	3	4	5	6	7	8	
AKR	100	40															[80]
$C_{57}Bl \times CBA$	100						10										[616]
$C_{57}Bl$	100								6								[172]
AKR	125								17								[175]
AKR	125		70	(50)[a]	50	35	24	17	12								[176]
−24 h endotoxin	125		2		1		0.4		0.1								
MF_1																	
Normal	150								1.3	1.7	3.0	4.1	10.6	22.1	35.6	62	[482]
−24 h endotoxin	150								0.8	0.8	0.9	1.0	1.5	2.6	6.2	15.2	
+4 h endotoxin	150								1.7	4.9	5.8		28.1	59.6	97.6		
MF_1																	
Normal	140									2	2.4	4	12	50		100	[478]
+ Erythropoietin (+8, +16, +24 h)	140									2	2.5	4.8	12	45		100	

[a] From other set of data in [176]

Since the CFU-C compartment is already actively proliferating under steady-state conditions, the sensitivity of CFU-C from regenerating bone marrow might be expected to be relatively less increased than that of regenerating CFU-S. This fact is clearly demonstrated by the study of Eaves and Bruce [176] where pretreatment with cyclophosphamide or with 150 rad TBI caused much smaller increments of drug sensitivity than in the CFU-S compartment. On the other hand, the influence of endotoxin given 24 h before 5-FU is quite marked [175, 176] (Table 34), and similar to the effect of *C. parvum* [204, 206] (Table 34) (for details, see page 165, 169).
The effect of repeated injections of 5-FU (40 mg/kg every 2 weeks) was studied by Foster [207]: 48 h after the fifth course, the surviving fraction of CFU-C was 26% (Table 34). These data indicate that there is no accumulated severe damage to the CFU-C pool during this particular treatment schedule. With a cumulative dose of 210 mg 5-FU given in seven divided doses every 24 h, the CFU-C content per femur was reduced to 1.1%. Concomitant administration of allopurinol reduced 5-FU toxicity to CFU-C [520] (Table 34).

CFU-C Sensitivity in Vitro and in Agar Difussion Chamber. The fact that human granulopoietic progenitor cells can be assayed in soft agar cultures as well as in agar-diffusion chambers offers the opportunity to compare the sensitivity of murine and human CFU-C to 5-FU directly. Two sets of data which relate to this question are listed in Table 35.
Ogawa [435] first compared the sensitivity of normal and of rapidly proliferating murine CFU-C by in vitro exposure (1 h at 37° C) to various concentrations of 5-FU. The $D_{1/2}$ value for rapidly proliferating CFU-C was considerably lower than that for normal bone marrow CFU-C (Table 35). In a subsequent paper, Ogawa [436] reported on the in vitro sensitivity of human CFU-C under similar experimental conditions. A twenty-fold higher concentration of 5-FU (1.5 m*M* versus 75 μ*M*) was necessary to reduce human CFU-C survival to 50% (Table 35). The in vitro sensitivity of the CFU-C from six tumor patients studied by Hillcoat et al. [285] exhibited a wide range of survival (Table 35).
Using the agar-diffusion chamber technique, Gordon [237] compared the sensitivity of murine and human CFU-C during an 18–20-h drug exposure in the primary recipient mouse. Again, human CFU-C were less sensitive to 5-FU than mouse CFU-C (Table 35). In these experiments, a direct comparison was made between the exposure of CFU-C to 5-FU in situ and in agar-diffusion chambers, and murine CFU-C exposed in situ (i.e., in the femur) were somewhat more sensitive (see Table 34, [237]).

CFU-C Recovery Studies. In the paper of Eaves and Bruce [176], a recovery study is reported for CFU-C after in vivo exposure to 125 mg/kg 5-FU. A rapid drop to values of around 10–20% occurred during the first 1–2 h. Subsequently, survival decreased more slowly to approximately 5% by 24 h. When endotoxin was given 24 h before 5-FU, the CFU-C compartment dropped to unmeasurable values within 1–2 h [176] (Table 34).

Bone Marrow Changes After 5-FU. Available data on the changes of bone marrow cellularity and of the functional bone marrow granulocyte reserve are summarized in Table 36.
Qualitative data from these studies indicate that regeneration of bone marrow is preceded by the reappearance of myeloblasts and proerythroblasts on day 6 after 5-FU [482].

Table 34. Effect of 5-FU on murine bone marrow CFU-C: Sensitivity studies in vivo

Strain, schedule pretreatment	Time of assay (h)	$D_{1/2}$ (mg/kg)	Shoulder	CFU-C survival (percent of controls) — Dose of 5-FU (mg/kg): 20–25	40–50	75	100	125	150	210	Reference
AKR, normal	24	22.5	–	46	21	10	5	2	1		[175]
Endotoxin −24 h		5.5	6	10	0.6						
AKR, normal	1–2							10–20			[176]
	24							5			
Endotoxin −24 h	1–2							0			
C_{57}Bl, normal	18–20	12	–	15	3						[237]
C_{57}Bl/6, normal	24			84							[204, 206]
C. parvum −24 h				35							
C_{57}Bl/6, normal	24	20	20	80–90	50	20	7				[207]
C_{57}Bl/6, five cycles every 14 days, assay after fifth cycle					26						[207]
CD_1, seven divided doses every 24 h	24 after last dose									1.1	[520]
Concomitant with allopurinol										17.1	

Table 35. Effect of 5-FU on stem cells: Sensitivity studies in vitro and in diffusion chamber

Source of target cells, incubation schedule	$D_{1/2}$	Stem cell survival (percent of controls)										Reference
		Concentration in incubation assay (μ*M*)										
		10	37.5	75	100	150	225	300	1,000	1,500	3,000	
CFU-S in vitro												
AKR mice, 1 h (37° C)	50 μ*M*			35		10	4	2				[80]
CFU-C in vitro												
BALB/c mice, 1 h (37° C)												
Normal	72 μ*M*			50		30		15				[435]
Rapidly proliferating	17.6 μ*M*		28	13		5						
Human bone marrow, 1 h (37° C)	1.65 m*M*								70	50	25	[436]
Human bone marrow[a], 1 h (37° C)		85 (40–100)			75 (25–100)				20 (1–50)			[285]
		Dose (mg/kg)[b]										
		12.5	**25**	**50**	**100**	**150**	**200**					
CFU-C in diffusion chamber (18–20 h)												
C_{57}Bl mice	23 mg/kg	61	33	15	3							[237]
Human bone marrow	59 mg/kg			60	40	25	15					

[a] Mean value and range from six patients
[b] Exposure to 5-FU in diffusion chambers in primary hosts

Table 36. Effect of 5-FU on bone marrow cellularity and functional bone marrow granulocyte reserve

	Cumulative dose (mg/kg)	Bone marrow cellularity (functional bone marrow PMN reserve) (percent of controls)										Reference
		Days after last 5-FU dose										
		1	2	3	4	6	8	10	12	14	18	
Bone marrow cellularity												
MF$_1$ mice, single injection	150		20		20	35	63	81				[482]
CBA/H mice, six divided doses every 24 h	140	42		56		60		75				[294]
ACI rats, single injection[a]	150	70	30		12	12	25	35	50	100		[289, 355a]
BALB/c × C$_{57}$Bl, single injection	150				12							[306a]
Functional bone marrow PMN reserve												
Rabbits												
Single dose	200				73			42		20	25	[573]
14 Divided doses every 24 h	280	50			63			63			50	

[a] Measured as DNA content/femur

The ^{3}H-TdR labeling index for myelocytes and promyelocytes was studied in rabbits [573]. Severe and long-lasting depletion of the labeling index occurred both after single high doses (one-third LD_{50}) and repeated low doses (one-thirtieth LD_{50} on 14 consecutive days) of 5-FU.

A morphological analysis of bone marrow specimens obtained during and after 5-FU chemotherapy (15 mg/kg/day × 5 followed by 7.5 mg/kg every 2 days to toxicity) in 58 patients was reported by Brennan et al. [74]. Twelve to 24 hours after the beginning of therapy, megaloblastic changes appeared in metamyelocytes, and cytoplasmic changes with peculiar vacuolization and multilobulated granulocytes developed. The M : E ratio rose from pretreatment values of 3 : 1 or 4 : 1 to values as high as 200 : 1. Bone marrow cellularity, as estimated from paraffin sections of bone marrow spicules, did not decrease appreciably during the time of these early morphologic alterations. Using the same schedule of chemotherapy, Stalzer et al. [554] described light- and electron-microscopic changes of human bone marrow in 16 patients during and after chemotherapy. There was a progressive decline of proliferating cells with a more severe depletion of the erythropoietic series, which led to an increase of the myeloid to erythroid cell ratio (M : E ratio) from 2.7 on day 0 to 20 on day 10. Thirty days after therapy, the M : E ratio had returned to 3.6. In addition, the ratio of proliferating and maturing granulocytic cells declined from a pretreatment value of 0.6 to approximately 0.25 on days 3 and 6. Morphological signs of megaloblastic changes also appeared on days 3–5 in the form of giant metamyelocytes. These authors could not confirm the experience of Brennan et al. [74] who reported that the extent of the increase of the M : E ratio correlated with the degree of subsequent granulopenia.

In a recent paper, Radley and Scurfield [471] give a detailed analysis of the morphological changes occurring in [(BALB/c × C_{57} Bl) F_1] mice following 150 mg/kg 5-FU. A severe depletion of cells in the extravascular space of the bone marrow was observed after 2 days, leaving only more mature cell elements intact. This decline in cellularity proceeded until day 5. The first evidence of granulocytic regeneration was apparent on day 7, and by day 9, there was an abundance of granulocytes. This sequence of events was accelerated by approximately 24 h when endotoxin was given 24 h after 5-FU.

Changes of Peripheral Blood WBC and PMN. Data on the changes of peripheral blood WBC and PMN in animal models following 5-FU administration are contained in Table 37. Bollag [60] states that the granulopoietic system of rats is somewhat more sensitive to 5-FU than that of mice. In mice, 40 mg/kg is equivalent to 30 mg/kg in rats with respect to the effect on hematopoiesis. From the data in table 37, the schedule-dependency of hematotoxicity is evident.

A schedule of intermittent short-term treatment with 5-FU was used by Foster [207], who gave 40 mg/kg every 2 weeks to C_{57}Bl/6 mice. After the first course, peripheral PMN declined to 35% of pretreatment values on day 7 and recovered to 122% on day 14. The values after the second and third course were between 80–126%. Thus, there is no evidence of cumulative toxicity to the granulopoietic system with intermittent administration of 5-FU.

From the litrature, it is difficult to derive satisfactory quantitative conclusions about the changes of peripheral WBC or PMN in man after the use of 5-FU. A great number of treatment schedules have been used in phase II and III studies and, as a rule, no serial follow-up of peripheral blood parameters is given. Instead, the fraction of patients experiencing a certain degree of hematotoxicity is reported. Table 38

Table 37. Effect of 5-FU on peripheral blood PMN (WBC): Recovery studies

	Cumulative dose (mg/kg)	Concentration of PMN (WBC) in peripheral blood (percent of controls)														Reference
		Days after last 5-FU dose														
		1	2	3	4	6	7	8	9	10	12	13	14	15	18	
MF_1 mice, single injection	150			33		2		20		67						[482]
$C_{57}Bl/6$ mice, single injection	100			110			0			40						[207]
	200			105			0			0						
	400			60			0			0						
	800			60			0			0						
C_3H mice, five divided doses every 24 h	90			1.5		25				35						[306]
	150			<1		5				27						
	250			<1		< 1				8						
CBA/H mice, six divided dcses every 24 h	140	40		45		40				60						[294]
Rats																
Single injection (WBC only)	150	90	80		65	60			50	90					100	[355a]
Four divided doses every 24 h	80	25			10	50				300	160				90	[60]
Four divided doses every 24 h	160[a]	7		0												
Eight divided doses every 24 h	240[b]	7		0		60			170			200		85		
Rabbits																
Single injection	200				29					15			25		25	[573]
Fourteen divided doses every 24 h	280	15			10						15				20	

[a] Ten of ten animals died in leukopenia
[b] Seven of ten animals died in leukopenia

Table 38. Depression of peripheral blood WBC after a standard 5-FU therapy (15 mg/kg/day × 5 followed by 7.5 mg/kg every 2 days to toxicity) in three studies

Reference	*n*	Definition of leukopenia	Percent with leukopenia
[315]	109	< 4,000	87
[11]	1091	2,000–3,000	22
		< 2,000	32
[397]	389	3,000–4,000[a]	20
		2,000–3,000	10
		< 2,000	6
		< 4,000[b]	46

[a] Estimated from graph
[b] Table

Table 39. Hematotoxicity of 5-FU in clinical studies comparing different schedules of administration

Schedule	*n*	Percentage of patients with hematotoxicity		Reference
		"None–light"	"Moderate–severe"	
"Loading" 12 mg/kg × 5 days, 6 mg/kg × 11 every 2 days, 15 mg/kg weekly	46	52	48	[12]
Weekly 15 mg/kg i.v.	69	77	23	
4 × 500 mg i.v., then 500 mg weekly	87	96	4	
15 mg/kg × 6, then weekly 15 mg/kg orally	66	73	27	
		WBC 3,900–3,000	WBC 2,900–2,000	
Weekly 15 mg/kg i.v.	14	7	7	[564]
Weekly 15 mg/kg orally	16	31	0	
		WBC 4,000–2,000	WBC 2,000	
12 mg/kg × 5 rapid injection	36	42	31	[527]
25–40 mg/kg × 5 continuous infusion	34	12		

summarizes some of the data on toxic effects of a frequently used schedule as reported in three studies with large numbers of patients, and a high incidence of leukopenia is generally observed. To illustrate these problems further, data on hematologic toxicity are summarized in Table 39 from three studies which compare different dose and time regimens of 5-FU in a randomized fashion. A different grading system to report leukopenia is used in each study. At any rate, hematotoxicity is dose-dependent, and the oral route did not decrease the degree of leukopenia. 5-FU, given by continuous infusion over 5 days, caused considerably less hematotoxicity than when the drug was given by rapid injection.

Modifications of 5-FU Hematotoxicity. The modifications of the cytotoxic effect of 5-FU by immune modulators, e.g., *C parvum* or endotoxin, are discussed elsewhere (see page 165).

Recently, attempts have been made to improve the therapeutic value of 5-FU by reducing its toxicity while preserving the antitumor effect. It is possible to influence the metabolism of 5-FU in various ways.

The concomitant administration of TdR increased the availability of 5-FU, probably by competing with the same pyrimidine-degradative enzymes [319]. While toxicity of 5-FU on normal murine CFU-S increased only 20% with TdR [499], the effect on AKR murine leukemia was augmented 100- to 1000-fold [498]. In two phase I studies in man [319, 625], hematotoxicity increased and became the limiting toxic factor, while, with 5-FU alone, mucositis is usually the limiting factor. Using a 5-day schedule, daily doses of 7.5–10 mg/kg 5-FU were tolerable in combination with TdR, as compared to 30 mg/kg/day (5-day continuous infusion) for 5-FU alone.

Allopurinol reduced toxicity in mice, presumably because pathways activating 5-FU in normal tissue were blocked [520]. The modifying effect of allopurinol was also apparent at the CFU-C level (Table 34) [520]. In a clinical trial, patients tolerated up to approximately 60 mg/kg/day 5-FU (5-day continuous infusion) when allopurinol (900 mg/day) was given during days 1–6 [210].

Finally, the modification of bioavailability by linking a furanosyl moiety to the 5-FU molecule (ftorafur) has attracted much attention. It is considered to be a slow-release form of 5-FU which undergoes metabolic activation in vivo [117]. The difference in toxicity between 5-FU and ftorafur is dose- and species-dependent. In mice, leukopenia after single doses roughly corresponded to equimolar or equitoxic doses, while the cumulative toxicity of ftorafur was much less with repeated-dose regimens [306].

Phase I studies in man [254, 542, 604] confirmed the experience reported from Russia [313] that the hematotoxicity of ftorafur is much less than that of 5-FU. However, marked neurotoxicity became apparent. In a phase II study, Buroker et al. [94] treated 84 patients with colorectal carcinoma with a total of 306 courses of ftorafur. While there was only mild hematotoxicity (WBC less than 4,000/mm^3 in 5% of the courses), the neurotoxicity of the compound and the lack of antitumor activity led the authors to conclude that ftorafur appears "not to make a significant contribution to the management of disseminated colorectal cancer".

4.10 Cytosine Arabinoside (Ara-C)

Ara-C is a synthetic nucleoside pyrimidine antimetabolite which exerts its cytocidal action by inhibiting the conversion of uridine to deoxyuridine nucleotides and competiting with deoxycytidine for deoxycytidine kinase. The plasma half-life is less than 9 min when given by i.v. rapid injection. The drug has little effect by the oral route. It has been utilized primarily for the treatment of adult acute myelogenous leukemia and for the control of meningeal leukemia.

Table 40. The effect of ara-C on CFU-S: Sensitivity studies in vivo

Species (strain)	Time of assay after ara-C (h)	Schedule of ara-C administration	CFU-S survival (percent of controls) Total dose of ara-C (mg/kg)									Reference
			0	50	100	250	500	1,000	1,500	2,000	2,500	
Normal CFU-S												
Mouse (–)	1	1×	100			100					90	[50]
Mouse (–)	1[a]	1×	100				75		70		70	[50]
Mouse [(C_3H × DBA/2)F_1]	24	1×	100	60								[177]
	24	1×	100	70								[178]
Mouse (CDF_1)	24	1×	100				70	50			50	[639]
Mouse (AKR/J)	1	Every 4 h × 6	100		40	20	20			20		[82]
Mouse (AKR)	24	Every 4 h × 6	100			30						[83]
Mouse (AKR/J)	1	Every 4 h × 12	100		20	0.7	0.7			0.7		[82]
Mouse (CDF_1)	24	Every 3 h × 8	100			15	10				10	[639]
Mouse ($C_{57}Bl$)	2	Every 2 h × 4	100		60	50						[43]
Mouse (CD-1)	2	Every 7 h × 3	100				90					[226]
Mouse (CD-1)	18	Every 7 h × 3	100				33					[127]
Mouse (AKR)	24	Every 8 h × 3	100			30	7	7				[175]
Rapidly proliferating CFU-S												
Mouse (–)	24[a]	1×	100				54			36	30	[50]
Mouse (–)	48[a]	1×	100				65			30	16	[50]

[a] Hours after bone marrow cell transfer into irradiated recipients

CFU-S Sensitivity Studies. In vivo dose-survival studies on the effect of single or repeated ara-C administration on normal or rapidly proliferating CFU-S are listed in Table 40. In vivo, the dose-survival curves of normal murine CFU-S regularly reach a plateau of more than 50% at single doses of over 500 mg/kg. A plateau of the dose-survival curve was also observed after in vitro exposure of CFU-S to ara-C [390]. Rapidly proliferating CFU-S, after bone marrow transplantation [50] or endotoxin [175], were considerably more sensitive to the drug than normal CFU-S, reflecting the greater fraction of CFU-S being in the ara-C-sensitive S-phase of the cell cycle under these experimental conditions. In general, repeated administration of ara-C at 3–4-h intervals resulted in considerably greater CFU-S kill than when the same total dose was given as a single injection. However, in one study [639], this increased CFU-S kill was reported to be marginal. For further details, the reader is referred to Table 40.

CFU-S Recovery Studies. Following ara-C (100 mg/kg × 3 every 7 h) bone marrow CFU-S declined to 30% on days 1 and 2, and recovery of the CFU-S compartment was noted by day 7 [127, 226, 441a].
The recovery within the bone marrow CFU-S compartment following a single dose of ara-C (1,000 mg/kg) was studied by Preisler et al. [466]. The number of CFU-S per femur dropped to 70% one day after ara-C treatment; a reduction to 50% after 16–24 h was also reported by Frindel et al. [222]. Thereafter, rapid CFU-S recovery (to 100% by day 2) and overshoot by day 3 was observed. The proliferative activity of CFU-S on day 2 was increased. A more detailed study of the changes in the proportion of CFU-S in S-phase after a single administration of ara-C was reported by Nečas et al. [420] who found that 15 h after doses of 25 mg/kg and 50 mg/kg, respectively, the proliferative activity of bone marrow CFU-S began to increase above control values. The extent and duration of this increased proliferative activity appeared to be dose-related, suggesting that the extent of damage to S-phase CFU-S may play a role in the regulation of the entry of nonproliferating (G_0) CFU-S into cell cycle.
A more rapid recovery was observed by Seidel et al. [523]. Following repeated administrations of ara-C (40 mg/kg × 6 every 4 h) to CBA/Ca mice, CFU-S per femur decreased to 25% of controls by the end of the treatment period. Two days after completion of treatment, CFU-S/femur were within the normal range and a transient increase of this value was determined 3 days after ara-C.

CFU-C Sensitivity Studies. The sensitivity of murine and human CFU-C to ara-C has been studied with different methods (Tables 41 and 42). When ara-C was injected i.p. into mice (33, 100, or 300 mg/kg as single or triple injections), the number of CFU-C per femur (day 1) showed a dose-dependent decline. Furthermore, identical daily doses were more effective in reducing the size of the femoral CFU-C compartment when given as three injections than when given as a single injection [602]. The in vitro sensitivity of CFU-C to ara-C was measured either by short-term incubation of CFU-C with the drug [247, 390], or by addition of ara-C in culture for the entire culture period [247, 425]. After short-term (60 min) incubation of murine CFU-C with ara-C, the dose-survival curve (0–40 μg/ml) showed a plateau at 80% CFU-C survival [390]. Similar data were reported by Greenberg et al. [247], who observed enhanced toxicity to CFU-C when the exposure period was extended to 4 or 8 h, respectively. The dose-survival curve of human CFU-C, determined in the same way, showed a dose-related decrease after 1 and 4 h of drug exposure. Again, this decrease was

Table 41. Effect of ara-C on CFU-C: Sensitivity studies in vitro

Species (strain)	Duration of incubation	CFU-C survival (percent of controls)											Reference
		Concentration of ara-C (μg/ml)											
		0	0.01	0.02	0.04	0.06	0.1	1	10	20	40	100	
Mouse ($C_{57}Bl$)	1 h	100							85		80		[390]
Mouse ($C_{57}Bl$)	1 h	100					90	85	70			80	[247]
	4 h	100					85	80	60			55	[247]
	8 h	100					85	82	40				[247]
Human	1 h	100					100	90	82			70	[247]
	4 h	100					87	60	55			45	[247]
Mouse ($C_{57}Bl$)	In culture[a]	100	80	50			0	0					[247]
Human	In culture[a]	100	75				20	~ 2	0			0	[247]
Human	In culture[a]	100	35	20		8							[549a]
Human	In culture[a]	100	8–70	1–30	0.1–15	0–8							[425]

[a] Ara-C added to the culture medium

Table 42. Effect of ara-C on murine CFU-C: Sensitivity studies in vivo

Mouse strain	Time of assay after ara-C (h)	Schedule of adminis-tration	CFU-C survival (percent of controls) Total dose of ara-C (mg/kg)				Refer-ence
			0	100	200	300	
C_3H	24	1×	100	100			[601]
BDF_1	24	1×	100	90		60	[602]
BDF_1	6	Every 6 h × 3	100	45		22	[602]
$C_{57}Bl$	2	Every 2 h × 4	100	60	50	50	[46]
CD-1	2	Every 7 h × 3	100			35	[226, 441]
CD-1	6	Every 7 h × 3	100			6	[127]

greater after 4 h than after 1 h of incubation with ara-C. When ara-C was added to CFU-C cultures directly for the entire culture period, sigmoid-shaped dose-survival curves were obtained for human and murine CFU-C [247], the latter displaying a somewhat greater sensitivity (abrogation of colony growth for murine CFU-C at doses greater than 0.1 μg/ml and for human CFU-C at doses greater than 1.0 μg/ml). Using a similar experimental approach, Niho et al. [425] determined exponential dose-survival curves of human CFU-C at low concentrations of ara-C (0–0.06 μg/ml), with considerable individual variability.

CFU-C Recovery Studies. The recovery pattern of murine bone marrow CFU-C following repeated doses of ara-C (40 mg/kg every 4 h × 6) was studied by Seidel et al. [523]. The CFU-C compartment was depleted to approximately 20% after the last ara-C injection and recovery to normal was not yet completed 4 days later. Following 100 mg/kg × 3 every 7 h, the number of CFU-C/tibia declined earlier and relatively more than that of CFU-S assayed in parallel [441a]: The nadir of CFU-C/tibia (6% of normal) was observed 2 h after the last dose of ara-C and recovery of the tibial CFU-C compartment to its normal size was noted on day 5.

Bone Marrow. When the marrow cellularity was determined 24 h after increasing doses of ara-C, it was reduced to about 50% at doses greater than 100 mg/kg [420] while, with 25 and 50 mg/kg, approximately 85 and 70% of the cells were killed, respectively. Other authors [602] observed a lesser reduction in the femoral cellularity, but Preissler et al. [466] reported the femoral cell count to be 30% of normal 24 h after 1,000 mg/kg ara-C. In this study, the recovery of mouse bone marrow cellularity was measured, and an initial phase of rapid recovery (70% of controls by day 3) was followed by a more gradual return to normal (control values reached by day 21). Others [523] observed a more rapid recovery of the femoral cell content: Following 6 × 40 mg/kg (every 4 h), the nadir (20% of normal) occurred 24 h after the last dose of ara-C and the cellularity had returned to normal values within 5 days.
Finally, Page et al. [441a] observed the lowest tibial cellularity (25% of normal) at 24–48 h after 3 × 100 mg/kg ara-C every 7 h. Return to normal tibial cellularity was seen by day 7.
The same authors studied the morphologically identifiable granulocytic marrow compartments. The recovery of the promyelocyte compartment and of the

Table 43. Effect of ara-C on peripheral blood WBC: Recovery studies. Changes of WBC count due almost exclusively to changes in PMN concentration

	Dose and schedule	WBC count (percent of controls)											Reference
		Day											
		0	2	4	6	8	10	12	14	16	18	20	
Mouse (BALB/c × DBA)F_1	100 mg/kg × 1	100	60	75					75			100	[466]
Human	50 mg/kg 1 × per week	No changes											[577]
Human	Up to 100 mg/kg × 1	No changes											[217]
Human	10 mg/kg by continuous infusion over 24- or 48-h period	Nadir day 8–20[a]											[217]
Human	0.4 mg/kg every 8 h × 30	Nadir day 14 after discontinuation of ara-C											[92]
Human	30 mg/m^2/day × 7 by continuous infusion; 60 mg/m^2/day × 3.5 by continuous infusion	Nadir day 14 after ara -C (~ 30%)											[182]
	120 mg/m^2/day × 1.75 by continuous infusion; 240 mg/m^2/day × 0.85 by continuous infusion; 480 mg/m^2/day × 0.44 by continuous infusion	No changes											[182]

[a] Later with greater WBC depression

myelocyte-metamyelocyte compartment followed that of the CFU-C compartment, but preceded that of the pool of band and PMN granulocytes.
Biro [40] studied the effect of five daily injections of 60 mg/kg upon the granulocytic system. One day after treatment, the M : E ratio was increased more than eight-fold and, within the granulocytic system, a considerable shift towards immature cells (myeloblasts to myelocytes) was apparent during this early period. Four days after completion of ara-C treatment, erythroid regeneration was marked and a return towards the normal distribution of the granulocytic cells was seen.
Megaloblastic changes of human erythroid and granulocytic marrow cells may be seen as early as 48 h after ara-C [447, 576]. By electron-microscopy, the formation of nuclear blebs occurs at the same time [4].
In mice, the functional bone marrow granulocyte reserve reached a nadir 3 days after 1,000 mg/kg ara C and returned to normal levels by day 7 [466].

Peripheral Blood White Cells. In several studies, the effect of various dosages and schedules on the peripheral blood WBC count was studied in man (Table 43). Changes in the WBC count after ara-C exposure were regularly found to be caused by the effect of the drug on granulocytes, lymphocytes being remarkably unaffected [182, 217].
After a single injection of as much as 100 mg/kg ara-C, the peripheral blood WBC count showed minor or no changes and this was also true when the injections were repeated every 7 days [182, 217, 577]. When ara-C was given by continuous infusion for 7 days, doses greater than 0.75 mg/kg/day reduced the peripheral blood WBC count to 30% of pretreatment values. The same total dose, given over a period of only 3.5 days, exerted similar toxicity on the peripheral blood WBC count. However, when an identical total dose of ara-C was administered over 1.75 days, 0.875 days, or 0.44 days, no effect on the peripheral blood WBC count was noted [182]. Other authors [93, 217, 577] similarly noted the effect of ara-C to be dose- and schedule-dependent: In man, hematopoietic toxicity became evident only after repeated administration or after continuous infusion.
In mice, the peripheral blood granulocyte count dropped to a nadir 2–3 days after a single injection of ara-C (100 mg/kg) [466] or after repeated exposure to the drug [60 mg/kg/day × 5 [40]; 100 mg/kg every 7 h × 3 (P. Page, personal communication).

4.11 6-Mercaptopurine (6-MP)

CFU-S and CFU-C. With increasing doses of 6-MP, murine CFU-S survival curves (assayed at 24 h) formed a plateau both after single [611] and after six divided doses of the drug [83]. The plateau level was at 50% CFU-S survival with single doses greater than 100 mg/kg, and at 70% CFU-S survival with four doses of 40 mg/kg each given every 4 h. The sensitivity of rapidly proliferating CFU-S or CFU-S recovery following 6-MP exposure have not been reported. Three and 5 days after 6-MP (100 mg/kg), the number of CFU-S per femur was 25% and 40%, respectively [223].
After 6-MP 4 × 40 mg/kg every 12 h, the number of murine bone marrow CFU-C declined to 30% of normal between days 2–5 after initiation of treatment and CFU-C recovery to normal was noted by day 8 [472].

Bone Marrow. Two recovery studies of the cellularity of mouse bone marrow after 6-MP exposure were reported. Following a single dose of 100 mg/kg, marrow cellularity declined gradually and the nadir (30% of pretreatment values) was reached by day 5. By day 10, the marrow cellularity had returned to 50% of control values [223]. Following 4 × 40 mg/kg every 12 h, the marrow cellularity was reduced to 75–90% of normal 3–8 days after the start of treatment [472].

Peripheral Blood. In the guinea pig, ten daily doses of 70 mg/kg 6-MP led to early disappearance of peripheral blood granulocytes. After cessation of 6-MP administration, rapid and rebounding recovery of peripheral blood PMN counts occurred [509]. After 4 × 40 mg/kg every 12 h mouse peripheral blood WBC declined to approximately 50% of pretreatment values by day 6 [472].

4.12 6-Thioguanine (6-TG)

CFU-S and CFU-C. After single doses of 6-TG, the dose-survival curve of murine CFU-S (assay performed 24 h after drug administration) formed a plateau at doses greater than 5 mg/kg with approximately 40% of CFU-S surviving [611]. Three and 5 days after 6-TG (30 mg/kg), the number of CFU-S per femur was 33% and 50% of controls, respectively [223].
Following in vitro incubation of bone marrow cells with 6-TG (0.01–1,000 μg/ml), a plateau of the dose-survival curve at approximately 70% for both murine and human CFU-C was found at concentrations greater than 1 μg/ml. Human CFU-C appeared to be slightly more sensitive to the drug than murine CFU-C [247]. No differences in CFU-C survival were observed after 1 or 4 h of drug exposure.

Bone Marrow. A recovery study for murine bone marrow cellularity has been reported [223] where 30 mg/kg 6-TG reduced cellularity to its lowest values (approximately 50% of controls) between days 3–5. By day 10, cellularity had returned to pretreatment values.

4.13 Vinblastine (VLB)

The vinca alkaloid VLB is used mainly in the treatment of Hodgkin's disease, but is also useful for the control of non-Hodgkin's lymphomas, testicular tumors, or breast cancer. Besides bone marrow toxicity, VLB has neurotoxic side effects.
With respect to its hematopoietic toxicity, VLB certainly is one of the most extensively studied cytotoxic agents. One of the reasons for this high experimental and clinical interest may be its activity in a variety of malignancies. More likely, however, this interest comes from the fact that VLB turned out to be a cytotoxic drug with a well-defined cycle-specificity of its cytocidal action. This unique feature has led to the widespread use of VLB as an experimental tool for elucidation of structure and regulatory mechanisms of the hematopoietic system. As a result of these studies, considerable insight into the action of VLB on different granulocytic compartments has been obtained.

Table 44. Effect of VLB on murine CFU-S: Sensitivity studies. Conversion of doses on the basis of an assumed body weight of 20 g/mouse

Strain	Time of assay (h)	CFU-S Survival (percent of controls) Dose of VLB (mg/kg)							Plateau of dose-survival curve	Reference
		0	2	4	6	8	10	20		
Bone marrow										
Normal CFU-S										
$C_{57}Bl$	20	100		60			20	20	+	[391]
$C_{57}Bl$	20–24	100			40		30	30	+	[46]
$(C_{57}Bl \times CBA)F_1$	24	100	70	25	15	8	6	2	(+)	[266]
AKR/J	24	100	60	35			20	15	+	[81]
AKR/J	24	100	61	33			20	19	+	[608]
AKR	24	100	60	40			30	30	+	[175]
AKR/J	24	100	65	35			20	15	+	[82]
$(C_3H \times C_{57}Bl)F_1$	24	100			28		23	18	–	[539]
$C_{57}Bl$	24	100						10	–	[172]
Rapidly proliferating CFU-S										
$C_{57}Bl$	20	100		8			5	5	+	[391]
AKR/J	24	100	6	1.5			1.5	1.5	+	[605]
Spleen										
AKR/J	24	100	30	18			5	1	–	[608]

Table 45. Effect of VLB on murine CFU-S: Recovery studies

	Dose (mg/kg)	CFU-S (percent of controls)									Reference
		Day									
		0	1	2	3	4	5	6	7	8	
Bone marrow											
NMRI	1	100[c]	92								[421]
AKR/J	1	100	Details for 0–14 h post-VLB for normal and rapidly proliferating CFU-S								[605]
C_3H/Cum	1.6	100	40	90	130	120	95	100			[107]
(C_3H × DBA/2)	4	100	35	50	105	90	50	100			[73]
(BALB/c × DBA/2)F_1	4	100	75	80	130	160		200			[548]
–	4	100		40			100				[58]
CD-1	4	100	71	42	94	144				44	[445]
C_{57}Bl[a]	10	100[b]	< 1			~1		~ 10		100	[43]
(C_3H × C_{57}Bl)F_1	50	100	6								[539]
Spleen											
(BALB/c × DBA/2)F_1	4	100	40	25		100		600			[548]
–	4	100		54			200				[58]
CD-1	4	100	38	55	83		193			288	[445]

[a] Continuously irradiated for 2–3 weeks (38 rad/day)
[b] On day 0, the CFU-S pool was 10% of normal
[c] Detailed time course for 0–24 h given

Table 46. Effect of VLB on CFU-C: Sensitivity studies

	Time of assay (h)	CFU-C survival (percent of controls)							Plateau of dose-survival curve	Reference
		Dose (mg/kg)								
		0	2	4	5	6	10	20		
Normal CFU-C										
Mouse ($C_{57}Bl$)	18–20[b]	100		60			40	30	+	[237]
Mouse ($C_{57}Bl$)	20	100		60			20	20	+	[391]
Mouse ($C_{57}Bl$)	18–20[a]	100		40			8	1	–	[237]
Human	18–20[a]	100		40			10	5	(+)	[237]
Mouse ($C_{57}Bl$)	20–24	100			40		30	30	+	[46]
Mouse [($C_{57}Bl \times CBA)F_1$]	24	100	30	9			0.8		(+)	[266]
Mouse (AKR)	24	100			15		5		–	[175]
Mouse ($C_{57}Bl/6N$)	24	100				18	12	7	(+)	[78]
Rapidly proliferating CFU-C										
Mouse ($C_{57}Bl$)	20	100		10			0.6		–	[391]
Mouse (AKR)	24	100			0.5		< 0.1		–	[175]

[a] Agar-diffusion chamber assay in secondary hosts; exposure to VLB in diffusion chambers in primary hosts
[b] Agar-diffusion chamber assay; exposure to VLB in situ

Table 47. Effect of VLB on mouse CFU-C: Recovery studies

Strain	Dose (mg/kg)	CFU-C (percent of controls)									Reference
		Day									
		0	1	2	3	4	5	6	7	8	
Bone marrow											
C_3H/Cum	1.6	100	22	50	110	105	100	100	100		[107]
CD-1	4	100	9.75	25			63			25	[445]
–	4	100		70			70			90	[58]
C_{57}Bl	10[a]	100	< 0.1	1		1		10			[43]
Spleen											
CD-1	4	100	30	100			463			354	[445]
–	4	100		100			500			400	[58]

[a] Given to animals that had been continuously irradiated for 2–3 weeks at 38 rad/day

CFU-S Sensitivity Studies. In any interpretation of the studies on effects of VLB on murine pluripotent stem cells (CFU-S) it must be kept in mind that the seeding efficiency of CFU-S, i.e., their capability for "homing" in an irradiated host's spleen, may decrease after exposure to VLB [212]. The experimental data obtained with the spleen colony assay may, therefore, underestimate CFU-S survival fractions.
The most comprehensive dose-survival studies of bone marrow- and spleen-derived CFU-S following exposure to VLB are listed in Table 44. In most studies, a plateau of the dose-survival curve (at 10–30% CFU-S survival) is reached at doses greater than 10 mg/kg. The relative size of the surviving fraction clearly is proliferation-dependent, proliferating CFU-S being more sensitive to the drug than normal CFU-S with little proliferative activity [391, 605, 608]. Spleen-derived CFU-S were found to be more sensitive to VLB than bone marrow-derived CFU-S (Table 44) [608].

CFU-S Recovery Studies. A number of authors described the recovery of the bone marrow CFU-S compartment after single doses of VLB (Table 45). Changes within the marrow CFU-S compartment during the first 24 h after VLB have been described in two studies [421, 605]; they are not included in Table 45. Usually, maximal CFU-S depletion was observed on day 1 with return of the CFU-S compartment to pretreatment pool size by day 3. In most studies, some overshooting and minor oscillations around the pretreatment pool size were subsequently noted. In continuously irradiated mice, 10 mg/kg VLB reduced the CFU-S pool to less than 1% of normal between days 1–4, and return to the pretreatment size was noted on day 8 [45].
Studying the proliferative activity of marrow CFU-S following VLB exposure in vivo, Nečas et al. [421] observed a transient increase of the fraction of CFU-S in S-phase 12–25 h after VLB administration.
In the spleen, recovery studies revealed somewhat greater VLB-induced CFU-S pool-size depletion. The nadir occurred by day 2; return to normal values by day 4, and overshooting recovery was noted on days 5–8 (Table 45).

CFU-C Sensitivity Studies. CFU-C appeared to be more sensitive to VLB than CFU-S (Table 46), although one paper [391] described identical sensitivity of both cell types to the drug. Rapidly proliferating CFU-C were more sensitive than normal CFU-C [391]. There is no agreement on the shape of CFU-C dose-survival curves following larger doses of VLB (Table 46). With doses of VLB greater than 10 mg/kg, a plateau of the dose-survival curve at 10–20% has been described [78, 237, 391]. However, others have reported exponential [175] or near exponential [266] dose-survival curves.
Human CFU-C have been studied by one group [237] (Table 46). Comparing the sensitivity of human and mouse bone marrow-derived CFU-C to VLB by means of the agar-diffusion chamber technique, these authors observed only minor differences in the dose-survival curves of CFU-C from the two species.

CFU-C Recovery Studies. The recovery of CFU-C compartments of bone marrow and spleen, respectively, after a single injection of VLB has been studied in mice (Table 47). In bone marrow, dose-dependent nadirs were reached on day 1. With low doses of VLB (1.6 mg/kg), return to pretreatment pool size was completed by day 3, whereas with higher doses (4 mg/kg), recovery appears to have taken considerably longer. A single dose (4 mg/kg) of VLB led to a brief reduction of the splenic CFU-C compartment size (on day 1), followed by an excessive pool-size repletion (up to 400–500% of normal on days 5–8) (Table 47).

Bone Marrow. The dose-effect of VLB on the murine bone marrow cellularity (determined 24 h postdrug) has been studied repeatedly (Table 48). From these investigations, it appears that marrow cellularity decreases with increasing doses of VLB until a plateau is reached with doses greater than 10 mg/kg. Recovery studies (Table 49) indicate that minimal marrow cellularity is not reached by day 1, but nadirs of bone marrow cellularity were determined on days 2 or 3 after VLB. Recovery of normal cellularity rapidly occurs and pretreatment values are observed 5–8 days after administration of VLB.

The changes in the different maturation stages of the morphologically identifiable granulocytic cells of the bone marrow were studied in mice [73]. Immediately after VLB (4 mg/kg), the cells of the proliferating granulocytic compartment (myeloblast to myelocyte) disappeared almost completely, only to recover to normal by day 3. In contrast, nonproliferating granulocytic cells of the marrow (metamyelocytes, granulocytes) reached lowest values by day 3 and recovered by day 6. In dogs, the percentage of marrow myelocytes dropped to near zero 1 and 2 days after VLB (0.2 mg/kg) and recovered with considerable overshoot (approximately two-times normal by day 6). Stable return to pretreatment percentage values was registered 10 days after VLB administration [52]. The same group of authors [51] later provided a more comprehensive view of changes in the granulocytic bone marrow of dogs following VLB (0.2 mg/kg). From this work, early (day 1) destruction of the early proliferating granulocytic cells (myeloblasts, promyelocytes) becomes apparent. Myelocytes reach lowest percentage values by days 1–2, metamyelocytes by day 3, and bands by days 4–6. Of interest is the observation that soon after VLB, the percentage of mature segmented neutrophils in the marrow increased dramatically (from 5 to 35%). This increase is the result of a destruction of VLB-sensitive cells, particularly of early granulocytic cells and, more importantly, of erythroid precursors. In agreement with these data, the M : E ratio in man was reported to rise threefold after VLB exposure [603].

A morphologic sequel of the mitotic spindle-blocking activity of VLB is the accumulation of proliferating cells in arrested metaphase of mitosis [51, 329]. In man, the percentage of arrested mitoses in granulocytic cells rises sharply after VLB, maximum values (3.5–4.8%) being reached 8 h [329, 330] to 24 h [603] after VLB.

In dogs, the "functional bone marrow granulocyte reserve", determined from the increase of the peripheral blood neutrophil concentration following endotoxin injection, was no longer existent 2 days after VLB [53].

Peripheral Blood. The recovery of peripheral blood WBC or neutrophils after VLB has been studied in several species (Tables 50 and 51). It appears that peripheral blood PMN are initially little affected though, in some studies, a transient increase in the PMN concentration of the peripheral blood has been observed within the first few hours after drug administration (perhaps an effect of the stress situation caused by drug administration). Later, a rapid decrease to a dose-dependent nadir occurs. In mice, this nadir is reached 3–4 days after VLB, in dogs it occurs by day 4, whereas in man it is seen 6–8 days after VLB. In rats, peripheral blood lymphocytes appear to react much more than PMN to VLB [137]. Recovery to pretreatment PMN concentrations is completed by day 5 in mice and by day 8 in dogs.

Table 48. Effect of VLB on mouse bone marrow and spleen cellularity: Sensitivity studies

Strain	Time of assay (h)	Cellularity (percent of controls)									Reference
		Dose of VLB (mg/kg)									
		0	0.1	0.5	1.0	2.0	2.5	4.0	5.0	10	
Bone marrow											
NMRI	24	100	115	76	52		43		30		[421]
AKR/J	24	100				100			75	60	[608]
$C_{57}Bl/6N$	24	100							~ 50	~ 40	[78]
$(C_3 \times C_{57}Bl)F_1$	24	100							~ 35	~ 25	[539]
Spleen											
AKR/J	24	100				70		66		45	[608]

Table 49. Effect of VLB on bone marrow and spleen cellularity in mice: Recovery studies

Strain	Dose (mg/kg)	Cellularity (percent of controls)								Reference
		Day								
		0	1	2	3	4	5	6	8	
Bone marrow										
$(C_3H \times DBA/2)F_1$	4	100	60	30	38	85		110		[548]
$(C_3H \times DBA/2)F_1$	4	100	60	30		85		110		[544]
–	4	100	110	35	12		100		105	[58]
CD-1	4	100	66	28	80		110		135	[445]
$(C_3H \times DBA/2)F_1$	4	100	35	15	30	80	85		100	[73]
$C_{57}Bl$	10[a]	100	37	30	27	25		22		[43]
$(C_3H \times C_{57}Bl)F_1$	50	100[b]	23							[539]
Spleen										
$(C_3H \times DBA/2)F_1$	4	100	150	90		115		120		[548]
$(C_3H \times DBA/2)F_1$	4	100	40	50	45	50	85	100		[73]

[a] Given to animals that had been continuously irradiated for 2–3 weeks at 38 rad/day
[b] Detailed time course for 0–24 h given

Table 50. Effect of VLB on WBC: Recovery studies

Species (strain)	Dose (mg/kg)	Peripheral blood WBC (percent of controls)								Reference
		Day								
		0	1	2	3	4	5	6	8	
Mouse (CD-1)	4	100	70	22	40		45		50	[445]
Mouse (–)[a]	4	100	55	58	35		71		47	[58]
Mouse [(C_{57}Bl × DBA/2)F_1]	4	100		15		60				[310]
Mouse [(C_3H × DBA/2)F_1]	4	100	60	35	50	65	85	100	100	[73]
Rat (Fischer, Sprague-Dawley)	6	100		40		< 20				[137]
Human	Dose-dependent toxicity for 0.1–0.4 mg/kg									[215]

[a] Bled 48 h before VLB

Table 51. Effect of VLB on blood granulocytes (PMN): Recovery studies

Species (strain)	Dose (mg/kg)	Peripheral blood PMN (percent of controls)									Reference
		Day									
		0	1	2	3	4	5	6	7	10	
Mouse (CF_1)	3	100		10–20		10–20		140	> 100	~ 150	[597]
Mouse [($C_3H \times DBA/2)F_1$]	4	100	110	10		30			250	100	[544]
Dog (–)	0.2	100	110	115	85	15	25	50	70	140	[51, 52]
Human	0.1–0.4	100	100	100					Nadir day 6–8		[329]
Rat (Fischer, Sprague-Dawley)	6	100		~ 60		~ 10					[137]

4.14 Vincristine (VCR)

Just as the other vinca alkaloids, VCR exerts its cytotoxic effect by binding to microtubular proteins of the cell, thereby interfering with the function of the mitotic spindle of dividing cells and, thus, causing mitotic arrest.
VCR has attracted considerably less attention from experimental researchers than its sister compound vinblastine. Nevertheless, the data available from the literature provide a sufficiently good insight into the effect of VCR upon the granulopoietic system to warrant inclusion of the drug into this survey.

CFU-S Sensitivity Studies. A dose-survival study of CFU-S after a single dose of VCR has not been reported. When VCR was given every 4 h for 24 or 48 h, respectively, the plateau in the dose-survival curve at 24% and 1% was reached at daily doses of 10 mg/kg and 1.25 mg/kg, respectively [82]. When 0.18 kg/24 h was administered for various periods of time, the CFU-S survival curve was exponential with an initial shoulder [82].

CFU-S Recovery Studies. Following 2 mg/kg VCR, a decrease in the size of the mouse pluripotent stem cell compartment to 69% of normal by day 1 was reported [548]. By day 3, the compartment had returned to pretreatment size. When VCR (0.5 mg/kg) was administered twice 6 days apart, the femoral CFU-S compartment was reduced to 57% and 42%, respectively, in two different strains of mice [304].

CFU-C. The effect of VCR on granulopoietic progenitor cells (CFU-C) has not been studied.

Bone Marrow. The femoral cellularity of mice was 58%, 64%, and 71% of controls at 1, 2, or 3 days after VCR (2 mg/kg) [548]. Twenty-four hours after two administrations of VCR (0.48 mg/kg given 6 days apart), the marrow cellularity of mice was 79% and 76% of controls, respectively, in two different strains of mice [304]. In rabbits, only erythroid depression was noted 48 h after 0.1 mg/kg VCR [424]. In rats, Frei et al. [216] reported a rapid decrease of the marrow cellularity. Twelve hours after 0.9 mg/kg VCR, the cellularity had dropped to 70% of normal and decreased even further to a nadir of 30% 3 days after VCR. Normal marrow cellularity was reached by day 14. The same investigators determined the mitotic index of rat bone marrow following VCR, but no discriminations between the mitotic indices of erythroid or granulocytic cells were made. In rats, accumulation of arrested myeloid mitoses was determined by Morse et al. [407] who found that 8 h after 0.3 mg/kg VCR, 23% of the cells in the proliferating granulocytic pool were in mitosis, at 24 h this value had decreased to 9%, and at 48 h to 3%. Morphological examination disclosed that all cells were arrested in metaphase [216]. Differential counts on bone marrow smears disclosed striking changes in the proportion of granulocytic cells: The initial rise (maximum by 48 h) was followed by rapid decrease. Both changes reflected the initial destruction and the subsequent rapid regeneration of cells of the erythroid series [424].

Peripheral Blood. The changes in the peripheral blood granulocyte concentration after VCR have been studied in several species. In mice, granulocyte counts decreased early, the lowest counts (approximately 30% of normal after 2 mg/kg VCR) were seen on day 3 and recovery to pretreatment levels was completed between days 4 and 5

[544]. In hypertransfused rats, VCR-induced neutropenia (0.3 mg/kg drug) was seen until day 6, with lowest counts (approximately 30% of normal) recorded on day 5 [407]. In man, weekly doses of 75 μg/kg of VCR exerted "almost no hemopoietic toxicity" [129]. With 10–75 μg/kg given weekly, other authors [99] observed leukopenia (WBC ≤ 2,000/μl) in 7 of 28 patients.

4.15 Actinomycin D (Act-D)

Act-D, an antibiotic with cytotoxic activity, binds to deoxyguanosine residues of the DNA molecule, thus, inhibiting DNA-directed RNA polymerase [230]. At very low doses, synthesis of ribosomal RNA is preferentially inhibited. In laboratory studies, the effect of daily low doses of act-D to eradicate erythropoiesis almost completely while leaving other hemopoietic systems intact has found useful application [477].

CFU-S Sensitivity Studies. Data on the changes of murine CFU-S after various doses of act-D are summarized in Table 52. Dose-response curves for normal and for rapidly proliferating bone marrow CFU-S showed an exponential cell kill 24 h after the drug, while rapidly proliferating CFU-S were more sensitive [175] (Table 52). Quite similar results were obtained by Bruce et al. [81] who gave act-D in six divided doses every 4 h and measured the surviving fraction of CFU-S 24 h after the first drug dose. Again, the dose-survival curve was exponential [81] (Table 52). In a study on the interaction of act-D with irradiation, survival data of CFU-S at 72 h after act-D are reported [545] (Table 52). Scaro [504] studied hematopoietic reconstitution in mice in which one leg had been shielded during lethal irradiation. These animals had been treated with 150 rad TBI and were given act-D (time of administration not stated). The dose-survival curve is exponential, the $D_{1/2}$ being 100 μg/kg [504] (Table 52). This value is much lower than that observed for normal bone marrow CFU-S, perhaps due to the high rate of proliferation of CFU-S observed in the endogenous spleen colony assay [462].
Single low doses of act-D (80 μg/kg) did not change the CFU-S content of normal murine bone marrow after 3, 24, and 48 h [192] (Table 52). Proliferating bone marrow CFU-S, on day 8 after isologous bone marrow transplantation or on day 6 after 336 rad sublethal irradiation, showed delayed regeneration at 24 h after act-D with a significantly lower CFU-S content per femur as compared to transplanted or irradiated animals not receiving act-D [192] (Table 52). This difference disappeared by 48 and 72 h. The fraction in S-phase of these rapidly proliferating CFU-S (measured by ^{3}H-TdR suicide on day 8 posttransplant) was depressed to 14.7% as compared to 47.9% in control animals. The depression of the proliferative state protected rapidly proliferating CFU-S from the cytotoxic effect of hydroxyurea in an experimental model where act-D was followed by hydroxyurea 2 h later, and CFU-S content was assayed 2 h after hydroxyurea. The reduction of CFU-S was only one-half of that observed after hydroxyurea alone [192].
The effect of single act-D doses is dependent upon the time of analysis. Valeriote et al. [610] reported data on the survival of bone marrow CFU-S at various time points after three dose levels of act-D [610] (Table 52). For doses of 500 and 1,000 μg/kg, CFU-S kill was first seen about 10 h after the drug and, thereafter, an exponential decline of CFU-S was observed. The intensity of CFU-S kill, the time of nadir, and the extent of CFU-S recovery after 3 days were dose-dependent. At 2,000 μg/kg, an immediate

exponential CFU-S kill was observed with values below the limit of assay after 12 h. From these kinetic observations, the authors postulated a double mechanism for the action of act-D: At low doses, act-D may act as a phase-specific agent killing only cells in S-phase. Such a phase-specific mechanism has been found in other systems [16]. S-Phase-specific depletion of the proliferating precursor compartments then triggers originally resting CFU-S into cycle, at a time when the level of act-D is still high enough to cause subsequent CFU-S kill. At higher dose levels, the cytotoxic activity of act-D appears to be independent of the phase of cell cycle, although proliferating cells were more sensitive, indicating cycle-specificity. These data on the dose-time interaction of the cytotoxic effect of act-D illustrate the complexity of factors that may influence CFU-S survival data.

The effect of act-D on the ability of transplanted spleen cells to form CFU-S in the recipient was studied by Sensenbrenner et al. [531] (Table 52) who gave 625 μg act-D at various times after transplantation. Up to 24 h after transplantation, the number of colonies developing in the spleen of treated animals was 60–84% of controls. Drug administration at 36 and 48 h after transplantation led to a progressive decline of spleen colonies with a nadir of around 1% at 72–96 h, while some recovery was evident when the drug was given 120 h after transplantation.

Seidel and Opitz [524] (Table 52) gave two injections of 120 μg/kg each on 2 consecutive days, and there was no change of the bone marrow CFU-S compartment 48 h later. A slight reduction on day 5 after the second dose was probably not significant; at this time, an expansion of the splenic CFU-S pool was observed.

Considering the dose and time observations discussed above, it is not surprising that repeated low doses do not exert considerable toxicity at the CFU-S level. In several studies [465, 483, 647], daily low doses of act-D were used to selectively eliminate erythropoietic precursor cells as originally described by Reissmann and Ito [477]. Preisler et al. [465] observed a slight increase in bone marrow CFU-S during 14 days of treatment (cumulative dose of act-D was 840 μg/kg). However, with other types of manipulations (hypertransfusion) to stop erythropoietic acitivity, the CFU-S pool expanded more than in act-D-treated animals. The authors suggest, therefore, a slight effect of act-D on CFU-S even at this dose level. An increase of CFU-S after five daily injections (75 μg/kg) to 170% of control values was observed by Zuckerman et al. [647]: In these experiments, splenic CFU-S remained unchanged. Rich et al. [483] observed normal values of CFU-S on day 4 after daily act-D doses. The relevant data are included in Table 52. In a long-term experiment (120 μg/kg every 2 days to CBA/CA mice), a constant CFU-S level was observed for up to 48 days of act-D treatment (I. Rich and B. Kubanek, personal communication).

After in vitro exposure of bone marrow cells to a concentration of 0.2 μg/ml act-D for 40 min, the survival rate of CFU-S was 74–84% [358].

Changes of CFU-C. Few data are available on the effect of act-D on CFU-C. Foster [206] included act-D in the group of drugs tested on normal C_{57}Bl/6 mice and animals treated with *C. parvum* 24 h before the cytotoxic agent. When CFU-C survival was measured 24 h after act-D in control mice, doses of 40, 200, and 400 μg/kg did not reduce the number of granulopoietic precursor cells (112%, 99%, 94% survival, respectively). It is somewhat surprising that this actively proliferating cell population was not more susceptible to act-D than CFU-S. Pretreatment with *C. parvum* did not significantly increase cytotoxicity of act-D at the lower dose levels (CFU-C survival 87% at 40 μg/kg and 86% at 200 μg/kg) but, on the other hand, the highest dose

Table 52. Effect of act-D on murine CFU-S: Dose-time response

Strain	Source of CFU-S, experimental schedule	Time of assay	$D_{1/2}$ µg/kg	Shoulder µg/kg	CFU-S survival (percent of controls)		
					Dose of act-D (µg/kg)		
					80	160	200–250
AKR	Normal bone marrow	24 h	650	–			70
	Endotoxin – 24 h		< 100	375			80
AKR	Every 4 h × 6	24 h[a]	≈ 500	–			80
BALB/c × DBA_2	Normal bone marrow	72 h					
–	Internal repopulation from shielded leg	8 days[b]	100		58	31	
AKR	Normal bone marrow	5 h					
		10 h					
		24 h					
		48 h					
		72 h					
(BALB/c × CBA)F_1	Normal bone marrow	3 h			96		
		24 h			99		
		48 h			93		
	Posttransplant bone marrow	3 days			148		
		6 days			166		
		24 days			71		
		48 days			83		
	Postirradiation bone marrow (336 rad)	3 days			106		
		24 days			74		
		48 days			106		
		72 days			91		

[a] Measured 24 h after first dose
[b] Measured on day 8 in spleens of treated animals
[c] Below the limit of assay

Table 52 (continued)

CFU-S survival (percent of controls)										Reference
Dose of act-D (μg/kg)										
300 −320	400	500	625	700 −750	1,000	2,000	2,500	60 μg/kg daily	75	
		70			30					[175]
		20	1		0.06					
		50			15		2			[81]
90				30						[545]
13										[504]
		100			100	20				[610]
		100			100	3				
		20			3					
		80			1	c				
		80			3					
										[192]

Table 52 (continued)

Strain	Source of CFU-S, experimental schedule	Time of assay	$D_{1/2}$ µg/kg	Shoulder µg/kg	CFU-S survival (percent of controls)		
					Dose of act-D (µg/kg)		
					80	160	200–250
CD_2F_1	Transplanted spleen cells; act-D given after transplantation 12 h	[b]					
	72 h						
	120 h						
NMRI	Two divided doses, days 0 and 1, bone marrow	48 h[d]					100
		120 h					69
	Spleen	48 h					70
		120 h					180
BALB/c × DBA_2	Normal bone marrow	72 h					
		7 days					
		14 days					
CF_1	Bone marrow	5 days					
	Spleen	5 days					
CBA/Ca	Bone marrow	4 days					
CBA/Ca	Bone marrow (120 µg every 2 days)	16 days					
		24 days					
		35 days					

[b] Measured on day 8 in spleens of treated animals
[d] After first dose

Table 52 (continued)

CFU-S survival (percent of controls)										Reference
Dose of act-D (μg/kg)										
300 –320	400	500	625	700 –750	1,000	2,000	2,500	60 μg/kg daily	75	
			84							[531]
			1							
			17							
										[524]
								126		[465]
								121		
								123		
									170	[647]
									100	
								100		[483]
								≈ 100		[I. Rich and B. Kubanek, personal communication]
								≈ 100		
								≈ 100		

(400 μg/kg) reduced the CFU-C bone marrow compartment to 13% of control values.

Rich et al. [483] observed a normal CFU-C content in bone marrow of mice treated with daily doses of 60 μg/kg when measured on day 4. Similarly, Zuckerman et al. [647] found normal CFU-C in bone marrow after 5 days of 75 μg/kg act-D. Seidel and Opitz [524] observed an expansion of the femoral CFU-C pool (198%) 2 days after 2 × 120 μg act-D given 1 day apart, which persisted on the following day (158%) and returned to 73% by day 5 after the first dose. In the spleen of these animals, the CFU-C pool, calculated as weight x incidence of CFU-C, declined to 36% on day 2 and showed slight expansion on day 3 (140%). In mice treated with 120 μg/kg act-D every 2 days over a prolonged period of time, the CFU-C level remained constant for 30 days, and decreased to approximately 50% by day 35 (I. Rich and B. Kubanek, personal communication).

Bone Marrow and Peripheral Blood. Bone marrow cellularity in mice decreased to 85% of pretreatment values at 72 h after 300 μg/kg act-D and to 48% after 700 μg/kg [548]. In other experiments, bone marrow cellularity decreased slightly (66%) 1 day after two doses of 120 μg/kg act-D and normal levels were found on the following day [524].

Scaro et al. [502] determined bone marrow cellularity and differential counts after various doses of act-D in FW mice. At 80 and 160 μg/kg, cellularity was reduced to 75% within 24 h. This cell loss was due to the almost complete disappearance of erythroid elements. After 400 μg/kg, bone marrow cellularity fell to a minimum of about 50% of pretreatment values at 72 h, and granulopoietic elements were also reduced.

During repeated administration of low act-D doses, erythroid precursor cells disappeared from bone marrow while total cellularity was little affected (~ 90% of control on day 21). In pretreatment marrow, erythropoiesis had accounted for about one-third of the recognizable cells. The loss of erythroid cells was compensated for by expansion of granulopoietic cells [477]. Similar changes were observed by Zuckerman et al. [647] in CF_1 mice after 5 days of 75 μg/kg act-D/day.

The bone marrow granulocyte reserve has been measured in rats by Constable and Blackett [125] after single doses of 300 μg/kg act-D, showing an increased response of PMN to endotoxin throughout the observation period of 18 days. An increased functional bone marrow granulocyte reserve was also observed in mice given repeated injections of low doses of act-D [477].

In the study of Reissman and Ito [477], in which the schedule for selective eradication of the erythropoietic precursors in mice is described, daily injections of 60 μg/kg act-D caused a marked constant increase of circulating PMN over 21 days from approximately 3,000/mm^3 to more than 10,000/mm^3.

In guinea pigs [509], daily doses of 15 μg/kg for 10 days induced a progressive rise of circulating PMN from pretreatment values (3,000 PMN/mm^3) to approximately 14,000/mm^3 at the end of treatment. After discontinuation of act-D, PMN fell to below 2,000/mm^3 on day 14 and returned to normal levels 4 days later. In the bone marrow of this species, the M : E ratio changed from a pretreatment value of 6 to 67. Thus, the reaction of the hemopoietic system of guinea pigs is quite similar to that of mice under repeated low doses of act-D, showing a severe depletion of erythropoietic elements and an elevation of circulating PMN.

In man, cumulative doses of 75 μg/kg given within 5 or 10 days led to a depression of WBC below 3,000/mm^3 in about 30% of 45 patients, with less than 1,000/mm^3 in two cases. Morphological changes of circulating PMN were observed, consisting of foamy appearance or large vacuoles in the cytoplasm [398].
Humphrey et al. [296] studied two dose levels of act-D (65 and 75 μg/kg), given in five divided doses every 24 h. The lower dose did not cause depression of WBC in ten of ten patients. Two of eleven patients treated with the higher dose of act-D showed leukocyte depression of 3,000–4,000/mm^3, and 1 of 11 showed 1,000–2,000/mm^3, the nadir occurring around day 15.

4.16 Anthracyclines

The cytostatic antibiotic daunomycin (dauno) was isolated from cultures of *Streptomyces peucetius* and introduced into clinical use in the early sixties by di Marco et al. [156], who later gave a comprehensive account on its mechanism of action [157]. In an attempt to improve the therapeutic index, several biosynthetic analogues containing the anthracycline structure were developed, of which adriamycin (ADR) has gained the widest application.
The list of anthracycline derivatives for which data on granulopoietic toxicity are available and presented in this chapter are given in Table 53.
In an attempt to enhance selectivity of these cytostatic drugs, Trouet et al. [593] have coupled dauno with DNA (dauno-DNA). This complex is taken up by pinocytosis and transferred to an active form by lysosomal enzymes, a mechanism which improved the therapeutic index for treatment of murine L 1210 leukemia [594]. Toxicity data on DNA complexes are also reported here.
The primary target of interaction for the anthracyclines is nuclear DNA: By intercalation, template activity is decreased and DNA and RNA synthesis are

Table 53. Anthracyclines relevant to this discussion

Generic name	Description	LD_{50} in the mouse (mg/kg)	Reference[a]
Daunorubicin = daunomycin (dauno)	Original anthracycline antibiotic isolated from *S. peucetius*	15.5 26	[150] [62]
Daunomycin-DNA	DNA complex with daunomycin		
Adriamycin (ADR)	14-Hydroxydaunorubicin isolated from *S. peucetius caesius*	21 20.2 11.3	[35] [62] [150]
Adriamycin-DNA	DNA complex with adriamycin		
Rubidazone	Benzol-hydrazol-hydrochloride- daunorubicin (semisynthetic)		
AD 32	N-Trifluoroacetyladriamycin-14-valerate	> 300	[448]

[a] References refer to LD_{50} data in mice

Table 54. Effect of anthracyclines on murine CFU-S: Sensitivity studies. $D_{1/2}$ values are reported when the data or a graphic documentation of the exponential dose-survival curve are given in reference. Percent survival at various doses are taken from experimental points in respective figures

Drug	Strain, experimental system	Time of assay (h)	Characteristics of dose-survival curve		CFU-S survival (percent of controls)										Reference
					Dose (mg/kg)										
			$D_{1/2}$ (mg/kg)	Shoulder (mg/kg)	4	5	6	8	10	12	20	30	40	80	
ADR	AKR, i.p.	24	13.5	None							40		8		[475]
ADR	DBA_2, i.p.	24 72	6.4	Extrapolation number ~ 0.5	50					15					[8]
ADR	DBA_2, i.v.	24	3.6/4.0	Extrapolation number ~ 0.8			70	50	30						[9]
	DBA_2, i.v., pre-treatment with α-tocopherol acetate	24	0.9	None			50	15	1						
ADR	$C_{57}Bl/CHF_1$	24						89							[370]
	$C_{57}Bl/CHF_1$, after bleeding (−48 h)	24						35							
ADR	$C_{57}Bl$, i.p.	20–24	7	None					27		18	9	2		[46]
ADR	C_3H/HeJ, i.v.	3	20	< 5							60		35	7	[279]
ADR	$C_{57}Bl/6J$, i.v.	24	3.1	< 2.5		60			15		1				[297]
ADR-DNA	$C_{57}Bl/6J$, i.v.	24	3.6	< 2.5		60			25		3				
Dauno	$C_{57}Bl/6J$, i.v.	24	3.4	< 2.5		60			15		2				
Dauno-DNA	$C_{57}Bl/6J$, i.v.	24	2.5	None		40			5		0.4				
Dauno	AKR, i.p.	24	5	None					30		10				[475]
Dauno	C_3H/DBA_2	24								25					[177]
Rubidazone	DBA_2, i.p.	72	12.4	15								56	20		[8]

inhibited [395]. The effect of anthracyclines is not dependent on the specific phase of the cell cycle. Thus, an exponential dose-response curve is regularly obtained when the effect on well-defined cell populations is measured.

CFU-S Sensitivity Studies. The sensitivity of pluripotent hemopoietic stem cells to anthracycline antibiotics has been tested almost exclusively in the mouse. Consistently, exponential dose-effect relations have been found without or with a shoulder of variable degree at low drug doses. From the available data, $D_{1/2}$ values have been estimated and the relevant results are summarized in Table 54.

Among the anthracyclines, ADR has been studied most extensively. A comparison of the $D_{1/2}$ values indicate that the experimental design greatly influences CFU-S sensitivity in that the slope of the survival curve is much steeper after i.v. [9, 297] than after i.p. administration [8, 475]. CFU-S survival differs according to the time of assay. When the assay was performed 3 h after ADR [297], a much higher value for $D_{1/2}$ is obtained than after a 24-h interval, which is consistent with the time-survival curve described below.

The mouse strain also appears to play a role: with comparable experimental systems, CFU-S of DBA_2 mice were twice as sensitive [8] than those of AKR mice [475] to ADR.

The evaluation of the graph given in the paper of Alberts et al. [8] shows that the exponential line crosses the abscissa at a value of 50% of survival. Such a low extrapolation number indicates that the drug is more toxic at low dose levels, a phenomenon also described for bleomycin [76].

The data of Massa et al. [370] differ from results of other authors: They found CFU-S to be unusually resistant to ADR. Only after stimulating the proliferation rate of the bone marrow (by bleeding the animals 48 h before ADR), the $D_{1/2}$ value was in the range observed by other authors.

Several studies are concerned with the comparison of different anthracyclines or the influence of modifying factors.

Since a protective effect against the cardiotoxicity of anthracyclines has been ascribed to vitamin E [414], it was important to test its influence on anthracycline-induced hematotoxicity. α-Tocopherol and α-tocopherol acetate, given 24 h before adriamycin, significantly enhanced the sensitivity of CFU-S [9] (Table 54).

The two most widely used anthracyclines, ADR and dauno, have been compared for their cytocidal action on CFU-S. Given i.p., ADR was much less toxic against CFU-S than dauno [475] (Table 54), but i.v. ADR was more toxic than i.v. dauno [297] (Table 54). The ADR-DNA complex was less toxic than ADR, while the dauno-DNA complex was more toxic to CFU-S than dauno [297] (Table 54).

Since cumulative cardiotoxicity is the limiting factor for repeated clinical use of anthracyclines, a great number of derivatives are being developed to overcome this problem. Such a derivative, rubidazone, was less toxic to CFU-S than ADR [8] (Table 54).

CFU-S Recovery Studies. Time-survival curves for CFU-S after anthracycline antibiotics are available from the study of Huybrechts [297] (Table 55).

For the various drugs tested, a rapid exponential decrease of femoral CFU-S is observed over the initial 24–33 h. For the two DNA complexes, a slowing or plateau phase occurred after 24 h. The pattern of recovery was biphasic, with a rapid partial restitution of the CFU-S compartment during the first 3–4 days and a slowing or

Table 55. Effect of anthracyclines on murine CFU-S: Recovery studies. Data from reference [297]

Drug	Strain	Dose (mg/kg)	CFU-S survival (percent of controls)								
			Time after anthracyclines								
			Early phase	24 h	33 h	2 days	3 days	4 days	6 days	9 days	12 days
ADR	C_{57}Bl/6J	20 i.v.	Exponential for 33 h	1.5	0.4	0.6	1.5	2	18	18	25
ADR-DNA	C_{57}Bl/6J	20 i.v.	Exponential for 24 h, then slowing	3	1.8	1.5	2	5	40	60	60
Dauno	C_{57}Bl/6J	10 i.v.	Exponential for 33 h	17	8	45	60	100	90	70	90
Dauno-DNA	C_{57}Bl/6J	10 i.v.	Exponential for 33 h, then plateau	5	5	15	20	40	40	25	55

Table 56. Effect of anthracyclines on murine CFU-C: Sensitivity studies. $D_{1/2}$ values are reported when the data or a graphic documentation of the exponential dose-survival curve are given in reference. Percent survival at various doses are taken from experimental points in respective figures

Drug	Strain, experimental system	Time of assay (h)	Characteristic of dose-survival curve		CFU-S survival (percent of controls)							Reference
					Dose (mg/kg)							
			$D_{1/2}$ (mg/kg)	Shoulder (mg/kg)	10	20	25	30	40	50	100	
ADR	C_{57}Bl, i.v.	20–24	12	None	60	30		18	14			[46]
	C_{57}Bl, i.v., agar-diffusion chamber	20–24	7	None	30	12		5	2			
ADR	C_{57}Bl, i.p.	24			67							[206]
	C_{57}Bl, i.p., *C. parvum* at −24 h	24			33							
ADR	C_{57}Bl/6J, i.v.	24	2.5	< 5	30	0.9		0.1				[297]
ADR-DNA	C_{57}Bl/6J, i.v.	24	2.5	< 5	30	1.5		0.1				
Dauno	C_{57}Bl/6J, i.v.	24	3.9	< 5	50	6		1.5				
Dauno-DNA	C_{57}Bl/6J, i.v.	24	3.1	< 5	22	1		0.3				
ADR	CD_1, i.v., agar-diffusion chamber	18	8	None	45	10		5				[368]
AD 32	CD_1, i.v., agar-diffusion chamber	18	25	None			65			30	7	[368]

plateau phase thereafter. The CFU-S pool returned to pretreatment values by 12 days only after dauno, whereas incomplete CFU-S recovery by this time was noted for the other compounds.

CFU-C in Vivo Sensitivity Studies. Data on the in vivo sensitivity of murine CFU-C to anthracyclines are summarized in Table 56. As for CFU-S, the dose-response curves of CFU-C are exponential and a shoulder is seen in some studies. In a simultaneous assay by six methods for hemopoietic precursor cells, the effect of ADR was studied on granulopoietic-determined precursor cells by the in vitro agar colony assay and by the agar-diffusion chamber assay [46] (Table 56). In this experiment, the granulopoietic-determined progenitor cells appeared to be more sensitive when assayed in the agar-diffusion chamber than in the in vitro agar colony assay. The administration of *C. parvum* 24 h before ADR significantly increased the sensitivity of CFU-C [206] (Table 56).

CFU-C Recovery Studies. The experiments of Huybrechts [297] comparing ADR, ADR-DNA, dauno, and dauno-DNA give detailed information on the time course of CFU-C after these drugs (Table 57). In their free form, both ADR and dauno caused excessive regeneration of CFU-C, while CFU-C returned to pretreatment values without rebound after administration of the DNA-bound drugs.

CFU-C Sensitivity in Diffusion Chambers or in Vitro. Marsh [368] (Table 58) performed a series of experiments in which granulopoietic progenitor cells of three species (mouse, dog, and man) were exposed to ADR and its analogue AD 32 in agar-diffusion chambers. Murine CFU-C were similarly sensitive, whether exposed in situ [368] or in the diffusion chamber (in situ data, see Table 56). The rank of toxicity for the three species, from highest to lowest sensitivity, was dog-mouse-man for ADR and dog-man-mouse for AD 32 [368] (Table 58). This reversal of relative toxicity to murine and human CFU-C for the two anthracycline derivatives illustrates the difficulties in extrapolating animal data to man.
Two reports deal with the in vitro sensitivity of human CFU-C to ADR (Table 58). We [350] have reported the dose-response of human CFU-C exposed to ADR for 30 min at 37° C before plating, and for the entire culture period. To reduce CFU-C to the same level, approximately 100-times higher concentrations of ADR were needed during the 30 min incubation than when the drug was added to the culture dishes. This difference is in agreement with studies on other mammalian cell lines [20]. We also

Table 57. Effect of anthracyclines on murine CFU-C: Recovery studies. Data from reference [297]

Drug	CFU-C survival (percent of controls)		
	Minimum	Maximum	12-Day recovery
ADR (10 mg/kg)	0.3 (Day 2)	130 (Day 9)	60
ADR-DNA (10 mg/kg)	1.3 (Day 1)	80 (Day 6)	70
Dauno (20 mg/kg)	55 (Day 1)	150 (Day 4)	75
Dauno-DNA (20 mg/kg)	23 (Day 1)	80 (Day 4)	55

studied human bone marrow CFU-C for their in vitro sensitivity to ADR before and after five intensive courses of chemotherapy containing ADR. The in vitro sensitivity remained unchanged after repeated in vivo exposure to the drug, indicating that no CFU-C subpopulation with a different resistance to ADR had emerged [350].

Buick et al. [89] reported in vitro toxicity data of CFU-C from a few individual patients, comparing ADR and dauno [89] (Table 58). There was a somewhat wide range of sensitivity, with an average $D_{1/2}$ of 1.8×10^{-3} g/l ADR for the four patients. For a comparison of these data with ours, the different experimental design (in vitro agar culture versus methyl cellulose culture) must be considered.

Droz et al. [164] describe the changes of CFU-C in one patient with metastatic thyroid carcinoma who received seven courses of 40 mg/m^2 ADR at 3-weekly intervals; CFU-C were expressed per kg body weight using the incidence per metamyelocytes for this estimation [449]. Prechemotherapy values were 12% of normal due to previous irradiation. Before the fourth and seventh courses of ADR, CFU-C per kg body weight were severely depressed (≈ 20% of prechemotherapy values), and 3 months after ADR, they had recovered to the pretreatment value.

Comparison of Stem Cell Toxicities. For a comparison of stem cell toxicity of various anthracyclines, the $D_{1/2}$ values for CFU-S and CFU-C, discussed above, are expressed as relative values with the $D_{1/2}$ of ADR as reference point. This was possible, since all reported studies comparing various anthracyclines contain ADR as one drug. These relative data are contained in Table 59. Values below 1 indicate higher toxicity and values above 1 indicate a lower toxicity of the respective compound to the tested stem cell population.

Dauno is more toxic than ADR on CFU-S of mice when the drug is given i.p. [475] (Table 59) and on human CFU-C in vitro [89] (Table 59). On the other hand, dauno is less toxic to CFU-S and CFU-C of mice when the route of administration is i.v. [297] (Table 59).

Huybrechts [297] has tested ADR, dauno, and their respective DNA complexes on murine CFU-S and CFU-C [297] (Table 59). The differences in toxicity of the parent compounds and their DNA derivatives and the possible mechanisms underlying these differences are thoroughly discussed in the paper.

Other tested analogues, rubidazone and AD 32, are significantly less toxic to the respective cell system than ADR [8, 368] (Table 59).

The sensitivity of CFU-C from three different species to ADR and AD 32 has been compared in diffusion chambers [368] (Table 59). For both drugs, the dog is the most sensitive species, though, the order of sensitivity is different for murine and human CFU-C, the latter being less sensitive to ADR and more sensitive to AD 32 than murine CFU-C.

Bone Marrow Cellularity. Some data are available on anthracycline-induced changes of bone marrow cellularity in mice and rats (Table 60). In mice, the decline of bone marrow cellularity proceeds more slowly than that of stem cell compartments, reaching a nadir between days 2–4, depending on the drug [297] (Table 60). This agrees with the data on the changes in bone marrow cellularity occurring during the initial 18 h after ADR and AD 32 [368] (Table 60).

A morphologic description of changes in rat bone marrow [444] (Table 60) suggests a very rapid decline of the bone marrow cellularity in this species. At a somewhat lower dose, the depletion and recovery of the bone marrow cellularity in rats was similar to

Table 58. Effect of anthracyclines on CFU-C: Sensitivity in diffusion chamber and in vitro

Drug		Experimental system	Characteristics of dose-survival curve		CFU-C survival (percent of controls) (agar-diffusion chamber progenitor cells)									Reference
			$D_{1/2}$ (mg/kg)	Shoulder	Dose to primary recipient (mg/kg)									
					5	10	15	20	25	30	40	50	100	
ADR	Mouse (CD_1)	Agar-diffusion chamber, exposed for 1 h in primary recipient	5.3	None		65				7	0.6			[368]
	Dog		2.3	None	25	1.5	1							
	Human		6.3	None	120	40	20							
AD 32	Mouse (CD_1)		25	None					65			30	4	
	Dog		11	None					25			2	0.4	
	Human		15	None					23			10	4	
			(g/l)		Concentration of drug (g/l)									
					2×10^{-6}	6.6×10^{-6}	2×10^{-5}	$2-2.5 \times 10^{-4}$	$5-6.6 \times 10^{-4}$	$1-1.3 \times 10^{-3}$	3×10^{-3}			
ADR	Human	ADR added to cultures	4×10^{-6}	Slight	79	60	6.8							[350]
	Human	Exposed for 30 min at 37° C before culture	3×10^{-4}				88	76	29	7.8	1			
ADR	Human	Methyl cellulose culture, exposed for 10 min at 37° C	$7-33^{a} \times 10^{-4}$	None					80	30	10			[89]
Dauno	Human		$1-3^{b} \times 10^{-4}$	None				50	12	4				

[a] Range of four reported individual values; one "representative" survival curve is given, the data of which are included as percent of survival
[b] Range of three individual values

Table 59. Comparison of stem cell toxicity of anthracyclines. $D_{1/2}$ are given relative to that of ADR. For the interspecies comparison, $D_{1/2}$ in mice are used as reference point

	Species	Relative values of $D_{1/2}$ (ADR = 1.0)						Interspecies comparison ($D_{1/2}$ mouse = 1.0)		Reference
		ADR	ADR-DNA	Dauno	Dauno-DNA	Rubidazone	AD 32	ADR	AD 32	
CFU-S, i.p.	Mouse	1.0		0.4						[475]
CFU-S, i.v.	Mouse	1.0				1.9				[8]
CFU-S, i.v.	Mouse	1.0	1.2	1.1	0.8					[297]
CFU-C, i.v.	Mouse	1.0	1.0	1.6	1.2					[297]
CFU-C, i.v.	Mouse	1.0					3.0			[368]
CFU-C, agar-diffusion chamber	Mouse	1.0					4.7	1.0	1.0	[368]
	Dog	1.0					4.7	0.4	0.4	
	Man	1.0					2.4	1.2	0.6	
CFU-C, agar in vitro	Man	1.0		0.12						[89]

Table 60. Effect of anthracyclines on bone marrow cellularity: Recovery studies

Drug		Dose (mg/kg)	Bone marrow cellularity (percent of controls)			Reference
			Initial phase	Overshoot	Recovery	
ADR	C_{57}Bl/6J mice, i.v.	10	Nadir 10 (Day 3–4)	–	85 (Day 12)	[297]
ADR-DNA		10	Nadir 13 (Day 3–4)	–	70 (Day 12)	
Dauno	C_{57}Bl/6J mice, i.v.	20	Nadir 30 (Day 2–3)	130 (Day 6)	100 (Day 12)	
Dauno-DNA		20	Nadir 20 (Day 3)	–	75 (Day 12)	
ADR	CD_1 mice, i.v.	40	Nadir 56 (18 h)			[368]
AD 32	CD_1 mice, i.v.	100	Nadir 44 (18 h)			
AD 32	CD_1 mice, i.v.	200	Nadir 50 (18 h)			
ADR	Wistar rats	15	"Very scarce" within 12 h		Beginning day 4–5, complete day 7	[444]
ADR	ACI rats	10	Nadir 40 (Day 4–6)[a]	130 (Day 14–16)[a]	110 (Day 20)[a]	[290]

[a] Bone marrow cellularity measured as DNA content per tibia

that observed in mice [290] (Table 60). In this latter study, the total dose of 10 mg/kg was given either as a single injection, or, divided in three and five doses given every 24 h. The decrease in bone marrow cellularity (measured as DNA content per tibia) was identical for the three schedules, while after the divided dose schedules the nadir of bone marrow cellularity was delayed for 8 days [290].

Peripheral Blood WBC and Granulocytes. There are few systematic data in experimental animals. Following administration of ADR (50 mg/kg) to Wistar rats, the WBC count fell from 12,000/mm^3 to a nadir around 1,000/mm^3 on day 2 and recovered to pretreatment values by day 8 with some overshoot by day 11 [444]. In a study on hepatoma-bearing ACI rats treated with 10 mg/kg ADR, the WBC count fell to 60–70% on days 4 and 7. This later development is influenced by the fact that the hepatoma caused leukocytosis in the untreated animals [290].

A description of the effects of anthracyclines on human peripheral granulocytes is usually contained in reports on phase I or phase II clinical trials. These data are given in more general terms. Patients have usually received pretreatment with chemotherapy and/or radiotherapy. In addition, most series contain patients with hematologic diseases, lymphomas, or with bone marrow infiltration by the tumor. Dauno has been used almost exclusively for the treatment of leukemias; and this discussion will, therefore, review some experiences with ADR only.

Early experience with ADR has been summarized in an international symposium [100]. In this symposium, Bonadonna et al. [62] reported on approximately 300 patients treated with five dose schedules of ADR. The least toxic schedule (20–25 mg/m^2 given on 3 consecutive days) caused myelosuppression in 45% of the cases. In 27 patients with lung cancer, single doses of 75 mg/m^2 ADR caused leukopenia with a nadir of 2,500 mm^3 on day 11 and revovery was completed on day 25 [62]. In a study comparing three dose levels (3×30 mg/m^2, 3×25 mg/m^2, 3×20 mg/m^2), the degree of leukopenia was dose-dependent with a nadir of 2,100 WBC/mm^3 on day 14 after the highest dose [385]. Benjamin [28] summarized the clinical experience with ADR in 88 patients, about half of whom had systemic disease of the hemopoietic or lymphatic system. The dose was 60 mg/m^2 as a single injection. The nadir of WBC was 2,000/mm^3 (range 200–6,200), the median day of nadir 12 (4–15), and recovery occurred around day 19 (12–41). Pretreatment with chemotherapy and/or radiotherapy did not influence hematotoxicity, while bone marrow infiltration with tumor or liver disease markedly enhanced the toxic effect of ADR.

In a clinical study of patients with primary liver cancer, pulse doses of 60 mg/m^2 produced leukopenia of 3,000–4,500/mm^3 in 27% of the patients, 2,000–3,000/mm^3 in 46%, and 1,000–2,000 in 9% [191]. ADR (75 mg/m^2) given in 3-weekly intervals caused leukopenia of from less than 4,000 to 2,500/mm^3 in 8 of 19, and less than 2,500/mm^3 in 3 of 19 patients with advanced ovarian carcinoma [149].

From these clinical studies, ADR given in high single doses with a sufficient rest period is the treatment schedule that exerts the lowest granulopoietic toxicity. Under these conditions, peripheral leukopenia is dose-dependent, with a nadir around day 14 followed by a rather rapid recovery.

4.17 Bleomycin

Bleomycin, a group of closely related antibiotics isolated from *S. verticillus*, shows "virtually no bone marrow toxicity" in clinical studies, as Blum [47] formulated in a clinical review.

CFU-S Sensitivity and Recovery Studies. The data summarized in Table 61 indicate a high resistance of normal murine CFU-S to bleomycin. The induction of a higher proliferative state increased the sensitivity of CFU-S to bleomycin. These findings are confirmed by in vitro experiments [596] (Table 61).
The dose-survival curve of proliferating CFU-S reported by Briganti et al. [76] shows a biphasic shape with a marked initial upward concavity. Rapid induction of resistance [580] or differential sensitivity of subpopulations [21] are discussed by the authors as possible causes of this biphasic curve. Another interesting finding in the study of Briganti et al. [76] is the induction of a parasynchronous state (Table 61). Twenty-four to 28 h after bleomycin, the fraction of CFU-S in S-phase, as measured by hydroxyurea kill, increased to 60%. This was followed by a doubling of the population size within 48 h. In the same series of experiments, there was no change in sensitivity of normal CFU-S when the bleomycin dose was split into two doses 4 h apart; in contrast, the split-dose regimen caused greater kill of rapidly proliferating CFU-S [76].
Weekly low doses of bleomycin (21 mg/m^2 in $CBA/C_{57}Bl$ mice, equivalent to 0.7 mg/kg in man) did not reduce femoral CFU-S content over a period of 44 weeks [430a]. The proliferative state of CFU-S, as measured by their sensitivity to hydroxyurea, was not altered.

CFU-C Sensitivity and Recovery Studies. Briganti et al. [77] reported on the dose-response and time course of murine CFU-C after bleomycin (Table 62). The $D_{1/2}$ of CFU-C is similar to that of proliferating CFU-S (Table 61) in that the initial upward slope of the dose-response curve is even higher than for CFU-S (extrapolation number 0.66). The killing action of bleomycin on CFU-C is very rapid, with excessive recovery by 24–28 h. Dividing the dose led to increased sensitivity of CFU-C.
In the above-mentioned long-term experiments of Nowrousian et al. [430a], the CFU-C compartment of murine bone marrow remained unchanged with respect to size and proliferative activity over 44 weeks of weekly low-dose bleomycin.

4.18 Hydroxyurea (HU)

HU selectively kills cells in S-phase and prevents progression of cells from G_1- into S-phase [540a]. HU is cleared from plasma of mice with a short half-life of 13 min [188] and 48 min [288], respectively. As soon as HU concentration has fallen below the effective dose level, the cells blocked at G_1-S immediately start to enter S-phase [37].
These pharmacologic characteristics have made HU a valuable tool in studying the proliferative state of hemopoietic precursor cells. A technique to selectively kill cells in DNA synthesis by in vivo exposure to HU has been introduced by Morse et al. [408] as an alternative to ^{3}H-TdR suicide. HU has also been used for the in vitro determination of proliferative activity [96].

Table 61. Effect of bleomycin on murine CFU-S: Sensitivity studies in vivo and in vitro

Strain	Source of CFU-S	Time of assay (h)	$D_{1/2}$ (mg/kg)	n[a]	CFU-S survival (percent of controls)						Reference
					Dose of bleomycin (mg/kg)						
					50	100	200	400	800	1,600	
BALB/c or $C_{57}Bl$	Normal bone marrow	24			100		80				[596]
	Proliferating (endotoxin; regenerating bone marrow)	24			40		20				
$C_{57}Bl \times C_3H$	Normal bone marrow	2						30			[76]
		4	440	0.84			60	40	20		
		12						40			
		20						40			
		40						60			
		48						80			
		60						80			
	Proliferating (endotoxin); bone marrow	4	670	–	50	30	15	10	7		
					in vitro		50		200 µg/ml		
BALB/c or $C_{57}Bl$	Normal bone marrow						60		35		[596]
	Proliferating, bone marrow						35		20		

[a] Extrapolation number

Table 62. Effect of bleomycin on $C_{57}Bl \times C_3H$ murine bone marrow CFU-C: Sensitivity and recovery study [77]

Treatment schedule	Time of assay (h)	$D_{1/2}$ (mg/kg)	n[a]	CFU-C survival (percent of controls)								
				Dose of bleomycin (mg/kg)								
				40	80	160	200	300	400	600	800	1,200
Single injection	2								26			
	4	670	0.66	65	55	57	60	43 (55)[c]	34 (50)[c]	35	28	18
	8								43			
	12								44			
	20								80			
	24								145			
	28								170			
	48								120			
Split into two doses 4 h apart	8[b]								19			

[a] Extrapolation number
[b] After first dose
[c] From different set of data in [77]

In addition to its usefulness in determining the proliferation rate of hemopoietic precursor cells, its ability to block proliferating cells at G_1-S has led to the widespread use of HU for synchronization experiments.

In general, the effect of HU on stem cell level has attracted great interest, whereas its effects on differentiating cells of the bone marrow and on circulating PMN have not been reported in detail. One reason for this discrepancy may be that the action of HU on stem cell level is of considerable theoretical interest, while researchers appear to expect little information from looking at later compartments. The primary clinical use of HU is in the treatment of chronic granulocytic leukemia, a disease characterized by a malignant transformation in the hemopoietic system. Clinical toxicity data on patients with normal hemopoiesis are, therefore, scarce.

Sensitivity of Normal Murine Bone Marrow CFU-S After Single Injection of HU. Data on CFU-S survival after single doses of HU are presented in Table 63. There is little effect of HU on an unperturbed CFU-S population of normal bone marrow, as expected from the mode of action of the drug, since there is only a small proportion of normal bone marrow CFU-S in cell cycle. In view of the small CFU-S kill, the problem of statistical significance is of critical importance, since the spleen colony technique is subject to a rather large SD. Therefore, the data should be interpreted with caution. At any rate, within the reported range, the dose of HU does not appear to influence CFU-S survival. Most groups used a dose of 900–1,000 mg/kg, but a dose as high as 4,500 mg/kg killed no CFU-S in a study for which the authors do not report the exact conditions of their experiment [374].

The mean for the 22 values listed in Table 63 is 85.0 ± 10.8% (1 SD) survival. The three values below 70% were found in experiments in which 4- and 24-h intervals were chosen between HU application and assay. However, there is no difference if one averages only the 13 1- and 2-h values (85.3 ± 6.5%).

There appear to be differences depending on the type of experimental animals used. Benestad [25] reports a 20% kill of CFU-S in 5-week-old mice, whereas CFU-S were completely resistant to the same dose of HU in 22-week-old animals (Table 63). CFU-S from two mouse strains showed a definite difference in the in vivo sensitivity to HU: CFU-S of C_{57}Bl mice were resistant to a 4-h exposure to HU, while the bone marrow CFU-S pool of C_3H mice was reduced to 80% by 1 h and to 68% by 4 h [619, 620] (Table 63).

Sensitivity of Murine CFU-S in Various Proliferative States. HU has been used to define the proliferative state of murine CFU-S in a number of experimental systems (Table 64).

During the embryonic phase, the development of the hemopoietic system is accompanied by an increased proliferation rate of CFU-S. Kubanek et al. [327] determined the surviving fraction of CFU-S from fetal liver on day 12 of gestation: approximately two-thirds of CFU-S were sensitive to HU (Table 64).

A widely used experimental source of rapidly proliferating hemopoietic precursors is the lethally irradiated mouse after syngeneic bone marrow transplantation. In elaborate studies on the effect of HU on the murine hemopoiesis, Hodgson et al. studied the sensitivity of rapidly proliferating CFU-S 7 days after bone marrow transplantation, and approximately 50% were in DNA-synthesis, as concluded from their sensitivity to HU [288] (Table 64). Similar results were reported by Chaffey and Hellman [106] who injected the primary recipient mice with low doses of HU

Table 63. Effect of HU on normal murine bone marrow CFU-S: Sensitivity studies

Strain	Time of assay (h)	CFU-S survival (percent of controls)					Reference
		Dose of HU (mg/kg)					
		250	450–500	900–1,000	2,500	4,500	
CF_1	1			84			[396]
CF_1	2			90			[468]
HSB	2			84			[69]
CF	2			76			[486]
CF	2			86			[409]
$C_3H \times DBA$	2			82			[308]
BALB/c	2			94			[288]
ND2	2			88			[629b]
BALB/c	9			95			[286]
$C_{57}Bl \times CBA$	16		60				[618]
CBA/OLA	24	65					[165]
Swiss	24			100			[501]
NMRI	24			98			[419]
$C_{57}Bl \times C_3H$	24			68			[370]
–	–					100	[374]
CBA (plethoric)	2			90			[328]
$(C_3Bl \times DBA_2)$ 5-weeks old	2			79			[25]
22-weeks old	2			98			
C_3H	1		80		78		[619, 620]
	4		68		73		
$C_{57}Bl$	4		95				

(150 mg/kg) 18 h after bone marrow transplantation and counted the developing spleen colonies in these animals on day 9 posttransplant: HU reduced the number of colonies to about 50% [106] (Table 64). Six days after sublethal irradiation, about one-third of femoral CFU-S were sensitive to HU [192] (Table 64).

Cytotoxic drug-induced damage to hemopoietic tissue triggers the hematopoietic cell lines into regeneration. Utilizing the S-phase-specific cell kill by HU, the increased proliferative activity of CFU-S during this regeneration phase has been studied for VLB [25] and for bleomycin [374] and, in both instances, the sensitivity of CFU-S increased markedly (Table 64).

When HU is followed by a second dose of HU under suitable experimental conditions, high sensitivity of CFU-S to the second dose is observed. As an example, the data of Hodgson on the 7-day posttransplant spleen are shown in Table 64 [288]. A more thorough discussion of synchronization studies with multiple doses of HU is given later (see page 131).

The effect of yet another agent of interest for its stimulatory influence on granulopoiesis, bacterial endotoxin, has been studied in this way [468]. Twenty-four hours after endotoxin, bone marrow CFU-S of CF_1 mice showed an increase in proliferation rate, with about one-third of CFU-S in DNA synthesis (Table 64).

In the experiments of Fehér and Gidali [192] (Table 64) act-D was used to prevent CFU-S from entering a state of active proliferation. In this way the toxic effect of HU was reduced by approximately 50%.

Sensitivity of Murine CFU-S Under Selected Experimental Conditions. From the data in Table 65, it appears that the effect of HU on murine CFU-S is largely independent of the dose. However, under selected experimental conditions, dose-response curves can be obtained which exhibit a marked correlation between dose and cell kill.

When a first dose of HU is used to trigger CFU-S into proliferation, a second dose of HU 7 h later exerts a dose-dependent effect [288] (Table 65). This dose-response curve approaches an exponential shape.

In the reverse situation, a variable first dose of HU was followed by a constant second dose 12 h later and, again, the efficacy of the first dose of HU to trigger CFU-S into active cell cycle was dose-dependent [421] (Table 65).

From these observations it can be concluded that with doses greater than 450–500 mg/kg, the maximum possible effect on the murine CFU-S compartment is achieved. Since most studies using HU experimentally are performed with doses of 900–1,000 mg/kg, maximum efficiency of HU is assured.

An interesting observation has been reported by Nečas et al. [423] on the number of circulating CFU-S in ICR mice. This population was highly sensitive to HU even at low doses (Table 65). At the same time, bone marrow CFU-S were minimally or not affected by HU. The meaning of this phenomenon is not clear, but it may become apparent when the function of the circulating stem cells is more completely understood.

CFU-S Sensitivity Studies in Vitro. In contrast to its wide application in vivo for estimation of the fraction of CFU-S in S-phase, few authors have utilized the drug in vitro for this purpose.

Byron [95] used 1 m*M* HU for 2 h to assay the fraction of CFU-S in S-phase: in cultures from normal B_6AF_1 mice, no in vitro CFU-S kill occurred (Table 66). When the donor

Table 64. Effect of HU on rapidly proliferating murine CFU-S: Sensitivity studies

Strain	Source of CFU-S, experimental conditions	Dose of HU (mg/kg)	Time of assay (h)	CFU-S survival (percent of controls)	Reference
DBA	Fetal liver, day 12 of gestation	1,000	12	35	[327]
BALB/c	Spleen, day 7 posttransplant	1,000	2	50	[288]
C_3H/HeJ	Spleen, 18 h posttransplant	150	[a]	50	[106]
(BALB/c × CBA)F_1	Femur, day 6 after 300 rad	900	2	71	[192]
C_3H × DBA/2	Bone marrow, VBL (4 mg/kg) −4 h	900	2	36	[25]
BALB/c	Bone marrow, bleomycin (400 mg/kg) −20 h	4,500	–	45	[374]
BALB/c	Spleen, day 7 posttransplant, HU −7 h	1,000	2	17	[288]
CF_1	Bone marrow, endotoxin −24 h	900	2	63	[468]

[a] Colonies counted in primary recipient on day 9 after transplantation

Table 65. Effect of HU on murine CFU-S under special experimental conditions: Sensitivity studies

Strain, experimental conditions	Time of assay (h)	CFU-S survival (percent of controls)						Reference
		Dose of HU (mg/kg)						
		10	50–67.5	100–125	250	450–500	900–1,000	
BALB/c, first dose of HU (1000 mg/kg) 7 h before variable second dose	2		85	50	35	23	17	[288]
ICR, first dose of HU variable, 12 h before second dose of 1000 mg/kg	2	81	53	42		25	24	[421]
ICR, circulating CFU-S	24	90	25	15		0	0	[423]

mice had been injected with 0.5 mg/kg neostigmine 2 h before bone marrow removal, the in vitro CFU-S kill by HU was almost complete. The author concludes that neostigmine causes a rapid transition of CFU-S from the G_0 state into DNA synthesis, possibly by the action of acetylcholine when the activity of cholinesterase is blocked by neostigmine. Using in vitro HU on CFU-S triggered into proliferation by testosterone, a time lag for the killing action of HU was observed, with no cell kill during the first hour, while the CFU-S were reduced to about 50% after 2 h [96] (Table 66). Such a time lag was not observed when ^{3}H-TdR suicide was used to kill cells in S-phase. Possibly, resting CFU-S may contain a pool of DNA precursors which render the cells resistant to the action of HU for a period of time.

Wu [642] studied the proliferation rate of CFU-S after several days of continuous TBI. Despite an in vitro exposure period of only 30 min, 15% cell kill by HU was observed for normal bone marrow CFU-S and a 35% CFU-S kill was measured after 10 days of continuous irradiation (Table 66).

CFU-S recovered from 2-day diffusion chambers showed a proliferation rate of 24–35% as measured by in vitro sensitivity to HU [26] (Table 66).

CFU-S Recovery Studies. Data on the recovery of the CFU-S compartment in mice after HU are summarized in Table 67.

When bone marrow CFU-S are followed after a single injection of HU (Table 67, upper part), CFU-S survival is regularly greater than 80% during the first 12 h. Thereafter, some studies report a slight to moderate depression, usually during days 2 and 3, with recovery by day 6, and an indication of rebound by day 8.

These changes in the bone marrow CFU-S pool are strain-specific, as illustrated by the studies of Vassort et al. [619, 620] (Table 67). In C_3H mice, a moderate decline to

Table 66. Effect of HU on murine CFU-S: In vitro sensitivity studies [95]

Source of CFU-S	Concentration of HU	CFU-S survival (percent of controls)				Reference
		Time of incubation (min)				
		30	60	120	180	
B_6AF_1, normal bone marrow	1 mM			100		[95]
in vivo treatment with neostigmine				1		
$C_3H \times AKR$, stimulated by testosterone	1 mM		100	55	50	[96]
$C_3H \times AKR$ or BDF_1,	1 mM[a]					[642]
normal bone marrow		85				
10 days irradiation (70 rad/day)		65				
NMRI or $C_3D_2F_1$, from 2-day diffusion chambers	10–20 mM			63–77		[26]

[a] Technique of [95] quoted

Table 67. Effect of HU on murine CFU-S: Recovery studies. The data are usually taken from graphs and should be considered as approximations

Strain	Source of CFU-S, experimental conditions	HU dose[a] (mg/kg)	CFU-S survival (percent of controls)									Reference
			Time after HU									
			1 h	2–3 h	4 h	5–6 h	8–10 h	12–14 h	16 h	19–20 h	24 h	
CBA/OLA	Normal bone marrow	250									65	[165]
BALB/c	Normal bone marrow			100			100					[286]
BALB/c	Normal bone marrow			94			95					[288]
CF_1	Normal bone marrow			90								[468]
HSB	Normal bone marrow			84								[69]
CF_1s	Normal bone marrow			80								[486]
Swiss	Normal bone marrow										100	[501]
CF_1	Normal bone marrow		84					81				[396]
(C_{57}Bl × C_3H)	Normal bone marrow										68	[370]
NRMI	Normal bone marrow						92	80		88	98	[419]
NRMI	Normal bone marrow			90							50–90	[422]
CF_1	Normal bone marrow			86	100			72			72	[408]
CBA	Plethoric bone marrow			90				85			85	[328]
C_3H	Normal bone marrow	500	80	60		69	74	60		56	67	[619]
C_3H	Normal bone marrow	2,500	78	80	73		55	45	67	72	76	
C_3H	Normal bone marrow	500	81		68		58	61	63	56	68	[620]
C_{57}Bl	Normal bone marrow	500			95	80	83	65	69			
CBA	Fetal liver, treated day 12 of gestation			70				35			38	[327]
NMRI	Normal spleen										50	[422]
NMRI	Spleen, endogenous CFU-S assay										80	
NMRI	Circulating CFU-S										0	[423]
BALB/c	Bone marrow	2× 1,000, 7 h apart					70				45	[288]
	Spleen						45					
DBA/2	Bone marrow Spleen[b]	4× 500 every 6 h										[526]
ND_2	Bone marrow	4× 500 every 6 h		5							4	[629a]

Table 67 (continued)

Strain	Source of CFU-S, experimental conditions	HU dose[a] (mg/kg)	CFU-S survival (percent of controls)									Reference
			Time after HU									
			2 days	3 days	4 days	5 days	6 days	7 days	8 days	10 days	26 days	
CBA/OLA	Normal bone marrow	250	41	175	260	120			165	90	140	[165]
BALB/c	Normal bone marrow											[286]
BALB/c	Normal bone marrow											[288]
CF_1	Normal bone marrow											[468]
HSB	Normal bone marrow											[69]
CF_1s	Normal bone marrow											[486]
Swiss	Normal bone marrow											[501]
CF_1	Normal bone marrow											[396]
($C_{57}Bl \times C_3H$)	Normal bone marrow											[370]
NRMI	Normal bone marrow											[419]
NRMI	Normal bone marrow		50				100		140			[422]
CF_1	Normal bone marrow											[408]
CBA	Plethoric bone marrow		75	85		70						[328]
C_3H	Normal bone marrow	500	120					95				[619]
C_3H	Normal bone marrow	2,500	140									
C_3H	Normal bone marrow	500										[620]
$C_{57}Bl$	Normal bone marrow	500										
CBA	Fetal liver, treated day 12 of gestation		87	137	163							[327]
NMRI	Normal spleen			100			150		270			[422]
NMRI	Spleen, endogenous CFU-S assay				200				100			
NMRI	Circulating CFU-S		100			300		130				[423]
BALB/c	Bone marrow	2× 1,000,	37	120	80		86					[288]
	Spleen	7 h apart	23	20	375		440					
DBA/2	Bone marrow	4× 500 every	20	40	60			100				[526]
	Spleen[b]	6 h	15	20	50			400				
ND_2	Bone marrow	4× 500 every 6 h	5	20	90	100	100	105	100			[629a]

[a] Only stated when other than 900–1,000 mg/kg
[b] Calculated as index of the splenic pool size (weight × incidence of CFU-S)

50%–60% becomes evident by 4 h. In contrast, the CFU-S of $C_{57}Bl$ mice do not change during the first 4 h after HU, but are reduced to 65–70% at 12 h. These differences are explained by the proliferative state of CFU-S in the two strains: While the pluripotent hemopoietic stem cells in $C_{57}Bl$ mice are virtually quiescent, a fraction of about 20% is in DNA synthesis in C_3H mice [620].

A recovery study of fetal liver CFU-S is reported by Kubanek et al. [327]. After 1,000 mg/kg HU given to pregnant mice on day 12 of gestation, the CFU-S pool of fetal liver shows some decrease by 2 h and a nadir by 12 h. Recovery commences on day 2 after HU, and regeneration is excessive during the following 2 days (Table 67).

In several papers, Nečas et al. [419, 420, 422, 423] report data on the changes of CFU-S after HU. In bone marrow, some degree of depression of the CFU-S pool by day 2 and slightly excessive recovery by day 8 occurs (Table 67). In the spleen, a depletion of CFU-S similar to that in bone marrow is seen on day 1, but recovery starts earlier and the overshoot on day 8 is more pronounced. In an endogenous spleen colony assay HU was given to sublethally irradiated mice: A smaller reduction of the number of colonies was observed on day 1, and an earlier, excessive regeneration by day 4 (Table 67).

Depending on the mouse strain and the dose of HU, some depletion of the bone marrow CFU-S compartment occurs during 1–2 days after single doses of HU (see Table 67). As an explanation for this phenomenon, Vassort [620] discusses several possibilities. The action of HU may persist long enough to kill some of the CFU-S which, despite the HU-induced block at G_1-S, may enter DNA synthesis. Alternatively, HU may cause a prolonged block of CFU-S at G_1-S, preventing effective replacement of differentiating pluripotent stem cells. Both explanations appear unlikely in view of the short plasma half-life of HU [188, 288] and the results of synchronization experiments discussed later (see below). Most likely, damage to more differentiated compartments of the hemopoietic system induces a wave of differentiation out of the CFU-S compartment, with efflux of CFU-S into the committed stem cell compartments which is not completely compensated for by the increased proliferation and self-replication of CFU-S.

In the recovery studies of Kubanek et al. [328], the effect of HU was compared with the effect of in vivo ^{3}H-TdR suicide, and the resulting depletion of CFU-S was prolonged as compared to HU, a difference that might be explained by reutilization of ^{3}H-TdR [514].

No CFU-S were demonstrated in circulation 24 h after HU. Recovery is rapid, and circulating CFU-S regain pretreatment levels by day 2 and a threefold overshoot is seen on day 5 [423] (Table 67).

There are considerable differences in the recovery of bone marrow and spleen CFU-S after repeated administration of HU. Following two doses of HU given 7 h apart, the reduction of the CFU-S pool in the spleen is more intensive. Recovery starts later, but leads to a four- to fivefold expansion of the splenic stem cell compartment [288] (Table 67). A very similar time course of changes in the bone marrow and spleen after four doses of HU (500 mg/kg) given every 6 h has been reported by Seidel et al. [526] (Table 67). This pattern of CFU-S recovery in bone marrow after four doses of HU has been confirmed by Wagemaker and Visser [629a] (Table 67).

Synchronization of Murine CFU-S with HU. In their recovery experiment, Vassort et al. [619, 620] determined the size of the femoral CFU-S compartment and the fraction of CFU-S in S-phase of the cell cycle at various time points after HU using the in vitro

Table 68. CFU-S/organ (percent of controls) and fraction in S-phase after HU (^{3}H-TdR suicide technique). Data from [619, 620]

		Control	Hours after HU																		
		0	1	2	3	4	5	6	7	8	9	10	11	12	14	16	18	20	22	24	39	48
C_3H, bone marrow (2,500 mg/kg)	CFU-S (%)	100	78		80	73				55		62		45	56	67	86	72	71	76		140
	Percent in S-phase	20			0	5				23		24		31	32	57	39	36	21	37		48
C_3H, bone marrow (500 mg/kg)	CFU-S (%)	100	80		60	68	69		58	58		74		60	67	65		56		67		120
	Percent in S-phase	20	0		0	0	21		25	25		38		50	31	15		37		38		26
$C_{57}Bl$, bone marrow (500 mg/kg)	CFU-S (%)	100				95		80	75	83				65		69						
	Percent in S-phase	0						2	12	20				50		30						

^{3}H-TdR suicide technique (Table 68). Two dose levels, 2,500 and 500 mg/kg, were used. CFU-S are transiently blocked from entering S-phase, although this block is lifted earlier after 500 mg/kg than after 2,500 mg/kg. A maximal fraction of CFU-S in S-phase was determined at 12 and 24 h (low-dose group) and 16 and 48 h (high-dose group). When C_{57}Bl mice were studied (whose CFU-S compartment is considered to be in almost complete proliferative rest under steady-state conditions), the increase of CFU-S in S-phase occurred later.

Thus, it appears that the block at G_1-S that exists in vivo, as long as effective concentrations of HU are maintained, can be utilized for synchronization of a CFU-S population. Sequential doses of HU given at different intervals have been used to establish a G_1-S block, and test doses of the drug were then given to assess the S-phase fraction of CFU-S in time-course experiments. From such investigations, a picture of the progression of CFU-S through the cell cycle phases and of their return to the unperturbed state can be drawn (Fig. 5).

In one experimental series [288] (Fig. 5 I) the survival of bone marrow CFU-S of BALB/c mice was determined after treatment with two injections of 1,000 mg/kg HU 7 h apart, and in parallel groups of mice these injections were followed by a third injection 2 h before CFU-S assay. Single injections, either 2 or 9 h before assay, did not reduce the survival rate of CFU-S. A moderate reduction of CFU-S is seen when two injections are given at 9 and 2 h before assay. A further decrease is observed when more time elapses between the two injections and assay. From 15–48 h after the dual dose, a third dose of HU is quite effective, indicating active proliferation in the CFU-S compartment during this time. When the interval between he two doses of HU and the third dose increases beyond 48 h, the surviving fraction returns to values around 60–70%.

Two doses of 1,000 mg/kg HU 3 h apart (Fig. 5 IIa) are not different from a single dose of HU (Fig. 5 I) with respect to CFU-S survival. This fact can be taken as evidence that one dose of HU establishes a G_1-S block for 3 h, during which time a second dose of HU is ineffective [286]. Following repeated doses of HU (at 31, 24, 10, and 7 h), a final dose of the drug (at 2 h before CFU-S assay) killed more than 80% of the remaining CFU-S, indicating a high degree of synchronization (Fig. 5 IIa). CFU-S of C_{57}Bl mice are more sensitive than those of BALB/c mice to the same schedule of HU treatment, due to the fact that there is already a certain degree of proliferation in the unperturbed state in C_{57}Bl mice (Fig. 5 IIa, IIb).

Using the model of actively proliferating CFU-S from posttransplant spleens, Hodgson et al. [288] studied the effect of two doses of 1,000 mg/kg HU given at varying intervals (Fig. 5 III). A single dose of HU given 2 h before assay reduced the CFU-S to about 50% of controls. When two doses were given at −5 and −2 h, there was virtually no additional CFU-S kill. CFU-S survival was reduced to 25% at −6 and −2 h. CFU-S kill was maximal when the first dose of HU preceded the second one by 5–7 h. These data indicate that the G_1-S block caused by 1,000 mg/kg HU persists for about 3 h. HU acts on a partially synchronized population of CFU-S when the interval between the two doses is extended to 5–7 h. Chaffey [106] reported very similar data on the effects of two doses of HU on endogenous CFU-S after sublethal irradiation given at different time intervals (Fig. 5 IV). Finally, the data reported by Monette [396] agree with the previous data (Fig. 5 V).

Nečas [422] found a single injection of HU, given at various times before CFU-S assay to NMRI mice, to be of little effect upon CFU-S survival. When two injections of HU were given, an interval of 11–14 h produced considerable CFU-S kill, while shorter or

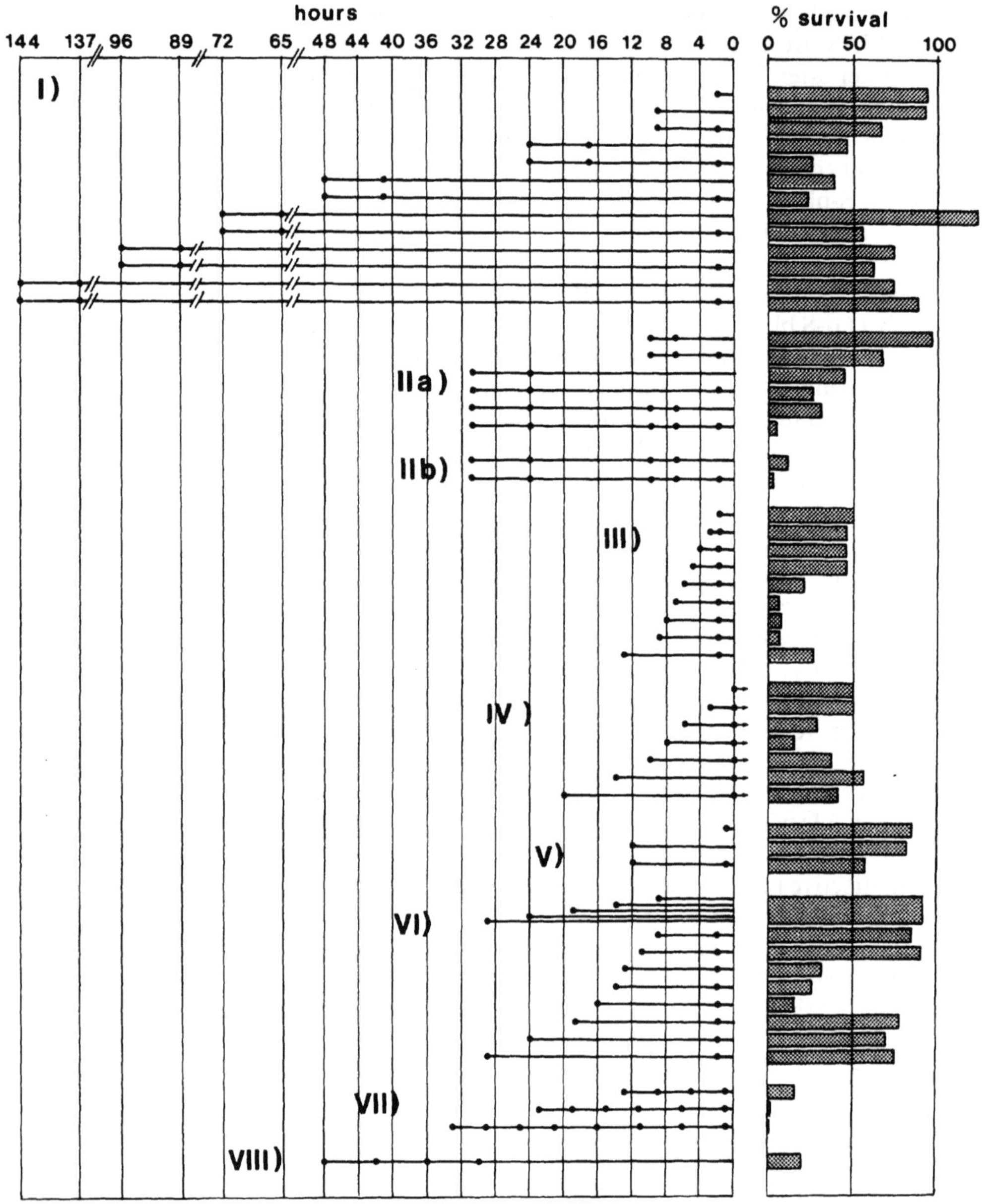

Fig. 5. (Legend see p. 135)

longer intervals were without effect. A second small peak of increased sensitivity of CFU-S to HU is suggested at intervals of 22–25 h between two doses of HU (Fig. 5 VI).

These kinetic data have been incorporated into drug regimens by which the CFU-S compartmet can be effectively depleted. Vassort et al. [619] used multiple doses of HU (500 mg/kg) at 4- to 5-h intervals and reduced the CFU-S pool to less than 5% (Fig.

Fig. 5. Synchronization experiments on murine CFU-S with repeated doses of HU. The *left side:* shows time schedule of HU application and the *right side:* shows survival of CFU-S (percent of controls). **I** Balb/c mice, normal femoral bone marrow, 1,000 mg/kg per injection [288]. **II a** Balb/c mice and **b** C_{57}Bl mice. Normal femoral bone marrow, 1,000 mg/kg per injection [286]. **III** Balb/c mice, rapidly proliferating spleen cells 1 week after bone marrow transplantation to lethally irradiated recipient mice, 1,000 mg/kg per injection [288]. **IV** C_3H/HeJ mice, first dose of HU (150 mg/kg) given 18 h after bone marrow transplantation into lethally irradiated recipients. Second dose (200 mg/kg) given at variable intervals after first dose. Assay of spleen colonies in the HU-treated recipients on day 9 after bone marrow transplantation [106]. **V** CF1 mice, normal femoral bone marrow, 900 mg/kg per injection [396]. **VI** NMRI mice, normal femoral bone marrow, 900 mg/kg per injection [419]. **VII** C_3H mice, normal bone marrow, 500 mg/kg per injection [619]. **VIII** DBA/2 mice, normal femoral bone marrow, 500 mg/kg per injection [526]

---

5 VII). Seidel and Opitz [525, 526] achieved an effective depletion of the CFU-S compartment with four doses HU (500 mg/kg) given every 6 h (Fig. 5 VIII).
The synchronization experiments with HU performed by Hodgson et al. [286, 288] present evidence that this treatment eliminates a subpopulation of "older" pluripotent hematopoietic stem cells while a "younger" CFU-S population stays intact [492]: CFU-S from fetal liver or adult bone marrow which survive pretreatment with HU produced spleen colonies with a higher content of CFU-S and CFU-C than those obtained from normal donors. This finding is interpreted within the framework of the generation-age hypothesis of the stem cell compartment [492].

CFU-C Sensitivity and Recovery Studies. Most data on the sensitivity of CFU-C to HU are reported after single doses of 900–1,000 mg/kg (Table 69). Under these conditions, the CFU-C compartment is reduced to about 50–60% of pretreatment values in the bone marrow of normal and plethoric animals within the first 3 h (Table 69, upper part). A similar sensitivity was observed 40 min after 4,500 mg/kg HU [77] (Table 69). This is well in accordance with the notion that the CFU-C compartment is in active proliferation. Pretreatment with endotoxin enhanced the killing effect of HU on CFU-C [77] (Table 69). Data on the recovery of the bone marrow CFU-C compartment are scarce, though it appears that at least partial recovery has occurred by 1 or 2 days after HU (Table 69).
After multiple-dose regimens [71, 525, 526, 602] (Table 69), the depression of the bone marrow and splenic CFU-C compartment appears to be dose- and schedule-dependent. Splenic CFU-C were more sensitive, but recovered with an impressive overshoot which peaked 4 days after the two-dose schedule and 10 days after the four-dose schedule. Even an eightyfold increase of splenic CFU-C has been reported [602] (Table 69).
In the fetal liver, 1,000 mg/kg HU given on day 12 of gestation caused a depression of CFU-C to approximately 50% by 2 h, and the CFU-C level recovered to pretreatment values by day 4 [327] (Table 69).

CFU-C Sensitivity Studies in Vitro. The extent of in vitro CFU-C kill by HU depends not only on the incubation procedure, but is also affected by the conditions of the subsequent CFU-C culture. Thus, Broxmeyer et al. [79] and Standen et al. [555] have pointed out that the apparent CFU-C kill by HU varies with the colony-stimulating activity (CSA) used for in vitro colony formation (Table 70). Data reported on the in

Table 69. Effect of HU on murine CFU-C: Sensitivity and recovery studies

Strain	Source of CFU-C, experimental conditions	Dose (mg/kg)	CFU-C survival (percent of controls)													Reference
			Time after HU													
			1 h	2 h	3 h	12 h	24 h	2 days	3 days	4 days	5 days	6 days	7–8 days	10 days	16 days	
ND2	Normal bone marrow	1,000		70												[629b]
CBA/OLA	Normal bone marrow	250					50	80	70	170	90		70	45	55	[165]
BDF_1	Bone marrow	900–1,000	55		42		63–95			96			120			[602]
	Spleen	900–1,000					30			30			1,360			
CBA	Plethoric bone marrow	900–1,000		57		72	85	90	90							[328]
CF_1	Normal bone marrow	900–1,000		51												[486]
	Day 5 after irradiation	900–1,000		70												[485]
	Day 5 after irradiation, in shielded leg	900–1,000		57												
$C_{57}Bl \times C_3H$	Normal bone marrow	4,500	49													[77]
	Bone marrow, endotoxin −20 h	4,500	21													
BALB/c	Normal bone marrow	1,000 × 2, 7 h apart						43		92		48				[71]
	Spleen							26		780		710				
CBA_2	Normal bone marrow	500 × 4 every 6 h						6	60	215			100	100		[525, 526]
	Spleen							1.7	1.3	40			200	900		
BDF_1	Normal bone marrow	333 × 3 every 6 h					13									[602]
	Spleen												7,981			
CBA	Fetal liver day 12 ofgestation	1,000		50		40	75	51	74	110						[327]

Table 70. Effect of HU on CFU-C: Sensitivity studies in vitro

Source of CFU-C	Duration of incubation (min)	CFU-C survival (percent of controls)													Reference
		Concentration of HU (m*M*)													
		0.1	0.3	0.5	1	1.6	2	4	4.4	5	8	13	17	20	
C_3D_2 bone marrow	180													85	[26]
BALB/c × CBA bone marrow	30				95										[600]
	60				90										
	90				65										
	120	100	80		60										
	240				60										
Human bone marrow	50				60 (36–73)[a]										[79]
Human bone marrow (concentration calculated per 10^6 cells)	60–120								——50–60——			——30——			[400]
Human bone marrow	90							60–70							[162]
Human peripheral blood															
0.25×10^6 cells in feeder layer	120				85–95										[555]
1×10^6 cells in feeder layer	120				77										
Human bone marrow, 1×10^6 cells in feeder layer	120				61										

[a] Depending on CSA

vitro sensitivity of CFU-C to HU have, therefore, to be interpreted with some caution. In general, about 40% of the murine and human CFU-C are killed by concentrations of 0.5–5 m*M*. Identical CFU-C survival was measured for exposure times of 1.5–3 h [600] (Table 70).

Bone Marrow Cellularity and Morphology. Despite the large amount of data on bone marrow CFU-S which require determination of the cell number per organ (femur, humerus), these latter data have only rarely been included in the reports. Therefore, information on the early quantitative events on bone marrow cellularity after HU is not available. Various single doses of HU reduce the cellularity of mouse and rat bone marrow (and probably spleen) to about 50% within 24 h (Table 71). Recovery of marrow and spleen cellularity rapidly occurs, pretreatment values being regained by days 3–5.

Multiple-dose regimens [59, 251, 526, 629b] (Table 70) cause a severe depletion of bone marrow cellularity which recovers after day 6. Morse et al. [408] observed cellular fragmentation and karyorrhexis starting 2 h after HU and persisting for the next 12 h. Erythroid precursors were more severely affected. HU induced megaloblastic changes in erythropoietic bone marrow cells [31].

Ben-Ishay [27, 29] described the morphological changes in rat bone marrow observed 9 h after 400 mg/kg HU. At this time, the cells of the hemopoietic series were severely depressed, while the bone marrow was composed predominantly of lymphocytes. The absolute lymphocyte number per organ had about doubled, while the cellularity had been reduced to 50%, thus, an influx of lymphoid cells into the depleted bone marrow was postulated. The ratio of erythroid : early myeloid : late myeloid : lymphoid cells was 1 : 0.26 : 0.51 : 0.32 before treatment and changed to 1 : 0.86 : 4.1 : 17.2. These ratios indicate that erythropoietic precursor cells and proliferating myeloid cells are primarily affected by HU treatment.

Philips et al. [455] reported on the quantitative changes of rat bone marrow after 1,840 mg/kg HU [455] (Table 71) and described the frequency of karyorrhectic cells and mitoses in bone marrow smears. Karyorrhectic cells appeared by 2 h, peaked at 3 h (approximately 6% of nucleated cells), and returned to normal values by 20 h. Virtually no mitoses were seen at 3–5 h but, subsequently, they increased to excessive values by 40 h.

In rat bone marrow, erythroid precursors were virtually absent on day 1 and 2 after 2,000 mg/kg HU. Proliferating myeloid cells were reduced to about 50% on day 1, recovered by day 2, and showed excessive values on day 6 [59, 251].

When 4 × 500 mg/kg were given every 6 h to DBA/2 mice, granulocytic cells dropped to about 1% of pretreatment values by day 2 and proliferating granulocytic cells reappeared from days 2–5, while nonproliferating granulocytic cells reappeared only by day 7 [526].

Peripheral Blood WBC and PMN. The moderate dose (250 mg/kg) used by Duménil [165] in CBA/OLA mice did not influence WBC for the first 8 days. However, by day 10, an overshoot to 170% was seen which returned to normal on day 16. No data on PMN are given in this study.

In rats [59, 251], 2,000 mg/kg HU led to a progressive drop of PMN to a nadir below 10% on day 4. Recovery was somewhat excessive on days 6–8. After 4 × 500 mg/kg every 6 h, the decline of PMN was more rapid; PMN were near zero at days 1–4 and recovered by day 8.

Table 71. Effect of HU on the cellularity of bone marrow and spleen: Recovery studies

Species, strain	Dose (mg/kg)	Bone marrow cellularity (percent of controls)																Reference
		Time after HU																
		2 h	6 h	9 h	12 h	24 h	2 days	3 days	4 days	5 days	6 days	7 days	8 days	10 days	12 days	14 days	16 days	
CBA/OLA mice	250					40	55	105	130	90			160	85			95	[165]
CF_1 mice	900					68	60	69	78	100								[408]
BDF_1 mice																		
Bone marrow	1,000						72		103			101						[602]
Spleen							55		96			97						
Rats	400			50														[421]
Rats, total cells	1,840					37	34	67	103			104						[455]
Rats, myeloid cells						40	95	60	64			90						
Rats	2,000				85	40	45	100	90		115		100					[59, 251]
Rats	4 × 500 every 6 h		40			15	15	15	20		35		42		60	100	95	
DBA/2 mice	4 × 500 every 6 h																	[526]
bone marrow							22	18	26			81		130				
Spleen (weight)							56	50	52			120		140				
ND_2 mice, bone marrow	4 × 500 every 6 h	45				14	16	30	90	90	60	70	90	125				[629b]

In a recent study, Belt et al. [24] presented toxicity data of continuous HU administration in patients with advanced nonhematologic malignancies. Oral HU (400 or 500 mg/m^2 every 4 h × 18; cumulative dose over 3 days, 7,200–9,000 mg/m^2, ≈ 200–220 mg/kg) did not induce leukopenia. At higher dose levels (800 mg/m^2 every 4 h × 18; cumulative dose 14,400 mg/m^2, ≈ 350 mg/kg) caused dose-limiting myelosuppression (WBC count in four courses was median 2,400/mm^3, range 100–4,000/mm^3). Because of marked variation of the plasma-concentrations after oral HU, the authors adopted a schedule of continuous HU infusion for 72 h where six dose levels with cumulative doses between 8,640 mg/m^2 (≈ 210 mg/kg) and 15,120 mg/m^2 (≈ 370 mg/kg) were studied. The degree of granulocytopenia was dose-dependent. In seven courses of 12,960 mg/m^2 (≈ 320 mg/kg), the nadir of PMN was from 500–2,300/mm^3.

4.19 DTIC (5-[3,3-dimethyl-1-triazeno]-imidazole-4-carboxamide)

The triazeno-imidazole DTIC exerts its cytotoxic action as an inhibitor of DNA synthesis, as an alkylating agent, and by interaction with sulfhydryl (SH) groups.

CFU-S, CFU-C Sensitivity and Recovery Studies. Data on the effect of DTIC on murine CFU-S are included in the extensive studies on cell cycle specificity of cytotoxic drugs reported by Van Putten [613, 617]: DTIC was given to $C_{57}Bl$ × CBA mice, and CFU-S survival was measured 16 h later. The $D_{1/2}$ was 260 mg/kg for normal resting murine CFU-S, and 170 mg/kg for rapidly proliferating CFU-S. A lower $D_{1/2}$ value of 72.6 mg/kg is reported by Vecchi et al. [621], measured in CD_2F_1 mice at 24 h. In these experiments, a nadir of approximately 35% survival was found 24 h after 160 mg/kg DTIC; slow regeneration of the CFU-S compartment occurred with 55% recovery on day 4 and 80% recovery on day 11 after the drug.

Foster [206] reported data on CFU-C survival after a single dose of DTIC; 24 h after 125 mg/kg of DTIC given to $C_{57}Bl/6$ mice, 28% of CFU-C survived; this fraction did not change when the animals received a dose of *C. parvum* 24 h before DTIC [206].

Thus, for both CFU-S and CFU-C, the cytocidal action of DTIC is little influenced by the proliferative state of the target cells.

Peripheral Blood. Hematotoxicity to man in phase I and II studies is usually described as mild at the dose levels used; few studies provide more detailed information on peripheral blood WBC, while data on peripheral blood PMN are usually not reported. Some of these clinical data are summarized in Table 72. A comparison of these data is made difficult by the variable end points reported. The mean nadir is usually observed at a later time than for most cytotoxic agents, with a nadir around days 21 [131] to 25 [361]. Cumulative doses of less than 800 mg/m^2 appear to be of no recognizable toxicity to WBC. Conflicting data are presented for dose levels of 1,000 to 2,000 mg/m^2: In the studies of Moertel [394] and Gottlieb [244], four of ten and six of eight patients experienced leukopenia below 2,000–2,500/mm^3. The same dose of DTIC caused a drop in WBC to less than 3,000/mm^3 in only 8% of more than 500 courses [630] (Table 72). Similarly, the dose of 1,250 mg/m^2 given by Luce [361] (Table 72) produced a drop of WBC below 3,000/mm^3 in only 4% of the treated cases. Cowan [131] provided more detailed information on circulating PMN after various doses of DTIC given as single

Table 72. Toxicity data from clinical phase I and II studies on DTIC

	Corresponding to approximate cumulative dose per m^2	*n* (courses or patients)	Toxic effect on WBC (percent of patients or courses) WBC/mm^3							Reference
			<2,000	<2,500	<3,000	2,900–3,400	<4,000	<4,500	<5,000	
200–275 mg/m^2/day × 5	1,000–1,375	13[a]	0				0			[394]
300–600 mg/m^2/day × 5	1,500–3,000	19[a]	35				50			
0.5–4 mg/kg/day × 10	200–1,500	131			5					[630]
4–5 mg/kg/day × 10	1,500–2,000	585			8					
5–6 mg/kg/day × 10	2,000–2,500	71			8					
2–3 mg/kg/day × 10	800–1,200							25		[100]
3–4 mg/kg/day × 10	1,200–1,500	160[a]						39		
4–5 mg/kg/day × 10	1,500–2,000							46		
150 mg/m^2/day × 5	750	96	2[b]		1[c]					[130]
3.5–5.5 mg/kg/day × 10	1,500–2,250	15				33				[225]
150 mg/m^2/day × 5	750	29[a]			3				21	[361]
250 mg/m^2/day × 5	1,250	91[a]			4				19	
350–400 mg/m^2/day × 5	1,750–2,000	7[a]			29				86	
150–200 mg/m^2/day × 5	750–1,000	15[a]		13						[244]
250–300 mg/m^2/day × 5	1,250–1,500	8[a]		75						

[a] Number of patients
[b] Described as severe
[c] Described as moderate

injections. A drop of circulating PMN below 1,000/mm^3 was experienced by one of 11 patients at doses of 650–950 mg/m^2, by six of 19 patients at 1,050–1,250 mg/m^2, and by five of six at 1,450 mg/m^2. Between individual patients, the changes in the granulocyte count varied widely. A very variable response of the WBC count after 1,800 mg/m^2 DTIC is also reported by Burke [93].

4.20 Nitrosoureas

One of the more recently developed groups of cytotoxic agents, the nitrosoureas, exert their cytocidal effects by alkylation and carbamoylation. The nitrosoureas have demonstrated a rather wide spectrum of cytotoxic activity in human neoplasias. CCNU, MeCCNU, and BCNU[1] have attracted a great deal of interest from pharmacologists and oncologists (for review, see [102, 439]). The vast majority of experimental and clinical papers on the hematopoietic toxicity of nitrosoureas deal with these three compounds. Therefore, this chapter will mainly summarize published data on the effect of CCNU, MeCCNU, and BCNU on the granulopoietic system of experimental animals and of man. Where available, similar work on other nitrosoureas (such as MNU, GANU[2], or streptozotocin) will be mentioned.

CFU-S Sensitivity Studies. When the survival of murine bone marrow CFU-S was measured 16–24 h after administration of BCNU, exponential dose-survival curves were regularly obtained (Table 73). From the data available, it appears that i.p. BCNU is more effective than the s.c. route of administration in terms of CFU-S kill. Rapidly proliferating CFU-S are more sensitive to BCNU than resting CFU-S both in vivo [616] and in vitro [435].
Although more limited data are available on the sensitivity of CFU-S to CCNU and MeCCNU, the effect of both drugs on CFU-S appears to be qualitatively identical to that of BCNU: Exponential dose-survival curves have been reported and rapidly proliferating CFU-S were found to be more sensitive than resting CFU-S (Table 73).

CFU-S Recovery Studies. Studies reporting quantitative changes with time of bone marrow CFU-S following nitrosourea treatment are listed in Table 74. As a rule, minimal values are reached early (day 1 or 2 after drug administration). This initial depletion of the CFU-S compartment appears to be dose-dependent. Recovery to pretreatment values is delayed: Normal values were not regained in several studies by day 21. The observation that the proliferative activity of marrow CFU-S is low during the first 14 days after BCNU treatment [466] fits well into this picture.

CFU-C Sensitivity Studies. In comparative dose-survival studies, nitrosoureas exerted identical toxicity on CFU-S and CFU-C [45, 435], with exponential dose-survival curves (Table 75). Like CFU-S, CFU-C in regenerating bone marrow were more

---

1 1-(2-Chloroethyl)-3-cyclohexyl-1-nitrosourea (CCNU), 1-(2-chloroethyl)-3-(4-methylcyclohexyl)-1-nitrosourea (MeCNU), and 1,3-bis(2-chloroethyl)-1-nitrosourea (BCNU)

2 1-Methyl-1-nitrosourea (MNU) and 1-(2-chloroethyl)-3-(B-D-glucopyranosyl)-1-nitrosourea (GANU)

Table 73. Effect of nitrosoureas on CFU-S: In vivo and in vitro sensitivity studies

Species (strain)	Time of assay (h)	CFU-S survival (percent of controls)						$D_{1/2}$ (mg/kg)	Reference
		Dose of drug (mg/kg)							
		0	20	40	50	60	80		
In vivo studies		BCNU							
Mouse [(C_{57}Bl/Rij × CBA/Rij)F_1]									
Normal, i.p.	16	100	65	40			15	30	[616]
Normal, s.c.	16	100	35	7	3			15	[616]
Rapidly proliferating, i.p.	16	100	15	2				NA[a]	[616]
Rapidly proliferating, s.c.	16	100	9	1	0.3			5	[616]
Mouse (–)									
i.p.	18	100	30	8		3		15	[45]
Mouse									
(AKR)	24	100	40	15		5	2	15	[606]
		CCNU							
Mouse (–)									
i.p.	18	100	40	8		3		12	[45]
Mouse [(C_{57}Bl/Rij × CBA/Rij)F_1]									
Normal, s.c.	16	100	60	30		15	6	30	[616]
Rapidly proliferating, s.c.	16	100	20	6		2	0.4	10	[616]

[a] Analysis not possible

Table 73 (continued)

Species (strain)	Time of assay (h)	CFU-S survival (percent of controls) Dose of drug (mg/kg) 0	20	40	50	60	80	$D_{1/2}$ (mg/kg)	Reference
		MeCCNU							
Mouse [(C_{57}Bl/Rij × CBA/Rij)F_1]									
Normal, s.c.	16	100	40	25		10	5	18	[616]
Rapidly proliferating, s.c.	16	100	20	6		1	0.5	NA[a]	[616]
Mouse (−)									
s.c.	18	100	25	2				12	[45]
Mouse (C_{57}Bl)	20–40	100	7	0.4				9	[45]
In vitro studies	Duration of incubation	Concentration of BCNU (μM/l) 0	10	20	30	40	50		
Mouse BALB/c	1 h, 37° C								
Normal		100	90	70			20	NA[a]	[435]
Rapidly proliferating		100	90	55			5	NA[a]	[435]

[a] Analysis not possible

Table 74. Effect of nitrosoureas on bone marrow CFU-S: Recovery studies

Species (strain)	Dose of drug (mg/kg)	Surviving CFU-S (percent of controls)									Reference
		Day									
		0	2	4	6	8	10	14	28	42	
	BCNU										
Mouse (CF_1)	35	100	25	45	40	55					[597]
Mouse[a]	35	100	40	65	80	85	90				[598]
Mouse [(BALB/c × DBA)F_1]	20	100	30		60			50	70	90	[466]
Mouse (−)	50	100	5		50		70	80	90		[45]
	CCNU										
Mouse (−)	40	100	5		50		70	80	90		[45]
	MeCCNU										
Mouse (−)	30	100	5		50		70	80	90		[45]
	MNU										
Mouse (CBA/J)	50	100	10		5–10			50	100		[522]

[a] Posthypoxic, polycythemic

Table 75. Effect of nitrosoureas on CFU-C: Sensitivity studies in vivo and in vitro

Species (strain)	Time of assay (h)	CFU-C survival (percent of controls)						$D_{1/2}$ (mg/kg)	Reference
		Dose of drug (mg/kg)							
		0	20	40	60	80			
In vivo studies		BCNU							
Mouse (–)	18	100	30	8	3			15	[45]
		CCNU							
Mouse (–)	18	100	40	8	3			12	[45]
		MeCCNU							
Mouse (–)	18	100	25	2				10	[45]
Mouse (C_{57}Bl)	20–24	100	7	0.4				8	[46]
	Duration of incubation (min)	Concentration of drug (µ*M*/l)							
		0	10	20	30	40	50		
In vitro studies		BCNU							
Mouse (BALB/c)									
Normal	60	100	90	70			20		[435]
Rapidly proliferating	60	100	90	55			5		[435]
Mouse (BALB/c)	60	100	80	50		20			[436]
Mouse (C_{57}Bl)	60	100		80			30		[433]
Mouse (C_{57}Bl)	120	100	90				75		[508]
Human	120	100	70				40		[508]
Human	60	100	60	40		15			[436]
		CCNU							
Human	120	100	45						[270]

Table 76. Effect of nitrosoureas on bone marrow CFU-C: Recovery studies

Species (strain)	Dose of drug (mg/kg)	Surviving CFU-C (percent of controls)								Reference
		Day								
		0	2	4	6	8	10	14	28	
	BCNU									
Mouse (–)	50	100	10–15				100			[45]
Mouse (CF_1)	35	100	35	70	100					[597]
Mouse[a]	35	100	25	75	100					[598]
	CCNU									
Rat (Wistar)	100	100		< 3		35		65	100	[253]
Mouse (–)	40	100	10–15				100			[45]
	MeCCNU									
Mouse (–)	30	100	10–15				100			[45]
	MNU									
Mouse (CBA/J)	50	100	~ 10			~ 50		~ 50		[524]

[a] Posthypoxic, polycythemic

Table 77. Effect of nitrosoureas on human granulopoiesis

Day	Peripheral blood PNM (per μl)		Peripheral blood CFU-C (per l)		Bone marrow CFU-C (per 10^5 cells)	
	MeCCNU[a]	BCNU[b]	MeCCNU	BCNU	MeCCNU	BCNU
0	6,610 ± 3,810	5,100 ± 2,400	38,100 ± 60,100	12,600 ± 12,000	27.5 ± 11.8	39 ± 28
7	5,290 ± 3,960	3,420 ± 1,550	1,700 ± 4,700	0	6.4 ± 7.2	11 ± 9.2
14	4,140 ± 2,990	3,080 ± 1,500	200 ± 500	0	6.8 ± 6.1	6 ± 1.8
21	2,110 ± 1,470	2,010 ± 1,370	110 ± 360	0	10.4 ± 9.6	6.2 ± 5
28	2,420 ± 1,040	2,940 ± 1,180	3,800 ± 7,500	1,440 ± 2,400	9.6 ± 5.2	7 ± 4
42–49	3,720 ± 1,930	3,580 ± 2,500	11,400 ± 1,680	1,470 ± 2,500	18.3 ± 5.5	NA

[a] Patients with metastatic gastrointestinal tumors were treated with oral MeCCNU (175 mg/m² day 1) VCR (1.4 mg/m² day 1 i.v.), and 5-FU (10 mg/kg days 1–5 i.v.)
[b] Patients with gastric cancer were treated with BCNU (40 mg/m² days 1–5 i.v.) plus 5-FU (10 mg/kg days 1–5 i.v.)

sensitive than normal CFU-C. Murine and human CFU-C had a similar sensitivity to nitrosoureas when tested in vitro (Table 75).

CFU-C Recovery Studies. The pattern of depletion and repletion of the bone marrow CFU-C compartment (Table 76) differs considerably from that described above for the CFU-S compartment. In general, the early depletion (nadir on day 1 or 2) was followed by prompt regeneration of the CFU-C pool. In mice, return to pretreatment pool size was regularly observed by day 6–10, with the exception of MNU [522]. In rats, normalization of the marrow CFU-C compartment following CCNU treatment was seen only by day 21 [253].

We [517a] have studied the granulopoietic toxicity of nitrosoureas in cancer patients treated with MeCCNU or BCNU as part of a combination chemotherapy protocol. Details of the treatment schedule are given in Table 77, and courses were repeated every 6–7 weeks. Administration of both drugs was followed by a long-lasting reduction of the incidence of marrow CFU-C, which showed no clear sign of recovery during the follow-up period of 6 weeks (Table 77). Interpreting these data, one must keep in mind that the bone marrow cellularity remained similarly depressed during the observation period (as judged from the marrow cell content of aspirates, and from histological sections of aspirated marrow spicules). Thus, the reduction of the CFU-C incidence incompletely reflects the degree of long-lasting exhaustion of the marrow CFU-C compartment.

In the peripheral blood, CFU-C disappeared almost completely following nitrosourea treatment. This disappearance of blood CFU-C persisted for the entire observation period (i.e., for 6–7 weeks) after BCNU, while there were signs of recovery of the peripheral blood CFU-C pool at 42 days after MeCCNU (Table 77).

Bone Marrow. A rather limited number of papers has dealt with changes of bone marrow cellularity following a single dose of a nitrosourea compound (Table 78). From these data, it can be concluded that the nitrosoureas reduce marrow cellularity

Table 78. Effect of nitrosoureas on bone marrow cellularity: Recovery studies

	Dose of drug (mg/kg)	Bone marrow cellularity (percent of controls)								Reference
		Day								
		0	3	7	14	21	28	35	42	
	BCNU									
(BALB/c × DBA)F_1 mice	20	100	35	65	65	65	90	85	95	[466]
	CCNU									
Wistar rats	100	100	40	55	75	100	100			[253]
	MNU									
CBA/J (♀) mice	50	100	60	65	75	90			80	[522]

Table 79. Effect of nitrosoureas on peripheral blood granulocytes (PMN): Recovery studies

	Dose of drug (mg/kg)	Peripheral blood PMN concentration (percent of controls)										Reference
		Day										
		0	2	3	4	6	7	8	10	12	14	
	BCNU											
CF_1 (♀) mice[a]	35	100	65		15	90		200	180			[481]
CF_1 (♀) mice	35	100	60		15	95		160	140	130		[597]
(BALB/c × DBA/2)F_1 mice	20	100		37								[209]
	30	100		12								
	CCNU											
Wistar rats	100	100	75		40			66			35 then overshoot	[253]
CDF_1 mice	~ 15	100		55								[443]
	~ 30	100		37								
	~ 40	100		25								
CD_2F_1 mice	40	100		25			50				60	[415]
	MeCCNU											
BDF_1 mice	21	100		25		130			150		100	[148]
	32	100		35		135			145		130	
	42	100		15		120			145		130	
	63	100		20		60					190	
	MNU											
CBA/J (♀) mice	50	100	35	70			120				60	[522]
BD_2F_1 mice	75	100		25			45				50	[442]

[a] Posthypoxic, polycythemic animals

promptly, and that it remains reduced for a prolonged period of time (i.e., 3–6 weeks) in both mice and rats.

Data reported by Udupa et al. [597] indicate that in mice the myeloblast and promyelocyte compartment is reduced in size during the first 4 days after BCNU (35 mg/kg), recovers to pretreatment size by day 6, only to be subnormal again 8 days after BCNU. The myelocyte compartment is severely depressed until day 6 and is normal thereafter. The nondividing granulocytic compartment (metamyelocyte and neutrophil) regains pretreatment values 8 days after BCNU administration. In agreement with these findings are data reported by Preissler et al. [466] on the functional bone marrow granulocyte reserve: It declines to its nadir on day 2 and returns to normal levels by day 7. Subsequently, the functional bone marrow granulocyte reserve shows a somewhat oscillating time course, with a second and third nadir on days 14 and 28, respectively.

Peripheral Blood Granulocytes. There appears to be early (nadir on day 3) dose-dependent toxicity of nitrosoureas to the peripheral blood granulocytes of mice (Table 79). In several studies, the return to normal values (in mice usually observed around day 6) was followed by a rebound up to twice normal values. However, this time course appears to be influenced by the dose of nitrosourea administered. With higher doses, the neutropenic phase appears to last longer, with a corresponding delay of the subsequent rebound [148]. There are no studies in mice with a follow-up longer than 14 days; therefore, the possibility of a second, longer-lasting neutropenic phase, such as that described after MNU [522], cannot be excluded after treatment with the other nitrosourea compounds.

In man, delayed leukopenia and granulocytopenia is a characteristic side effect following treatment with nitrosoureas [5, 152, 153, 196, 283, 393, 633, 646]. Granulocyte nadirs usually occur 30–40 days after administration of the agent (BCNU, CCNU, or MeCCNU), and persist for 5–21 days. For details, the reader is referred to the original papers and to review articles [102] (see also Table 77).

Cumulative toxicity of nitrosoureas to peripheral blood granulocytes has been repeatedly observed, requiring dosage reductions and/or extension of the interval between successive doses [196, 491, 633, 646]. Most likely, this cumulative toxicity reflects repeated perturbation of the slowly regenerating pluripotent stem cell pool, leading to progressive reduction of the pluripotent stem cell compartment. More important, however, may be the qualitative changes within the stem cell compartment referred to elsewhere (page 179), namely, that nitrosoureas preferentially kill the "youngest" pluripotent stem cells with the highest potential for self-replication. It is easily conceivable that such injury, if repeated, may lead to the failure of the pluripotent stem cell pool to fulfill the demand for input of a sufficient number of cells into the committed stem cell compartments.

4.21 cis-Diamminedichloroplatinum (DDP)

DDP, a square planar coordination complex, was recognized as a cytotoxic agent by Rosenberg et al. [490] in 1965, and since found acceptance as one of the major new anticancer drugs in clinical oncology. Its primary toxicity concerns renal function impairment which has been subject to extensive experimental and clinical evaluation.

On the other hand, hematotoxicity is of minor clinical importance at the usual dose range. Information on the changes of granulopoiesis after DDP is, therefore, rather limited.

CFU-C In Vitro Sensitivity Studies. One study by Ogawa et al. [437] provides useful information on the effect of DDP on murine and human CFU-C exposed to DDP in vitro. Dose-survival curves for murine CFU-C, both from normal and rapidly proliferating transplanted bone marrow, were exponential with a $D_{1/2}$ of approximately 4 μg/ml. An exponential dose-survival curve was determined for human CFU-C, which were less sensitive to DDP ($D_{1/2}$ ~ 10 μg/ml) than murine CFU-C.
Survival studies on murine CFU-C exposed to DDP in vitro at temperatures from 4°–37° C showed that low temperatures did not reduce the cytotoxic effect of DDP to a great extent. Apparently, membrane transport of DDP is by passive diffusion and not dependent on an active, temperature-sensitive transport mechanism [437].

Peripheral Blood PMN and WBC. Studies on preclinical toxicity including data on hematopoiesis and granulopoiesis are available for rats, dogs, and rhesus monkeys.
Kociba and Sleight [320] reported serial blood counts in male Spartan rats after i.p. 12.2 mg/kg DDP, equivalent to the LD_{50}. Peripheral PMN fell to near zero by day 3, recovered with more than a twofold overshoot by day 5, and normalized after day 9. Bone marrow cellularity was severely depressed on days 2–3 and recovered after day 5. In Sprague-Dawley rats, a strain closely related to the Spartan rats, no depression of circulating neutrophils at dose ranges of 7.5 and 15 mg/kg or 3 × 1 to 3 mg/kg occurred. In these animals, particular sensitivity of the lymphoid organs was noted [585].
An approximate LD_{50} of 3.75 mg/kg (5 × 0.75 mg/kg) was reported in dogs by Schaeppi [506]. At this dose level, three of five dogs showed severe granulocytopenia or agranulocytosis. Four dogs treated with lower doses did not show a depression of PMN counts. A dose of 3 mg/kg DDP reduced the WBC count to 40% in 17 dogs, with only minor variation induced by prehydration or mannitol infusion [138]. In rhesus monkeys, DDP doses compatible with survival (5 × 1.25 mg/kg) induced no significant changes of circulating PMN counts. Two monkeys that died after higher doses showed moderate to severe bone marrow hypocellularity, while one of them showed peripheral agranulocytosis [506].
Since DDP was introduced into clinical use at a time when standards for clinical trials were firmly established, one might expect a satisfactory body of data concerning toxicity of this compound in man. However, the data provided in phase I and II studies are very heterogeneous, comprising a great variety of doses and time schedules, as well as a diversity of reported limits of toxicity to human granulopoiesis. The clinical experience has been summarized in a review paper by Gottlieb [243] and in other literature [123]. The more recent studies have used combinations of DDP with other cytotoxic agents. Few studies report data on the changes of peripheral granulocytes. Usually, only WBC values are given, making a thorough analysis difficult.
The general impression form these clinical studies is that hematotoxicity is usually mild and not of limiting intensity when doses of 100 mg/m^2/course are not exceeded. A dose-response relationship appears to exist as evident from the data in Table 80, which

Table 80. Incidence of WBC depression in clinical phase I and II trials of DDP. "Severe" hematotoxicity is usually defined as WBC $< 2,000-2,500/mm^3$ and "moderate" as WBC $< 3,500-4,000/mm^3$

Degree of hematotoxicity at DDP doses[a]								Reference
$20\ mg/m^2$		$30-70\ mg/m^2$		$70-100\ mg/m^2$		$100\ mg/m^2$		
Severe	Moderate	Severe	Moderate	Severe	Moderate	Severe	Moderate	
			4/ 31					[325]
	0/11	2/ 11	1/ 11	4/ 21	2/ 21			[578]
	0/ 9		0/ 7	2/ 14	4/ 14			
						17/78	21/78	[284]
			0/ 9		0/ 17			[632][b]
	1/ 5		1/ 3		0/ 9		0/ 3	
				3/ 19	6/ 19	6/16	3/16	[326]
			4/ 23					[643]
			5/ 25		8/ 32		1/ 1	[495]
	1/25	2/106	15/106	9/112	20/112	23/98	25/98	
	4%	16%		26%		48%		

[a] DDP was usually given as a 5-day course, indicated is the cumulative dose per course
[b] Two regimens (single injection and 5-day course)

summarizes phase I and II studies in which data on WBC are given in a somewhat comparable fashion. In these studies, the cumulative dose was given between 1 day and 2–3 weeks and most regimens prefer a 5-day schedule. With weekly doses of 40 mg/m^2 DDP, no depression of WBC occurred up to a cumulative dose of 120 mg/m^2 [474].

In 26 courses with DDP at high-dose levels of 125–200 mg/m^2, the nadir of WBC reached 35% of pretreatment values at 12–19 days [269]. While the renal toxicity was ameliorated by mannitol infusion, the hematotoxicity of DDP was not altered.

5 *Granulopoietic Toxicity of Cytotoxic Agents: Pathogenesis, Pathophysiology, Methods of Modulation, and Clinical Aspects*

5.1 General Discussion of Cytotoxic Drug Effects on the Granulopoietic System

Ideal cancer therapeutic agents would combine high antitumor activity with little or no toxicity to normal cellular systems. Unfortunately, most cytotoxic agents that are clinically available at the present time are far from fulfilling this ideal. As outlined in the previous chapters, they exert a variable toxicity to the hematopoietic systems and, from a clinical point of view, the granulopoietic system is the most important one. Myelotoxicity is the predominant and therefore the limiting toxicity of a number of chemotherapeutic agents, such as cytosine arabinoside, vinblastine, the alkylating agents and the nitrosoureas; other chemotherapeutic agents (such as MTX, 6-MP, 6-TG, the anthracyclines) may exert limiting toxic effects other than their myelosuppressive action.

In modern oncology, cytotoxic agents are usually administered intermittently, and only rarely (e.g., in some hematologic disorders) is continuous administration of cytotoxic drugs utilized. In designing such intermittent chemotherapy schedules, clinicians are guided by duration of granulocytopenia, since, usually, a new course of treatment is given only after restoration of the peripheral blood granulocyte concentration to its original levels.

A discussion of mechanisms that lead to cytotoxic drug-induced development of peripheral blood granulocytopenia and the subsequent normalization of peripheral blood granulocyte counts requires knowledge of the effects of a cytotoxic drug upon sensitive granulopoietic cell populations. These data have been presented in detail in the preceding chapters. Furthermore, the proliferative state of the granulocytic system has to be taken into consideration, since the cytotoxic action of chemotherapeutic agents frequently is proliferation-dependent. This information has also been included, and a review article on this subject is also available [607].

There are a number of other factors that influence the overall toxicity of a cytotoxic drug upon the granulopoietic system. The physiology and kinetics of the granulopoiesis partly determine the time course of the damage to the various granulopoietic compartments. In addition, the kinetics of recovery of the granulopoietic system from cytotoxic drug-induced damage vary with the level at which a drug exerts its maximal cytocidal effect. Therefore, without knowledge of structure, kinetics, and physiology of the granulocytic system, any attempt to understand the changes of granulopoiesis following a single or repeated exposure to a cytotoxic agent remains incomplete. The physiology of the granulopoietic system is not reviewed here, but the reader is referred to a short survey elsewhere in this book (page 4), and particularly to excellent in-depth reviews [134, 197, 203, 337, 347, 488, 562, 563].

The mode of action of a drug (phase-specific, cycle-specific, or cycle-unspecific [80–82]), dosage and schedule of drug administration, and the pharmacokinetics of the drug are further variables that affect toxicity of an antineoplastic agent upon the granulopoietic system. The reaction pattern of the granulopoietic system may differ with the strain of laboratory animal used or with different routes of administration. Such differences will be disregarded here, but should nevertheless be kept in mind.

The experimental observation of a decline in size of a granulopoietic compartment following cytotoxic chemotherapy may be caused by one or a combination of several of the following factors:

- First, the cytotoxic agent may directly damage the cells of the respective compartment, thus leading to damage and possibly even to cell death. The mode of action of the cytotoxic drugs explains why this factor can only be operative in proliferating granulopoietic compartments, whereas the nondividing (maturing) granulocytic compartments cannot be affected directly by a cytotoxic agent.
- Second, a sustained cellular feed-out into the ensuing, more differentiated compartment may not be fully matched by cell influx from the preceding, less differentiated compartment. This mechanism can be operative in all granulopoietic compartments except the CFU-S compartment, which by definition has no preceding compartment.
- Third, if cells possess self-replicative capacity, this potential for self-replication may be reduced following cytotoxic drug exposure. Such a change of self-replicative capacity may be a direct result of drug action upon the cells, explained either by a change in the proliferation kinetics, or by a shift in the characteristics of the cell population. An example of the first mechanism is the nitrosourea-induced change of the growth fraction of a proliferating cell population [645], and an example for the latter is the shift from "young" to "older" pluripotent stem cells seen after several cytotoxic agents (for details, see page 179). Alternatively, reduced self-replication within a hemopoietic stem cell compartment may be caused by regulatory factors. In this case, a shortened transit time through the compartment must be postulated, favoring differentiation over self-replication ("differentiation pressure").

The immediate reduction of the proliferating compartments, seen after administration of most cytotoxic agents, can only be explained by direct damage to these cells. Similarly, a clear conclusion concerning the underlying mechanism can be drawn with respect to the cytotoxic drug-induced damage upon the nonproliferating granulocytic compartments. This damage can result only from the second of the mechanisms discussed above. Difficulties arise when one attempts to determine which mechanisms are responsible for the delayed decline of a compartment after a short-acting drug, such as the depletion of the bone marrow CFU-S compartment during the first 2 days after administration of short-lived cytotoxic drugs, such as cytosine arabinoside or hydroxyurea. The most likely explanation for this experimental observation is a continued outflow of CFU-S into the committed stem cell compartment, which is not fully compensated for by the increased self-replication of CFU-S during this early period after drug administration. Further examples for this phenomenon have been reported after busulfan: Increases in the morphologically identifiable granulocytic bone marrow compartment were observed before the repletion of the committed stem cell compartments [57, 308].

An analysis of the time course of recovery in the CFU-C pool and the successive granulocytic compartment does not allow discrimination between a misbalance of cellular influx and efflux or a more rapid compartment transit time as the cause of a reduced CFU-C compartment size. When near normal numbers of granulocytes are produced, although the CFU-C pool is depleted (c.f., busulfan-treated mice [401], or the nitrosourea-treated patient (page 149)), a more rapid transit of cells through the CFU-C compartment is likely.

The presentation and discussion of a model might be helpful in delineating important aspects of the development of granulopoietic toxicity following cytotoxic drug exposure. Let us consider the repeated administration of an S-phase-specific cytotoxic drug given to a mouse with an unperturbed hematopoiesis. Since, under such steady-state conditions, the proliferative activity of CFU-C is considerably greater than that of CFU-S, the committed granulopoietic stem cell compartment experiences greater damage from the first drug dose than the pluripotent stem cell pool. Therefore, the size of the pluripotent stem cell compartment declines minimally after the first dose of the phase-specific drug, whereas the committed stem cell pool and the proliferating granulocytic compartment are considerably reduced in size. The nonproliferating compartments of the granulocytic system, i.e., the maturing compartment and the granulocyte compartment in bone marrow and peripheral blood, do not experience direct toxic damage and are, therefore, not affected immediately. However, the damage to the proliferative granulopoietic compartments temporarily leads to reduced cell input into the subsequent compartment of maturing granulocytic cells, while the cellular efflux from the maturation compartment into the PMN compartments of bone marrow and blood continues at its normal rate. Therefore, the maturing granulocytic compartment experiences indirect damage with some delay after administration of the drug. This delay is determined by the kinetics of proliferation and maturation within the granulocytic system. Species-specific differences in these kinetics explain to some degree the species differences in the pattern of granulopoietic toxicity observed after cytotoxic drug exposure.

The last of the granulocytic compartments to be indirectly affected by the cytotoxic action of a phase-specific drug is the mature neutrophil (PMN) pool in bone marrow and peripheral blood. The extent and duration of cytotoxic drug-induced reduction of granulocyte production will determine whether peripheral blood granulocytopenia develops: The bone marrow granulocyte storage pool will, for a limited time, allow sustained efflux of normal numbers of granulocytes into the peripheral blood in spite of a reduced granulocyte formation. Peripheral blood granulocytopenia will, therefore, occur only if formation of granulocytes is reduced long enough to deplete the bone marrow storage pool, since it will then no longer be able to maintain a normal granulocyte feedout into the peripheral blood. From these considerations, it is important to realize that a normal peripheral blood granulocyte concentration cannot be interpreted to indicate an unperturbed state of the earlier granulopoietic compartments: A normal peripheral blood granulocyte concentration can exist even though earlier granulocytic compartments are reduced in size.

Regeneration of the granulocytic system originates in the pluripotent and, to some degree, in the committed stem cell compartment. Just as cytotoxic drug-induced damage, the granulopoietic regeneration proceeds from these early pools in a wave-like fashion through the successive granulocytic compartments, the granulocyte compartment of bone marrow and peripheral blood being the last to be restored.

Let us now assume that a second dose of the phase-specific drug is administered before complete normalization with return to steady-state conditions has taken place at all levels of the granulopoietic system. The effect of such a prematurely administered dose is different from that observed after the first one. The proliferating compartments (pluripotent stem cells, committed stem cells, and proliferating granulocytic pool) are still in regeneration and, therefore, in an increased proliferative state, which makes them relatively more sensitive to the drug. They will, therefore, be damaged to a greater extent by the second than by the first treatment course. Similarly, the nonproliferating compartments, having not fully recovered at the time of the second drug administration, will now shrink even further. When successive doses of the drug are given at the same short intervals, the size of all granulopoietic compartments will decline more and more, while the granulocyte storage pool of the bone marrow and then the peripheral blood granulocyte pool will be the last to shrink.

Let us now slightly modify the model by using a cycle-specific or a cycle-unspecific agent rather than a phase-specific drug. Agents belonging to both classes of drugs will exert cytotoxic action not only on proliferating cells, but on resting (G_0) cells as well, as exemplified by their exponential dose-survival curves. Therefore, the first administration of such a drug will damage the pluripotent stem cell pool to a greater extent than did the phase-specific agent. This has consequences for both the duration of granulocytic system perturbation and the potential for induction of late bone marrow damage (see below). Early readministration of cycle-specific or cycle-unspecific agents will lead to cumulative toxicity by mechanisms identical to those discussed above for a phase-specific agent.

According to these considerations, granulopoietic damage is rather late to appear in the most mature granulocytic compartments, and it is important to reiterate that a normal peripheral blood granulocyte count does not necessarily indicate that the early granulocytic compartments are normal. This is not only true after cytotoxic drug treatment, but also in patients with other disease conditions, such as in remission from aplastic anemia [316]. Measurement of the bone marrow compartment sizes would be a quite reliable indicator of granulopoietic perturbation, though such measurements cannot be performed in clinical practice. The clinician is thus left with a situation that can be monitored safely only to a limited degree. It is conceivable that even with rather extensively depleted bone marrow compartments, particularly with depleted committed stem cell pools, near normal peripheral blood granulocyte concentration can be maintained. This may be explained by a more rapid transit through the respective cellular compartments, in an attempt to fulfill the demand for cell input of the ensuing cell compartments, favoring differentiation at the expense of compartment reconstitution. In man, such a situation may exist following nitrosourea treatment (see page 149) and, in mice, it has been observed following busulfan administration [402]. Obviously, readministration of a myelotoxic agent in this situation must lead to cumulative toxicity, and this has been repeatedly observed following nitrosourea treatment (page 151).

Chervenick et al. [109] have put forth the hypothesis that a severely reduced pluripotent stem cell pool will not feed cells into the committed stem cell compartments until it is reconstituted to a certain size. In their radiation model, this threshold size was 10%. If this hypothesis is correct, severe reduction of the pluripotent stem cell pool by single or repeated doses of a cytotoxic drug transiently interrupts the inflow from that pool into the subsequent bone marrow compartments. This, of course, extends the duration of peripheral blood granulocytopenia. The priority of self-replication over differentiation at low pluripotent stem cell compartment sizes may be interpreted as a protective mechanism preventing the vital stem cell compartment from "burning out".

Aspects of the regulatory mechanisms underlying the regeneration of the granulopoietic system after cytotoxic drug-induced damage are poorly characterized in man.

We have therefore analysed our experimental data with respect to the regulation of the proliferation of human bone marrow CFU-C following cytotoxic drug-induced perturbation [353, 354, 517]. It is evident that the increase in the proliferative activity of CFU-C starts early after chemotherapy, at a time when the number of segmented granulocytes (PMN) in bone marrow and blood is reduced very little. More importantly, bone marrow CFU-C return to their original proliferative activity at a time when the number of PMN progressively decreases in bone marrow and peripheral blood, respectively (see Figs. 1 and 2). From this kinetic analysis, we have concluded [354, 517] that the number of mature granulocytic cells (particularly that of PMN) in bone marrow or blood is not a major factor for regulation of the proliferative activity of bone marrow CFU-C during granulocytic regeneration from cytotoxic drug-induced damage. Such a negative feedback control mechanism has been proposed [562]. Rather, our data suggest that local CFU-C population size control [366] or a negative feedback control from early granulocytic compartments (e.g., myeloblasts) regulates the proliferative activity of bone marrow CFU-C following in vivo exposure of the human bone marrow to cytotoxic agents.

The relationship between the mode of action of cytotoxic drugs and the resulting perturbation of the granulocytic system deserves some consideration. Bruce and coworkers [80–82] were the first to point out that cytotoxic drugs can be classified according to the degree of cytotoxicity they exert in different phases of the cell cycle. From this work and that of others, it has become clear that some cytotoxic agents act only during certain phases of the cell cycle, whereas they are without effect when the cells are in other phases of the cell cycle. By means of sensitivity studies (see page 10), these phase-specific agents are characterized by a plateau of their dose-response curve. Cytotoxic drugs such as ara-C, HU, VBL, VCR, and MTX belong to this class of agents. From the shape of their dose-survival curve, it becomes clear that an increase in the drug dose increases the cytotoxic effect only to a certain point since, at even higher doses, no further increment in the cytotoxicity ensues. A further feature of this class of agents is that, by virtue of their phase-specifity, they exert cytotoxicity only on proliferating cells, whereas resting cells (cells in G_0) are protected from the cytocidal action. This, however, has an immediate and clinically important consequence. Since pluripotent hematopoietic stem cells are mostly out of cycle under normal steady-state conditions the pluripotent stem cell pool, when exposed to phase-specific agents in the unperturbed state, will be little if at all damaged. Damage from phase-specific agents will, therefore, almost exclusively occur in the actively proliferating, committed granulocytic stem cell compartment and in the proliferating granulocytic compartment. The little-damaged pluripotent stem cell pool allows for a rapid regeneration of the damaged, more differentiated compartments and this in turn limits the maximal duration of a peripheral blood neutropenia. Therefore, the granulocytopenia caused by a single exposure of an unperturbed granulocytic system to a phase-specific cytotoxic agent is short-lived.

Furthermore, cytotoxic drug-induced residual bone marrow damage can develop only if the earliest pluripotent stem cells, which are almost exclusively resting cells, are damaged by a drug (see page 177). In theory, phase-specific agents spare these pluripotent stem cells and, therefore, do not induce residual marrow damage [67, 590].

The short duration of their acute hematopoietic toxicity and their negligible potential for the induction of late marrow failure renders the phase-specific cytotoxic agents a class of relatively "safe" chemotherapeutic drugs. It must be kept in mind, however, that the degree of cytotoxicity is quite different when phase-specific agents act on a perturbed granulopoietic system. For example, during recovery from cytotoxic drug-induced damage, cell populations, usually mostly out of cycle (such as the pluripotent stem cells), may be actively proliferating and, therefore, be quite vulnerable to a phase-specific drug. Other cell populations may proliferate much more intensively than under normal steady-state conditions, and they, too, may be affected more intensively by phase-specific agents in this situation.

If phase-specificity of a cytotoxic drug combines with a short in vivo half-life of its cytocidal action, the toxic effect of a single dose of the drug may be minimal. A good example of this is ara-C. With its short biologic half-life, the cytocidal action of a rapidly administered single dose is limited to cells in S-phase of the cycle at this time. Cells entering S-phase some time later will not be affected by the drug, since it has decayed in the meantime. Since, of any given cell population, only a fraction is in S-phase when ara-C is administered, the extent of damage to the sensitive cellular compartments of the granulopoietic system resulting from a single acutely administered dose of the drug will remain limited both in extent and in time. In other words, a rather narrow segment of the sensitive cell population will be killed and the resulting decrease in cell production will therefore be limited. In this situation, the bone marrow granulocyte storage pool will be able to dampen and possibly even completely abolish the effect of the transiently decreased cell production upon the peripheral blood granulocyte concentration.

If, however, ara-C is administered repeatedly at short intervals or if the drug is given continuously, its effect upon the granulocytic system may be quite different. Here, the proliferating cell populations may be killed almost completely. Even more, cell populations in a resting state (e.g., the pluripotent stem cells) may start to proliferate in reaction to the first drug dose, and may then be hit by a subsequent dose of ara-C. Thus, intermittent or continuous administration of ara-C may cause a profound depletion of the proliferating granulocytic pools. Such severe toxicity can no longer be dampened by the bone marrow granulocyte storage pool, which explains the remarkable hematologic toxicity of such a drug regimen (see page 85).

Two other groups of cytotoxic agents were classified as "cycle-specific" and "cycle-unspecific" by Bruce et al. [80–82]. The sensitivity of rapidly proliferating cells to a cycle-specific drug is greater than that of resting cells, whereas the sensitivity to cycle-unspecific drugs is independent of the proliferative activity of a cell population. More importantly, however, is the fact, indicated by the exponential dose-survival curve for these agents, that cells are sensitive to these drugs irrespective of their position in the cell cycle. Thus, cycle-specific and cycle-unspecific agents act not only on proliferating cells, but also on cell populations that are minimally or not proliferating (G_0 cells). Unlike phase-specific agents, they do not spare cells in any particular phase of the cell cycle. With respect to the granulopoietic system, this means that pluripotent stem cells may, under steady-state conditions, experience much more toxicity from a cycle-specific or cycle-unspecific drug than from a phase-specific agent.

The extent of the toxicity of these drugs to the granulopoietic system, the onset and duration of this toxicity, and the potential of these agents for induction of late bone marrow failure depend to some degree on the cellular level within the granulopoietic system at which they exert maximal cytotoxicity. Cyclophosphamide, for example, damages all proliferating compartments of the granulopoietic system from the pluripotent stem cell to the myelocyte. However, rapid regeneration of the CFU-S and CFU-C occurs in all species studied (for details, see pages 25, 28), indicating that cyclophosphamide causes little if any loss of proliferative potential of pluripotent stem cells (see page 180). The cytocidal effect of cyclophosphamide on myelocytes causes early onset of granulocytopenia, but the early regeneration in the CFU-S and CFU-C compartments allows early resumption of granulocyte production, and thus limits the duration of peripheral blood granulocytopenia.

The nitrosoureas, in contrast, display a late-onset and prolonged acute granulopoietic toxicity. As pointed out elsewhere (page 179), nitrosoureas preferentially kill pluripotent stem cells, particularly the earliest ones. Considerable time, determined by the kinetics of the granulocytic system, is required until this damage proceeds from the very early stem cell level to the granulocyte compartment of bone marrow and blood. Furthermore, since a substantial part of the granulocytic regeneration is carried by the pluripotent stem cells, the preferential damage to these cells explains the rather long duration of granulopoietic toxicity observed after nitrosourea treatment. Finally, nitrosoureas have been described to induce long-lasting reduction of the growth-fraction of a proliferating cell population [645]. This would provide an additional explanation of the long time period required for hematopoietic reconstitution following nitrosourea treatment. The existence of long-lived metabolites has been suggested as a possible cause of the delayed hematopoietic toxicity of nitrosoureas [439]. However, bone marrow transplanted within a few days after nitrosourea administration grafts without any problems in both animals [466, 561] and man [246, 634]. This, in our opinion, refutes the hypothesis that long-lived cytotoxic metabolites of nitrosoureas cause the delayed hematotoxicity typical of these agents.

The time course of granulopoietic toxicity seen after busulfan similarly exemplifies how the mechanism of action of a drug, the structure and kinetics of the granulopoietic system, and the level at which the drug exerts maximal cytotoxic effects all affect the pattern of toxicity. As pointed out elsewhere (pages 47 and 179), the drug exerts toxicity preferentially to the early pluripotent stem cells. This explains the delayed onset of peripheral blood granulocytopenia that is characteristic for busulfan. It appears justified to assume that the prolonged granulocytopenia typical of the drug most likely reflects the very gradual reconstitution of the pluripotent stem cell pool following busulfan exposure, and this may mirror the loss of proliferative potential of the pluripotent stem cell comparment.

The damaging effect upon the pluripotent stem cell pool makes the cycle-specific and cycle-unspecific cytotoxic agents good candidates for the induction of irreversible bone marrow damage. As pointed out elsewhere (page 179), BCNU and busulfan have been shown to cause residual marrow damage in mice, nitrosoureas are known to frequently cause cumulative hematopoietic toxicity, and a combination of cyclophosphamide and ADR has been shown to cause long-term (permanent?) damage to the human granulopoietic system [349a]. Thus, there is substantial evidence for a permanent stem cell defect caused by these agents (for review of this subject and discussion, see page 177).

Table 81. Effects of endotoxin on murine and human hematopoiesis. Arrows indicate migration or shifts between the compartments of granulopoiesis

Cellularity and morphology	CFU-S
Spleen 25 μg/mouse, 24 h; no difference in cellularity and morphology [547] 5 μg/mouse, 6 days; increase of cellularity (120%) [380] 20 μg/mouse, days 1–2; minimal depression of cellularity [335]	Endogenous CFU-S after sublethal irradiation Increase, maximum 20- to 25-fold; dependent on dose (maximum at 25 μg/mouse), time before irradiation (maximum at −24 to −6 h), and route of administration (s.c. < i.p. < i.v.). "Tolerance" after endotoxin pretreatment [259] Postirradiation dip 20-fold decreased after 20 μg/mouse [335] Exogenous CFU-S 50-fold expansion 2–8 days after 500 μg/mouse [629] Expansion via genetically determined mechanism [375] Proliferative activity increased (10%–60%) 24 h after 25 μg/mouse [175] Pretreatment of recipient Improved seeding (1.7-fold) after 20 μg/mouse [335] Migration from shielded leg to spleen doubled 4 and 8 h after endotoxin [259]
Bone marrow Cellularity 50 μg/mouse; no change at 24 h [259] 25 μg/mouse; no change at 24 h [547] 25 μg/mouse; reduction to 50% at 24 h [335] 5 μg/mouse; reduction to 75% days 2–4 [380] Increase of ^{3}H-labelling index days 2–4, decrease of maturation compartment, and increase of proliferation compartment [467]	Transient depression [335], no change [467, 547], and elevation [259] have been reported 500 μg/mouse; doubling by days 6–10 [629] Variation of f-fraction [212, 467] may contribute to conflicting data Proliferative activity increased on days 1 and 2 [375, 467, 482]
Peripheral blood Increase of peripheral blood PMN ("granulocyte repopulation ability") used as parameter for bone marrow regeneration after irradiation or cytostatic drugs [124, 125][a]	500 μg/mouse; biphasic increase (1 h, 7 d) 100 μg/mouse; less effect 10 μg/mouse; minimal effect [629]

[a] Data from rats

Table 81 (continued)

CFU-C	PMN
5 μg/mouse; first peak (170%) at 2 h, second peak (ten-fold) day 3 [467] 20 μg/mouse; rise up to 40-fold, peak on day 6 [13, 377, 379] "Tolerance"; less increase after pretreatment with endotoxin Pretreatment of recipient mice; increase in recovery in spleen [228] Migration from bone marrow to spleen likely [259]	Early sequestration (at 6 h); second rise (at 48 h) as consequence of CFU-C proliferation [468]
Early (20 min) decrease; nadir by 6 h [467]; Slight (insignificant) increase days 2–4 [380] "Tolerance" after pretreatment with endotoxin, no decrease by 6 h [467] Proliferative activity increased [467] Size shift to larger subpopulation [380]	PMN almost disappeared by 6 h [467] as consequence of release from bone marrow [132, 467, 546]. In "tolerant" mice mobilization still possible [470] Increase of circulating PMN established as parameter of functional bone marrow PMN reserve [132, 583]
Early depression (1–2.5 h), ten-fold increase by 6 h [468, 469] In "tolerant" mice, no increase [470] In man, transient increase of unstimulated CFU-C [114] CSF (colony-stimulating factor): Immediate increase in mice]108, 469] and man [114, 231]. In "tolerant" mice no increase [470]. In vitro induction in human macrophages by endotoxin [115] Stimulating effect not correlated with toxicity [3]	Acute drop followed by fivefold increase by 6 h [467] In man, depression of PMN during first hour, doubling by 4 h [114]. Neutrophil-releasing activity increased [54]

5.2 Modulation of the Granulopoietic Toxicity of Cytotoxic Agents by Bacterial Products or "Immunostimulants"

Any factor able to perturb the steady-state of hematopoiesis will, necessarily, influence the effect of cytotoxic agents on the system. Since infection is one of the primary stimuli of granulopoiesis, the modulation of hematopoietic toxicity of cytotoxic drugs by bacteria or bacterial products is of major interest. It is a common clinical experience that hematotoxic effects of cytotoxic chemotherapy can be unexpectedly severe. In some of these cases, occult infections may have perturbed the steady-state of hemopoiesis, thus rendering the system more vulnerable to the cytotoxic agents. With respect to these practical problems, experimental studies on the modulation of the effect of cytotoxic drugs by bacterial products may provide valuable information. In the following paragraph, the modifications of cytotoxic effects by endotoxin, *C. parvum,* Calmette-Guérin bacillus (BCG), other bacterial derivatives, and infection are described. Furthermore, a consideration of the "immune modulator" levamisole is included.

Endotoxin. Endotoxins, a group of bacterial lipopolysaccharides, may be derived from *Salmonella typhi, Escherichia coli, Pseudomonas,* and other gram-negative bacteria. They produce a wide spectrum of effects on all levels and compartments of granulopoiesis. A compilation of such effects described in the mouse system, including few corresponding data in man, is given in table 81.
With respect to the modulation of the granulopoietic toxicity of cytototix drugs by endotoxin, the following observations are of interest:

1) The proliferative activity of both CFU-S and CFU-C is increased one to two days after endotoxin; since most cytotoxic agents are more effective on cells in active proliferation (see the respective chapters of this book and reference [605, 614, 615]), the toxicity of cytotoxic agents on precursor cells will be increased.
2) Endotoxin induces shifts of hemopoietic cells between organ systems, i.e., bone marrow, spleen, and peripheral blood, and modifies the migration in the partially irradiated mouse [258]. Both CFU-S and CFU-C are increased in peripheral blood by endotoxin under suitable conditions [468, 469, 629], and migration from bone marrow to spleen plays an important role in the endotoxin-induced changes of hemopoiesis. Thus, a sequence of events is elicited on all the compartments of the granulopoietic system which will modify the action of a subsequent cytotoxic agent depending on the time interval between endotoxin and the drug.
3) The technical problems in evaluation of nonsteady-state hemopoiesis and its damage by cytotoxic drugs are illustrated by the change in seeding efficiency (*f*-fraction) observed after endotoxin [212, 467]. For instance, Quesenberry et al. [468] pointed out that an apparent decrease of the bone marrow CFU-S compartment could be explained by the reduction of the *f*-factor from 11.1% in control mice to 7.6% in mice treated with endotoxin 24 h earlier.
4) The increment of peripheral blood PMN after a dose of endotoxin has been utilized as a measure for the granulopoietic repopulating ability (GRA) of bone marrow transfused into lethally irradiated recipients several days earlier (see page 12 [124, 125]). Although dose-response curves with good correlation between transfused bone marrow and granulocytic response have been described, it is difficult to interpret these data with respect to the stem cell content of transfused marrow.

5) The changes in hematopoiesis induced by endotoxin follow different time courses for various parameters. For example, biphasic curves have been observed with early peaks during the first hours after endotoxin and second peaks during later days (e.g., CFU-S in peripheral blood [629] or CFU-C content of spleen [467]). Therefore, the effect of cytotoxic agents on endotoxin-perturbed granulopoiesis will critically depend on the time interval between the application of endotoxin and the cytotoxic agent(s).
6) The development of "tolerance", i.e., loss or mitigation of the endotoxin effect, when single or multiple injections precede the test dose, is observed for many, but not all parameters of granulopoiesis (see Table 81). While the mobilization of PMN into peripheral blood is still elicited in tolerant mice, the increase of CSA and circulating CFU-S is abolished by previous exposure to endotoxin. The induction of tolerance widens the spectrum of influences on the granulopoietic system, which can modify the effect of cytotoxic drugs.

In dogs, similar effects of endotoxin on the granulopoietic system have been observed [55, 108, 364]. Also, the induction of tolerance has been described in the canine system [365].

The general considerations made above are well illustrated by the data obtained for the effect of 5-FU in endotoxin-treated mice. Pretreatment with endotoxin increases the sensitivity of murine CFU-S and CFU-C to 5-FU. From data shown in Tables 32, 33, and 34 it is obvious that the timing of endotoxin in relation to the administration of 5-FU is of particular importance. This temporal relationship has been investigated by Reissman et al. [482] and by Eaves and Bruce [175, 176]. Both groups studied the changes in various compartments of granulopoiesis which occurred when the time schedule of the application of endotoxin and 5-FU was varied. A comprehensive view of these data is given in Table 82.

In all compartments studied, endotoxin is able to either enhance the toxicity of 5-FU or to accelerate recovery from cytotoxic injury, depending on the time of application. These two opposite effects may be explained by the ability of endotoxin to stimulate the proliferative activity of CFU-S and CFU-C (see Table 81). When endotoxin is given at suitable time points before 5-FU, a more sensitive, actively proliferating stem cell population is exposed to the cytotoxic drug. On the other hand, endotoxin following 5-FU can stimulate the regenerative potential of the hemopoietic system. These opposing effects may be operative simultaneously, the relative influence depending on the time schedule. Morphological evaluation of bone marrow changes induced by 5-FU shows that the drug-induced events are accelerated by 24 h when endotoxin is given 4 h after the cytotoxic drug [471].

Endotoxin is frequently used to trigger uncommitted or committed hemopoietic precursor cells into active proliferation and to compare the effect of cytotoxic agents under these conditions. Table 83 summarizes these data, and details are reported in the sections dealing with the specific drugs.

In general terms, pretreatment with endotoxin increases the sensitivity of hemopoietic stem cells, while the characteristics of the dose-response curves are maintained. The plateau phase seen in phase-specific agents is established at a lower level. In cycle-specific agents, the slope of the exponential curve is steeper, indicating an increased sensitivity after endotoxin.

C. Parvum. C. parvum by itself has been shown to have marked antitumor activity [201, 255, 521] which may be mediated by stimulation of the macrophage system [640].

Table 82. Interaction of 5-FU with endotoxin: **A** AKR mice, 25 μg/mouse *S. typhi* endotoxin; 125 mg/kg 5-FU [482] and **B** MF_1 mice, 25 μg/mouse *S. typhi* endotoxin; 170 mg/kg 5-FU [175, 176]

	Time of endotoxin administration (h)	Recovery of hemopoietic function (percent of controls)											
		Time after 5-FU											
		6 h	1 day	Days 1	2	3	4	5	6	7	8	9	10
CFU-S	Control	50	12	1.3	1.7	3	4	11	22	36	62		
	−96	50−60											
	−72	50−60											
	−60	20											
	−48	2											
	−36	0.5											
	−24	2	0.2	0.8	0.8	0.9	1	1.5	2.6	6.2	12.5		
	−12	10											
	− 6	20											
	+ 4			1.7	5	6		28	60	98			
CFU-C	Control	20	5										
	−96	20											
	−72	20											
	−60	1											
	−48	0.2											
	−36	0.1											
	−24	0.1	0										
	−12	0.7											
	− 6	2											
		A		B									

Table 82 (continued)

	Time of endotoxin adminis-tration (h)	Recovery of hemopoietic function (percent of controls)											
		Time after 5-FU											
		6 h	1 day	Days 1	2	3	4	5	6	7	8	9	10
Bone marrow cellularity	Control				20		20		35		63		81
	−48										66		
	−24				15		18		12		13		32
	−16										35		
	− 6										59		
	− 2										72		
	0										93		
	+ 4				18		28		63		94		107
PMN (peripheral blood)	Control					33			2		20		67
	−48										17		
	−24					49			1		1		9
	−16										1		
	− 6										20		
	− 2										56		
	0										98		
	+ 4					26			83		248		289
	+24								18		137		196
	+48								4		51		135
							B						

Table 83. Interaction of endotoxin with various cytotoxic drugs (except 5-FU) on the stem cell level. For details, see respective chapters dealing with individual drugs

System	Drug	Effect of drug		Reference
AKR mice; 25 μg *S. typhi* endotoxin, i.v., −24 h, assay 24 h after drug	VLB	CFU-S:	Rapid decrease at low doses, plateau or less steep decrease at higher doses; endotoxin-treated CFU-S more sensitive	[175]
	VLB	CFU-C:	No plateau; endotoxin-exposed CFU-C more sensitive	
	Ara-C	CFU-S:	Similar to VLB	
	Cyclophosphamide	CFU-S:	Exponential curves without shoulder; $D_{1/2}$ after endotoxin greatly reduced	
BALB/c or $C_{57}Bl$; 50 μg *S. typhi* endotoxin, i.p., −20 h, assay 24 h after drug	Bleomycin	CFU-S:	Little effect on normal CFU-S even at doses around LD_{50} (200 mg/kg); markedly increased sensitivity after endotoxin. Similar results in vivo and in vitro	[596]
$(C_{57}Bl \times C_3H)F_1$; 50 μg *S. abortus equi* endotoxin, i.p., −20 h, assay 4 h after drug	Bleomycin	CFU-S:	Biphasic curve; initial upward concavity much higher after endotoxin; final slope not different. Split doses of bleomycin not different in normal mice; increased sensitivity toward split doses after endotoxin treatment	[76]
$(C_{57}Bl \times C_3H)F_1$; 50 μg *S. abortus equi* endotoxin, i.p., −20 h, assay 40 min after drug	HU	CFU-C:	Surviving fraction (49% after HU alone) reduced to 21% after endotoxin	[77]

Its effect on hematopoiesis in the mouse system is in many respects similar to that described for endotoxin in the previous paragraph. These effects are remarkable for their long duration after single doses of *C. parvum*. For instance, the elevation of PMN in C_{57}Bl mice, injected with 0.55 mg *C. parvum* i.p., lasted for 33 days, and the bone marrow cellularity and the CFU-C content per femur were depressed for 21 days [179].

Reduction of bone marrow cellularity is a common finding in various studies [179, 180, 208, 363]. This effect is dose-dependent with a maximum effect at doses greater than 0.7 mg/mouse [208]. Spleen weight and cell content are three- to sixfold increased after *C. parvum*, with a maximum as late as 17 days afterwards [363].

The CFU-S content of the bone marrow is stable during the initial period, when an increase in the incidence compensates for the decrease in cellularity. Subsequently, depression occurs for up to 12 days, with normalization by day 17 [363]. In the spleen, a sixfold increase in CFU-S concentration and a 13-fold increase in absolute number was observed [363]. In the same experiments, a marked reduction of seeding efficiency, similar to that observed after endotoxin, was found for both bone marrow- and spleen-derived CFU-S. Also, the proliferative activity, as measured by the sensitivity to HU, increased after *C. parvum:* The surviving fraction for bone marrow and spleen CFU-S was 80–90% before, and about 50% at 3 and 7 days after *C. parvum*.

For bone marrow CFU-C, variable data are reported. Foster [206, 207] observed depression, stable content, and increase in various sets of experiments. Differences between the batches of *C. parvum* and between batches of mice are discussed as the reason for the observed variations. The author speculates that some undetected infection may have influenced the sensitivity to *C. parvum*. An oscillating pattern of the CFU-C content of bone marrow was seen by Eliopoulos et al. [179, 180]. In their experiments, the proliferative activity of CFU-C (measured by their sensitivity to HU) was also increased on days 1, 2, and 5 after *C. parvum*. The same effect was observed by Foster [206] using in vitro ^{3}H-TdR suicide.

A set of data has been presented by Foster [204, 206, 207] concerning the effect of killed *C. parvum* on granulopoiesis and its interaction with cytotoxic drugs, in particular with 5-FU (Table 84). The interaction between 5-FU and *C. parvum* with respect to bone marrow CFU-C is dose- and time-dependent. As for endotoxin, the most attractive explanation for this increased cytotoxicity of 5-FU is the induction of a higher proliferative state in the compartment.

An interesting observation concerns the changes in the spleen (Table 84). From the concentration of CFU-C/10^5 cells and the spleen weight, an index of the splenic CFU-C content is calculated which shows a peak on day 8 after *C. parvum*. The most impressive reduction of splenic CFU-C is seen when 5-FU is given 24 h after *C. parvum*, but there is still a marked effect when 5-FU is given on day 7 after *C. parvum*. At this time interval, 5-FU does not influence the femoral CFU-C compartment. Thus, it appears that there can be different proliferative rates for the spleen and bone marrow CFU-C at any particular time.

The schedule-dependent interaction between 5-FU and *C. parvum* on the peripheral blood PMN count (Table 84) is quite similar to that discussed above for endotoxin.

Foster [207] also reports experiments in which 40 mg/kg 5-FU was given every 2 weeks, without or with *C. parvum* either 24 h before or 24 h after 5-FU. In the animals given 5-FU only, a moderate degree of granulopenia (35% of controls) occurred after 7 days

Table 84. Interaction of *C. parvum* and 5-FU on murine hemopoiesis [206, 207]

	Percent of controls							
	Days after *C. parvum*-5-FU							
	2	3	4	7	8	10	15	22
CFU-C (femur)								
5-FU[a]	90							
C. parvum								
1,400 µg, day 0	160							
1,400 µg + 5-FU[a]	35							
C. parvum								
350 µg, day 0	90–110							
350 µg, + 5-FU[a]	50		65		90–100			
CFU-C (spleen)								
(1) *C. parvum*								
350 µg, day 0								
CFU-C index (conc. × weight)	116		530		1,240		380	24
(2) *C. parvum* + 5-FU[a] [in percent of (1)]	7%		25%		18%		75%	75%
Peripheral PMN								
C. parvum 1,400 mg day 0		230		240		285		
5-FU[b]		70		0.4		0		
C. parvum-5-FU[b]		35		0		0		
5-FU[b] – *C. parvum*		40		60		155		

[a] 5-FU (20 mg/kg) given 24 h before assay
[b] 5-FU (200 mg/kg) given day 0 or day 1 (alternating with *C. parvum*)

with recovery (120%) before the second course and, from that point on, PMN counts were from 80–120% throughout the second and third chemotherapy course. *C. parvum* given 24 h before each 5-FU dose enhanced both granulocytopenia on day 7 (15%) and excessive recovery on day 14 (440%) of the first course. During the following courses, PMN counts were usually two- to three-times normal. In the group receiving *C. parvum* 24 h after 5-FU, the PMN counts were three- to fourfold increased throughout the three treatment cycles. Thus, it appears that granulopoiesis can adapt to this type of cyclic 5-FU therapy after the first course, and that this adaptation is at a higher level when *C. parvum* is given before or after 5-FU. With respect to the changes of the peripheral blood PMN, it is only during the first cycle that the schedule-dependence of the interaction between 5-FU and *C. parvum* becomes apparent, i.e., increased toxicity when *C. parvum* is given before and decreased toxicity when given after 5-FU.

Foster [204, 206] also described the changes of CFU-C per femur after various cytotoxic drugs given 24 h after 350 µg/mouse C.p. (Table 85). A varying degree of increased sensitivity of the CFU-C was observed for some drugs; in some cases, this effect was dose-dependent.

Table 85. Changes of survival of murine CFU-C after pretreatment with *C. parvum*, (350 μg/animal) 24 h before cytotoxic drug. CFU-C were assayed 24 h after drug [204, 206]

Drug	Dose (mg/kg)	CFU-C survival after *C. parvum* pretreatment in percent of survival after the drug alone
Cyclophosphamide	80	102
L-Phenylalanine mustard	1.6	82
DTIC	125	105
MTX	16	120
	50	106
	400	67[a]
Azathioprine	40	25[a]
VBL	0.75	98
	5	3[a]
Adriamycin	10	53[a]
Act-D	0.04	77
	0.2	85
	0.4	13[a]

[a] Significant with $p < 0.05$

Mycobacterial Adjuvants: BCG and Freunds Complete Adjuvant (CFA). In the treatment of malignant diseases, mycobacterial adjuvants have attracted great interest since they have been shown to augment host resistance to cancer in animal models [18, 373, 438] and have been introduced into clinical use as adjuvants in the therapy of leukemias [372], malignant melanomas [410], and other solid tumors [158, 250]. Their role in clinical medicine remains highly controversial [19, 464, 581].

A major source of difficulties is introduced by the wide spectrum of mycobacterial adjuvants that are claimed to have unique properties not shared by equivalent preparations from other institutes. The following brief discussion is restricted to some basic aspects of the interaction of mycobacterial adjuvants with granulopoiesis and their ability to influence the toxic effect of cytotoxic drugs.

In mice, the CFU-S compartment was studied after 1 mg BCG given i.p. [463]. There was a short, statistically not significant increase in the bone marrow CFU-S compartment, with a peak at 8 h and return to control values by 20 h. In contrast to these minor quantitative changes, a significant increase in the proliferative rate of bone marrow CFU-S was observed. The fraction killed by ^{3}H-TdR suicide increased from 5% to around 40% and this increased proliferative rate was observed for 72 h [463].

In the same study [463], the bone marrow CFU-C compartment showed a first transient peak at 8 h, followed later by an increase to two-times normal numbers of CFU-C by 72 h. Buhles et al. [88] observed an approximately twofold expansion of the bone marrow CFU-C pool 10 days after i.p. BCG ($> 1 \times 10^7$ organisms, Philipp strain), and a 2.8- to 5-fold expansion after 0.1 ml CFA i.p. The s.c. application of BCG or CFA was less effective.

An early rise of CSA in mouse serum was observed to peak at 2 h after BCG with return to control values by 8 h [463]. This increase of CSA was much smaller than that

observed after 5 μg endotoxin in the same mouse strain. In a study by Ladisch et al. [333], no effect on CSA was found 8 days after 1×10^7 organisms BCG i.p.
There was no change in bone marrow cellularity of mice after mycobacterial adjuvants in a study of Buhles [88] on days 10, 20, and 30 after CFA.
PMN in peripheral blood of mice were unchanged for 4 days after CFA and increased through days 6–10 [88]. In the study of Pouillart [463], peripheral blood WBC showed a peak of 130% of control values on day 4 after BCG. No difference in circulating WBC on days 8 and 11 after BCG was found by Ladisch et al. [333].
While the data just reported for the effect of mycobacterial adjuvants on normal murine hematopoiesis vary somewhat, there is a rather uniform pattern for their interaction with cyclophosphamide. Generally, a similar rate and extent of granulopoietic depression is observed after cyclophosphamide with or without BCG, while recovery is accelerated after the adjuvant treatment. Pouillart [463] showed that the recovery of peripheral blood WBC occurred about 48 h earlier when a dose of 250 mg/kg cyclophosphamide was preceded by 1 mg BCG Pasteur i.v. Similarly, the recovery of peripheral blood PMN was faster and excessive when cyclophosphamide (250 mg/kg) was given on day 10 after CFA. In these experiments, daily doses of 75 mg/kg cyclophosphamide did cause less depression of peripheral blood PMN in CFA-pretreated animals.
Also, in the study of Ladisch [333], exponential recovery of peripheral blood PMN was observed after 300 mg/kg cyclophosphamide which occurred about 1 day earlier when BCG had been given to the test animals 8 days before the cytotoxic drug. In a subsequent study [334], the recovery of CFU-C was "twice as rapid" in BCG-treated animals. The increase in CSA induced by cyclophosphamide was augmented by BCG pretreatment.
From clinical studies in acute leukemia, it has been postulated that BCG may increase the regenerative capacity of human bone marrow after cytotoxic treatment, thus allowing a better tolerance to secondary chemotherapy after relapse [214]. However, a study directed at this question by Goldman et al. [234] found no difference in the incidence of bone marrow CFU-C of patients with or without BCG-containing immunotherapy in remission of acute myeloid leukemia. Both groups showed a similar incidence of CFU-C in bone marrow, comparable to that of control bone marrow from persons not pretreated with chemotherapy.
A contrary clinical observation is contained in the study of Pouillart [463]. In patients exposed to combination chemotherapy, in whom the time required for hemopoietic recovery was established, the recovery period could be shortened by BCG scarification in four of ten cases and by oral BCG in two of ten cases. Due to the small number of patients and the great variability of the observed parameters, these observations should be interpreted with caution.

Levamisole. In the context of cancer therapy, levamisole is considered as an antianergic immunotherapeutic agent which restores cell-mediated immunity in immunodepressed hosts [571] and may prolong the remission period after cytoreductive therapy [10, 489]. The short-term use of levamisole as an antihelminthic is virtually free of side effects [303].
While the changes of immunologic parameters after levamisole have been extensively studied in animal models, no toxic side effects on hematopoiesis were reported. It is only in clinical studies that levamisole has been connected with toxic effects on granulopoiesis. In a thorough study, Symoens et al. [572] reported on 88 cases of

Table 86. Changes of the functional bone marrow granulocyte reserve (ΔPMN/μl) and of bone marrow CFU-C after the sixth course of adjuvant ADR-cyclophosphamide [515]

	+ Levamisole		− Levamisole		p^a
	Mean	Confidence limit	Mean	Confidence limit	
Granulocyte reserve (ΔPMN/μl)					
Before sixth course	5,000	± 927	4,250	± 582	0.3
Day 4	3,700	± 527	3,900	± 543	0.3
Day 14	1,300	± 358	1,255	± 207	0.3
Day 21	3,800	± 697	3,280	± 837	0.3
Day 50	3,560	± 954	4,360	± 502	0.3
CFU-C per 10^6 bone marrow cells					
Before sixth course	40	± 6	35	± 8	0.3
Day 4	22	± 5	26	± 2	0.3
Day 14	44	± 16	59	± 12	0.3
Day 21	69	± 23	34	± 20	0.3
Day 50	35	± 5	32	± 8	0.3

[a] Value at which the confidence limits of the means are overlapping, see legend to Fig. 6

agranulocytosis and 43 cases of leukopenia retrieved from 3,900 cases on whom side effects were reported. Agranulocytosis had occurred predominantly in women, in rheumatic disease, and was associated with an increased incidence of HLA-B27. Several facts point to an immunologic mechanism, and leukoagglutinins have been found in the serum of four of eight tested patients.

The interaction of levamisole with cytotoxic chemotherapy has been described in two studies.

Vogel et al. [623] used a combination chemotherapy regimen described by Bonadonna [62a] for adjuvant therapy of breast cancer, and levamisole was added during the 6 months of chemotherapy and continued thereafter. During 4–8 weeks after discontinuation of chemotherapy, 6 of 25 patients on levamisole developed agranulocytosis. The authors discussed the possibility that a rebound recovery of immunocompetence may have led to an exaggerated production of leukoagglutinins in sensitive patients.

In a similar setting (adjuvant chemotherapy of breast cancer) we have studied the effect of levamisole upon the granulopoietic toxicity of a combination of ADR and cyclophosphamide [515]. All patients received six courses of chemotherapy at monthly intervals; half of the patients were randomly assigned to receive additional immunotherapy with levamisole during and after chemotherapy. A comparison of the changes in granulopoiesis during and after chemotherapy with or without levamisole did not show any differences on any of the studied parameters (Table 86 and Fig. 6). The reason for the controversial results of these two studies are unclear, since patient population, design of treatment, and dose of levamisole were quite comparable. The only obvious difference is the combination of cytotoxic agents.

Pyogenic Infection. An experimental model to study the effect of bacterial infection on the hematotoxicity of cytotoxic agents has been used by Harding and McLennan [263].

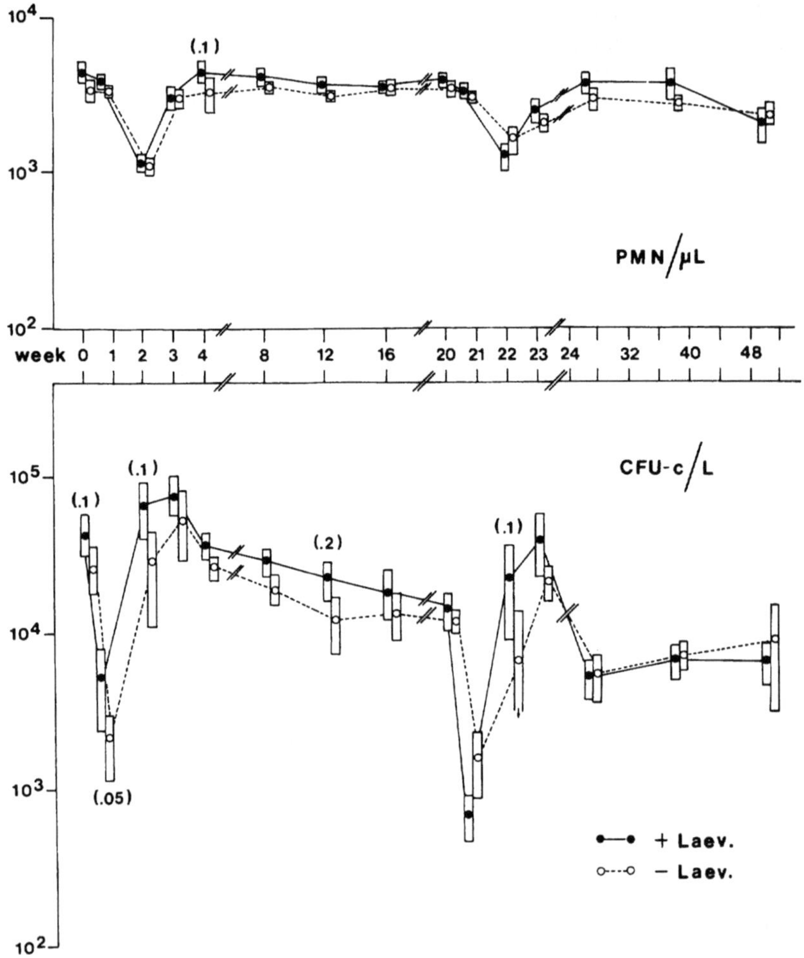

Fig. 6. Peripheral blood granulocytes (*upper panel, ordinate*) and peripheral blood CFU-C (*lower panel, ordinate*) in the levamisole-treated (●——●) and untreated (○——○) groups. The vertical bars give the confidence limits of the mean. Overlapping of these confidence limits is taken as an indication that no difference between the groups exists. This overlap occurs in most cases with P values ≥ 0.3. At time points where the confidence limits were overlapping at P values < 0.3, the respective P value is indicated in parentheses. From [515] with permission of the publisher

Pyogenic infection was induced by injecting *E. coli* i.v. into rats whose ureter had been ligated. MTX (15 mg/kg) was given at various time points before and after pyogenic infection. Neutropenia was greater and occurred earlier when MTX was given 1 day before, on the same day, or 1 day after infection. When given on later time points after experimental infection, the toxic effect of MTX on peripheral PMN was not consistently affected.

It is of clinical importance that infection, similar to the agents described above, is able to influence the cytotoxic effect of cytostatic agents under appropriate circumstances. As seen in the other systems, the temporal relationship between the modifying factor and the application of the cytotoxic drug is of major importance.

5.3 Effect of Lithium Upon the Granulopoietic System

Lithium carbonate causes granulocytosis in hematologically normal human beings [413, 432, 537] in connection with an increased circulating [557, 558] and marginated [496] peripheral blood granulocyte pool. The peripheral blood granulocyte turnover is considerably increased during lithium treatment [496]. Furthermore, lithium increases the unsaturated vitamin B_{12}-binding capacity of the serum, this value being an indirect measure of the total body granulocyte mass [588]. Thus, there is good indirect evidence that lithium causes increased granulocyte production. This conclusion is further supported by reports of elevated serum levels of CSF and its increased urinary excretion [249]. In vitro, lithium stimulated the production and/or the release of CSF by monocytes and macrophages [264, 551]. During lithium administration, the incidence of CFU-C in mouse and dog bone marrow was elevated [193, 310]. Recently, utilizing an in vitro liquid culture system for the long-term support of proliferation and differentiation of pluripotent hematopoietic stem cells, Levitt et al. [343] suggested the primary effect of lithium to be at the pluripotent stem cell level. The same conclusion may be drawn from the observation of an abrogation of the cyclic hematopoiesis in dogs during lithium treatment [257].

In the experimental animal, lithium administration reduced both the extent and the duration of a cytotoxic drug-induced neutropenia [310]. In man, this finding has been corroborated following cytotoxic drug treatment for acute leukemias and solid tumors [362, 556, 559]. Clinically, ameliorated and abbreviated leukopenia was reflected in a reduced incidence of infectious episodes and in reduced infection-related mortality [362]. Furthermore, the more rapid recovery of peripheral blood granulocyte concentrations from chemotherapy-induced leukopenia during lithium treatment necessitated less frequently a dose reduction of the cytotoxic agents [362], thus possibly permitting more effective anticancer treatment.

From the above, further studies on the clinical usefulness of lithium for the amelioration of the cytotoxic drug-induced damage to the granulopoietic system are certainly warranted. However, this type of treatment remains experimental at this time and, thus, should be limited to well-executed clinical studies. In theory, lithium treatment may, in addition to its well-known direct toxicity, cause increased hematopoietic damage: It is conceivable that lithium increases the proliferative activity of both pluripotent and committed hematopoietic stem cells, thus rendering them more vulnerable to chemotherapy-induced injury. Thus, intermittent lithium treatment starting postchemotherapy could be preferable to continuous lithium administration. These and other questions should be addressed in future clinical studies on the use of lithium for the stimulation of granulopoiesis postchemotherapy.

5.4 Prediction of Hematopoietic Toxicity of Cytotoxic Chemotherapy in Humans

The hematopoietic toxicity of cytotoxic drug treatment is determined, among other variables, by the mode of action of the drug, its dose, the route of administration, the time interval between successive courses, or abnormal pharmacokinetics due to diseases of, for example, the liver or the kidneys. However, one of the major variables that influence the hematopoietic toxicity of cytotoxic agents is the state of the hematopoietic system at the time of treatment. Thus, patients pretreated with cytotoxic agents or radiotherapy frequently exhibit increased toxicity after standard doses of cytotoxic agents. However, it is a common experience that, in spite of identical treatment conditions, wide variability in the extent of cytotoxic drug-induced hematopoietic toxicity can be observed even in patients who have not received marrow-ablative treatment before.

Clinically, the hematopoietic tolerance of an individual that has not been treated with cytotoxic drugs is "tested" by exposure to a dose known to be usually well tolerated. If major hematopoietic toxicity ensues, successive treatment courses will be administered at lower dosages. Clinical chemotherapists have long attempted to predict cytotoxic drug-induced hematopoietic toxicity to more rationally determine dosages of cytotoxic agents. There is a considerable amount of literature [144, 624] indicating increased hematopoietic toxicity in patients with decreased functional bone marrow granulocyte reserve. However, a normal peripheral blood granulocyte concentration did not exclude increased hematopoietic toxicity in these studies. On the other hand, a reduced functional granulocyte reserve did not necessarily allow prediction of an increased hematopoietic toxicity.

Both the functional marrow granulocyte reserve and the peripheral blood granulocyte concentration represent a measure of the two most mature granulocytic cellular compartments, namely of the granulocyte compartment in the bone marrow and the peripheral blood. Cytotoxic agents, on the other hand, exert direct toxicity not on these compartments, but on the immature proliferating granulocytic compartments. Since the compartment of committed granulopoietic stem cells (CFU-C) plays a major role in both the direct cytotoxic drug-induced damage and the granulocytic regeneration following cytotoxic drug treatment, the evaluation of the CFU-C pool as a predictive parameter of hematopoietic toxicity of cytotoxic agents appears warranted. To our knowledge, such studies have not been reported in the literature, although the in vitro sensitivity of human marrow CFU-C to 5-FU has been found useful for prediction of marrow toxicity of the drug [285].

In the course of studies reported elsewhere [354], we have attempted to answer this question. Patients pretreated with a combination chemotherapy (cyclophosphamide 500 mg/m^2 + ADR 50 mg/m^2, given every 4 weeks to a total of six courses) were analysed for the extent of granulopoietic toxicity following the first cytotoxic drug course. No patient had been pretreated with cytotoxic agents or with radiotherapy. Both the granulocyte nadir following chemotherapy (250–4,000 granulocytes per μl) and the maximal drop in the peripheral blood granulocyte concentration (Δ PMN) following chemotherapy were taken as a measure of granulopoietic toxicity. Both values were correlated with the pretreatment values for the functional bone marrow granulocyte reserve, the peripheral blood CFU-C compartment size (CFU-C/l of whole blood) and the CFU-C bone marrow compartment size (CFU-C per ml aspirate) [120, 240, 449]. The results are depicted in Table 87.

A significant inverse correlation was found only between the maximal decrease in the peripheral blood granulocyte concentration following chemotherapy (Δ PMN), and the pretreatment CFU-C bone marrow compartment size (CFU-C/ml aspirate). Since the decrease in the peripheral blood granulocyte concentration (i.e., the difference between pretreatment value and nadir) is a more suitable measure for the granulopoietic toxicity of cytotoxic agents than the minimal granulocyte concentration, and since tolerance to chemotherapy probably is greater with greater pretreatment CFU-C bone marrow compartments, this correlation appears meaningful.

Table 87. Prediction of hematopoietic toxicity of cytotoxic drugs in man. From reference [349]

x	*y*		*r*	*p*
Δ PMN[a]	Functional marrow PMN reserve before treatment	$y = 4{,}350 + 0.036\ x$	0.032	NS
Δ PMN[a]	CFU-C/l blood before treatment	$y = 14{,}900 + 6.54\ x$	0.15	NS
Δ PMN[a]	CFU-C/ml marrow aspirate before treatment	$y = 16{,}070 + 2.22\ x$	0.36	0.05
PMN nadir[b]	Functional marrow PMN reserve before treatment	$y = 3{,}700 + 0.42\ x$	0.17	NS
PMN nadir[b]	CFU-C/l blood before treatment	$y = 34{,}750 - 2.25\ x$	0.07	NS
PMN nadir[b]	CFU-C/ml marrow aspirate before treatment	$y = 7{,}470 + 2.25\ x$	0.17	NS

[a] Maximal reduction of the PMN count after chemotherapy
[b] Minimal PMN concentration after chemotherapy
NS, Not significant

The fact that the correlation coefficient ($r = 0.36$) is low is most likely explained by methodologic limitations on the measurement of the bone marrow CFU-C compartment size. The bone marrow cell concentration in bone marrow aspirates as a measure of bone marrow cellularity in man can be used with some reliability only in population studies, but not in individual cases [349].
Our data are in conflict with other reports [144, 198, 229, 624] that the pretreatment functional bone marrow granulocyte reserve is correlated with the degree of granulopoietic toxicity of cytotoxic agent treatment. This discrepancy may be explained by differences in patients studied: In the papers referred to above, patients with hematologic diseases have been studied in whom a severe disturbance of the normal hematopoietic system was present while, in our studies, only patients with a primarily normal hematopoietic system were included. In this situation, the "functional bone marrow granulocyte reserve" determination may not be sensitive enough to detect small differences in the size of the bone marrow granulocyte compartment. In patients with hematologic diseases, compartment size differences may be large enough to be measurable as a difference in the functional bone marrow granulocyte reserve.

5.5 Problem of Irreversible Bone Marrow Damage After Cytotoxic Drug Exposure

In a decade that has witnessed an enormous increase in the use of cytotoxic agents, the possibility of potentially harmful long-term damage of cytotoxic therapy to the self-renewal systems of the body has been increasingly appreciated. This is particularly true since in the past few years clinical investigators have begun to use these drugs prophylactically following cancer surgery, in an attempt to eradicate suspected micrometastases ("adjuvant chemotherapy") [307]. Since some of the patients treated by such adjuvant chemotherapy protocols will be long-term survivors, they are particularly at risk of developing the signs of late damage to their self-renewal systems.

Clinicians have become aware of potential long-term effects of repeated exposure to cytotoxic drugs. Persistent chromosomal aberrations have been observed [392] and cytotoxic drug-induced late damage to various organs has become apparent [507]. Furthermore, the risk of development of acute leukemias following cytotoxic agent therapy is now known to be considerably increased [476, 538]. The problem of possible long-term defects of self-renewal tissues has only recently gained attention. In the context of this work, the evidence for possible long-term defects of the hematopoietic system following cytotoxic drug exposure will be reviewed.

For the purpose of this review, the concept of an age-structure within the pluripotent stem cell compartment is of importance [67]. Evidence has been presented that pluripotent stem cells are not a uniform cell population, but a heterogeneous one. According to this concept, stem cells form a continuous spectrum in which the greatest potential for self-replication is found in cells that are mostly out of cycle. As these stem cells gradually lose their proliferative potential, their proliferative activity increases. It appears that under steady-state conditions most of the demand for cell input into the hematopoietic cell lines is fulfilled by the "older" stem cells with low proliferative potential. In this way, the "younger" stem cells with a high reserve for cellular divisions are protected, since they are only occasionally called upon to maintain the equilibrium between the hematopoietic cellular compartments.

In theory, cytotoxic drug-induced failure of the pluripotent stem cell compartment to feed a sufficient number of cells into the hematopoietic cell lines may result from a reduction of the size of the pluripotent stem cell compartment or a change within the stem cell compartment's age structure, i.e., a shift towards "older" stem cells. Thus, the question arises of what cytotoxic drugs do to the hematopoietic stem cell compartment.

Perturbing factors, such as exposure to a cytotoxic drug, may cause changes in both the size and the structure of the pluripotent stem cell compartment. The pattern of depletion and repletion of the stem cell compartment depends on the type of cytotoxic agent, as addressed previously here. It has been shown that after most cytotoxic agents the pluripotent stem cell compartment rapidly restores its pretreatment size by a transiently increased proliferative activity of those stem cells surviving exposure to the agent. However, it has also been shown that, after certain cytotoxic drugs, such as busulfan or the nitrosoureas, the stem cell compartment does not rapidly regain its pretreatment size, but rather remains depleted for a prolonged period of time. It is easily conceivable that premature readministration of these drugs may lead to cumulative toxicity to the stem cell compartments, i.e., to a progressive shrinking of their size (see page 157).

Even if the stem cell compartment returns to its pretreatment size after exposure to a cytotoxic agent, this does not necessarily indicate its complete normalization. Changes in the age structure may persist even after quantitative normalization of the pluripotent stem cell compartment. The following experimental evidence has been presented showing that such qualitative changes of the pluripotent stem cell compartment may actually occur following cytotoxic drug exposure.

Schofield [512], measuring the capacity of CFU-S for self-replication within individual spleen colonies, observed a decrease in this parameter after busulfan. Hellman et al., using the capacity to repopulate marrow of lethally irradiated mice in serial bone marrow transfer experiments as a measure of pluripotent stem cell potential for proliferation and replication, reported a decreased repopulating ability of marrow after short-term cytotoxic drug treatment (busulfan, melphalan) of the original marrow donors [65, 66]. Measuring the capacity of CFU-S to replicate within the femur of an irradiated recipient, the same authors could more clearly demonstrate "aging" of pluripotent stem cells (i.e., loss of proliferative capacity) after these two cytotoxic agentens [281]. The observation of a delayed repopulation of the bone marrow CFU-S compartment by bone marrow cells pretreated with cyclophosphamide (transfer of bone marrow, previously exposed to the drug, into syngeneic irradiated recipients) [218] similarly indicates a decreased proliferative potential of CFU-S following exposure to cyclophosphamide.

Taken together, these data document that stem cells lose proliferative potential after exposure to some cytotoxic drugs. In other words, "aging" of the stem cell population may follow cytotoxic drug treatment. Most likely, the non-physiologic cytotoxic drug-induced depletion of the stem cell compartment acts as a trigger for "young" stem cells to divide repeatedly in an effort to replete the compartment to its original size. By doing so, these "young" stem cells use up some of their total capacity for cellular divisions [67, 275]. An alternative hypothesis has been put forth by Schofield [512]: He postulated that under normal conditions stem cells with high proliferative potential occupy (nutritional?) "niches". When these cells are destroyed by exposure to a cytotoxic drug, stem cells with lower proliferative potential move into the empty niches; thus, the average capacity of the stem cells for divisions decreases, which means that a reduced number of committed stem cells will be produced per pluripotent stem cell. Both hypotheses agree that such loss of proliferative potential of stem cells may accumulate following repeated injury to pluripotent stem cells, and that such cytotoxic drug-induced loss of stem cell proliferative potential is irreversible, since these cells can only lose but not gain the capacity for self-replication.

When given repeatedly, busulfan, BCNU and, to a limited degree, cyclophosphamide, caused persisting residual marrow damage [202, 401, 590]. Recently, evidence was presented that repeated administration of melphalan, chlorambucil and mitomycin C may cause persistent marrow injury [591]. This damage could be most clearly demonstrated in the pluripotent stem cell compartment as a reduction in the size of the pluripotent stem cell pool [202, 218, 402, 590], but also as a qualitative defect [66, 218, 511]. Furthermore, in the busulfan-induced late bone marrow damage, a depletion of the committed stem cell compartments and, later on, also of the morphologically identifiable granulocytic compartments was seen [202, 401, 402, 406]. Finally, impaired in-vitro growth of erythropoietic colonies has been demonstrated following short-term busulfan treatment [592]. Other cytotoxic drugs, such as methotrexate, 6-mercaptopurine, 5-fluorouracil, or vinblastine failed to induce late marrow damage [590]. The effects of repeated administration of busulfan, BCNU, melphalan, chlorambucil and mitomycin C are thus in analogy to experimental data that the stem cell pool does not fully recover to pretreatment size after intermittent whole body irradiation [282].

It is of some interest that the same two drugs (busulfan and BCNU) that induce late marrow damage also cause the greatest degree of stem cell "aging" [67], whereas antimetabolites failed to exert both effects. These differences are most likely the result of a different drug action. Antimetabolites, killing cells preferentially or exclusively during certain phases of the cell cycle, act on proliferating cells only – with respect to the spectrum of pluripotent stem cells, this means that they preferentially kill the "older", more actively cycling cells which have little proliferative capacity left. By sparing the "young" (resting) stem cells which possess most of the proliferative capacity of the pluripotent stem cell compartment, the antimetabolites have little or no adverse effect on the structure of the stem cell compartment. In contrast, busulfan and BCNU both act on non-cycling cells, and may therefore seriously injure the "young" stem cells with high proliferative potential. In this regard, loss of stem cell capacity for self-replication reported after irradiation is comparable [512].

If the stem cell renewal potential is indeed restricted, as suggested by Hellman et al. [275], this could have far-reaching clinical importance. Experimentally, the stem cell proliferative potential considerably decreases during the fetal life span, but then remains identical throughout the extrauterine life period [383]. This means that under normal life conditions, there is no recognizable "aging" of the stem cell population. However, it is conceivable that repeated perturbation of the stem cell compartment, for example, by repeated administration of cytotoxic drugs, could repeatedly lead to loss of proliferative capacity and ultimately result in failure of the stem cell compartment. This, of course, would mean hematopoietic failure.

Experiments reported by Morley et al. [401, 402, 404, 406] do indeed demonstrate the possibility of late marrow failure following cytotoxic drug therapy: After a short treatment with busulfan, mice apparently recovered hematologically, only to die of marrow hypoplasia some time later. The overt marrow aplasia was preceded by a phase of "latent aplasia" which was characterized by normal mature hematopoietic compartments, but progressively shrinking stem cell pools. A defect of the hematopoietic microenvironment appeared to contribute little if any to this busulfan-induced late marrow failure. Trainor and Morley [590, 591] later extended these findings, demonstrating residual marrow failure after BCNU, chlorambucil, melphalan and mitomycin C as well, though they failed to detect late hematopoietic defects after cyclophosphamide, MTX, 6-MP, 5-FU, or VLB. With regard to cyclophosphamide, evidence has been presented more recently suggesting the development of late marrow damage after shortterm intermittent drug administration [218]. Similarly, late bone marrow injury has been documented following ADR but not after ara-C [72]. In man, there are few data on cytotoxic drug-induced persisting hematopoietic changes. However, it is a well-known fact to clinicians that in patients pretreated with multiple cytotoxic drug regimens, the hematopoietic system is frequently unusually sensitive to further administration of cytotoxic agents. This often requires dosage reduction and/or a longer time interval between successive treatment courses. Such cumulative toxicity has been particularly frequent during intermittent therapy with nitrosoureas [196, 491, 633, 646]. Since the sensitivity of the individual hematopoietic cell to cytotoxic agents appears to remain unchanged after repeated exposure in vivo [350], the observation of an increased sensitivity (i.e., of cumulative toxicity) is most likely the result of irreversible damage to the bone marrow caused by the preceding cytotoxic drug treatment. Indeed, a long-lasting marrow failure has been observed after meCCNU treatment [440]. In our own laboratory, we have demonstrated long-lasting defects of the granulopoietic progenitor cell compartments in bone marrow and peripheral blood after BCNU and meCCNU (see pages 148, 149).

There is further evidence of a long-lasting defect in the hematopoietic systems after chemotherapy. Following phenylalanine treatment, decreased granulocyte production and a reduced bone marrow granulocyte reserve have been reported [128]. We have described a long-lasting (persisting?) defect at all levels of the human granulopoietic system after discontinuation of adjuvant chemotherapy with cyclophosphamide-ADR [353, 517]. It is of great interest, and of some concern, that the changes we have described in these patients are qualitatively identical to those reported by Morley et al. [401] for the phase of the "latent aplasia" in their busulfan-treated mice. From this experimental model, we have hypothesized that a persisting stem cell defect is present in our patients following chemotherapy. Our failure to demonstrate anemia or thrombocytopenia in these patients does not refute this hypothesis, since in these two hematopoietic cell lines a defect of the stem cell pool is less easily expressed than in the granulopoietic cell line [323, 357, 401].

It remains to be seen what this cytotoxic drug-induced long-lasting defect of the hematopoietic system will mean for our patients. From the theoretical considerations and the experimental data discussed above, the development of late bone marrow failure does seem a serious possibility [275]. However, even if the residual marrow damage does not proceed to overt bone marrow failure per se, these patients may be prone to marrow failure when they are exposed to factors which usually possess little stem cell toxicity. It is conceivable that normal bone marrow can cope with such toxic factors without recognizable impact on blood cell production, but when the same factors act on a marrow with preexisting defect, overt marrow failure may ensue. This consideration is not merely hypothetical, since experimental data do indeed suggest unrecognized marrow damage as a possible etiologic factor in marrow failure following exposure to toxic substances [405].

Finally, nonapparent cytotoxic drug-induced late marrow failure may become clinically manifest in situations of hematopoietic stress. This has been documented experimentally during erythropoietic stress [72], whereas other authors failed to unmask cytotoxic drug-induced late marrow injury by short-term granulopoietic stress [202].

Although the development of irreversible stem cell damage appears to be inherent to the action of some cytotoxic agents, and therefore unavoidable, it can certainly be enhanced by inappropriate usage of the drugs (see page 158). As mentioned repeatedly in the respective sections, the return of the stem cell pool size to pretreatment levels following cytotoxic drug administration is accomplished by a transiently increased proliferative activity of pluripotent stem cells; "young" stem cells of which only few are in cycle under normal conditions will participate in this proliferative effort. Since in-cycle cells are more vulnerable to the cytotoxic action of anticancer agents (see the respective sections and reference [607]), such stem cells could well be killed by prematurely administered phase-specific or phase-unspecific agents which usually affect them only very little. These considerations suggest that permanent damage to the hematopoietic system can be minimized by allowing the pluripotent stem cell pool to regenerate between successive cycles of cytotoxic agents. But how to recognize clinically that such regeneration has indeed occurred? The normalization of peripheral blood granulocytes is usually interpreted to indicate return of the size of the various granulopoietic compartments to pretreatment values. However, this is not necessarily so (see page 149) since, following nitrosoureas, we have observed a return of peripheral blood granulocyte concentrations to near normal values, while CFU-C in bone marrow and peripheral blood were still considerably reduced (see Table 77).

To date, information on late bone marrow failure is scarce in both animal systems and clinical situations. This may change as more and more patients become long-term survivors of cytotoxic agent therapy. For the clinician, it appears prudent at this time to realize that anticancer chemotherapy may not only induce a short-lived damage to the hematopoietic system which is rapidly repaired, but that long-term and possibly permanent damage to the hematopoietic systems may be caused by such treatment. This consideration appears to be of particular importance in the setting of adjuvant chemotherapy studies in which patients are treated prophylactically with cytotoxic chemotherapy. From the present knowledge, studies of the hematopoietic system (including stem cell assays in bone marrow and blood) during and after treatment should, therefore, be a mandatory part of any investigational adjuvant chemotherapy treatment protocol, since the ultimate value of such a protocol is determined not only by its antitumor activity, but also by its potentially harmful long-term side effects.

6 References

1. Abb J, Netzel B, Rodt H, Grosse-Wilde H, Weger N, Thierfelder S (1977) Hematologic and immunologic studies in dogs given nitrogen mustard (HN_3). Blut 35: 51–56
2. Abb J, Netzel B, Rodt H, Thierfelder S (1977) Effects of busulfan (bu) on hemopoiesis and immune reactivity in dogs. Biomedicine 26: 403–408
3. Abdelnoor AM, Liang Chang H, Hong Pham P, Novotny A (1980) Lack of relationship between toxicity and bone marrow cell colony stimulating activity of endotoxin preparations. Proc Soc Exp Biol Med 163: 15–18
4. Ahearn MJ, Lewis CW, Campbell LA, Luce JK (1967) Nuclear bleb formation in human bone marrow cells during cytosine arabinoside therapy. Nature 215: 196–197
5. Ahmann DL, Bisel HF, Hahn RG (1974) A phase 2 evaluation of 1-(2-chloroethyl)-3-(4-methyl-cyclohexyl)-1-nitrosourea (NSC 95441) in patients with advanced breast cancer. Cancer Res 34: 27–30
6. Alberts DS, van Daalen T (1976) The effect of phenobarbital on cyclophosphamide antitumor activity. Cancer Res 36: 2785–2789
7. Alberts DS, van Daalen T (1976) The effect of allopurinol on cyclophosphamide activity. Cancer Res 36: 2790–2794
8. Alberts DS, van Daalen T (1976) Rubidazone vs. adriamycin: an evaluation of their differential toxicity in the spleen colony assay system. Br J Cancer 34: 64–68
9. Alberts DS, Peng YM, Moon TE (1978) Alpha-tocopherol pretreatment increases adriamycin bone marrow toxicity. Biomedicine [Express] 29: 189–191
10. Amery WK (1978) Final results of a multi-center placebo-controlled levamisole study of resectable lung cancer. Cancer Treat Rep 62: 1677–1684
11. Ansfield F, Schroeder JM, Curreri AR (1962) Five years clinical experience with 5-fluorouracil. JAMA 181: 295–299
12. Ansfield F, Klotz J, Nealon T, Ramirez G, Minton, J, Hill G, Wilson W, Davis H Jr, Cornell G (1977) A phase III study comparing the clinical utility of four regimens of 5-fluorouracil. Cancer 39: 34–40
13. Apte RN, Pluznik DH (1976) Evidence for different mechanisms controlling proliferation of hemopoietic colony forming cells after stimulation with endotoxin and particulate materials. Exp Hematol 4: 10–18
14. Asano M, Odell TT, McDonald TP, Upton AC (1963) Radiomimetic agents and X-rays in mice and AET protectiveness. Arch Pathol 75: 250–263
15. Ash R, Chaffey JT, Hellman S (1972) The effects of nitrogen mustard on the survival of murine hematopoietic stem cells. Cancer Res 32: 1695–1702
16. Bacchetti S, Whitmore GF (1969) Actinomycin D: Effects on mouse L cells. Biophys J 9: 1427–1445
17. Bagley CM Jr, Bostick FW, De Vita VT Jr (1973) Clinical pharmacology of cyclophosphamide. Cancer Res 33: 226–233
18. Baldwin RW, Pimm MV (1971) Influence of BCG-infection on growth of 3-methylcholanthrene-induced rat sarcomas. Eur J Clin Biol Res 16: 875–881
19. Baldwin RW, Pimm MV (1979) Tumor immunotherapy: Experimental and clinical prospects. In: Flad HD, Herfarth Ch, Betzler M (eds) Immunodiagnosis and immunotherapy of malignant tumors: Relevance to surgery. Springer, Berlin Heidelberg New York, pp 195–205
20. Barranco SC, Gerner EW, Burk KH, Humphrey RM (1973) Survival and cell kinetic effects of adriamycin on mammalian cells. Cancer Res 33: 11–16

21. Barranco SC, Humphrey RM (1971) The effects of bleomycin on survival and cell progression in Chinese hamster cells in vitro. Cancer Res 31: 1218–1223
22. Bateman JC, Klopp CT, Cromer JK (1951) Hematologic effects of regional nitrogen mustard therapy. Blood 6: 26–38
23. Becker AJ, McCulloch EA, Siminovitch L, Till JE (1965) The effect of differing demands for blood cell production on DNA synthesis by hemopoietic colony-forming cells of mice. Blood 26: 296–308
24. Belt RJ, Haas CD, Kennedy J, Taylor S (1980) Studies of hydroxyurea administered by continuous infusion. Cancer 46: 455–462
25. Benestad HB, Breivik H (1971) Properties of hematopoietic progenitor cells. Acta Physiol Scand 83: 389–398
26. Benestad HB, Warhuus K, Reikvam A (1977) Hydroxyurea (HU) in experimental hematology. I. Characterization of in vitro and in vivo effects on progenitor and transit cells. Exp Hematol 5: 408–414
27. Ben-Ishay Z (1975) The lymphoid bone marrow. An experimental model. Isr J Med Sci 11: 978–985
28. Benjamin RS, Wiernik P, Bachur NR (1974) Adriamycin chemotherapy: Efficacy, safety, and pharmacological basis of an intermittent single high-dose schedule. Cancer 33: 19–27
29. Ben-Ishay Z, Reichert F, Sharon S (1978) Migration of lymphoid cells to the bone marrow of rat following eradication of cells in DNA synthesis and in mitosis. Experientia 34: 1369–1370
30. Berenbaum MC, Calley M (1962) Effect of anti-tumor agents on non-dividing cells. Nature 196: 656–658
31. Bergsagel DE, Levin WC (1960) A prelusive clinical trial of cyclophosphamide. Cancer Chemother Rep 8: 120–134
32. Bergsagel DE, Frenkel EP, Alfrey CP Jr, Thurman WG (1964) Megaloblastic erythropoiesis induced by hydroxyurea. (NSC-32065). Cancer Chemother Rep 40: 15–17
33. Bergsagel DE, Robertson GL, Hasselback R (1968) Effect of cyclophosphamide on advanced lung cancer and the hematological toxicity of large, intermittent intravenous doses. Can Med Assoc J 98: 532–538
34. Berman J, McCabe B, Dauer MM (1969) Behavior of marrow stem cells in irradiated and nonirradiated mice after treatment with cytotoxic agents. Radiat Res 38: 296–306
35. Bertazzoli C, Chieli T, Grandi M, Ricevuti G (1970) Adramycin: Toxicity data. Experientia 26: 389–390
36. Bertino JR (1977) "Rescue" techniques in cancer chemotherapy: Use of leucovorin and other rescue agents after methotrexate treatment. Semin Oncol 4: 203–216
37. Bhuyan BK, Fraser TJ, Gray LG, Kuentzel SL, Neil LG (1973) Cell-kill kinetics of several S-phase-specific drugs. Cancer Res 33: 888–894
38. Bierbrauer U (1961) Die Einwirkung der Cytostatica Endoxan und Trisaethylenimino-benzochinon auf das Knochenmark und periphere Blut der Ratte. Folia Haematol (Leipz) 5: 143–161
39. Bierman HR, Kelly KH, Kundson AG, Maekawa T, Timmis GM (1958) The influence of 1,4 dimethylsulfonoxy-1,4-dimethylbutane (CB 2348, dimethylmyleran) in neoplastic disease. NY Acad Sci 58: 1211–1221
40. Biro V, Goldenberg DM (1971) Hematological toxicity of 1-β-D-arabinofuranosylcytosine, and its prevention by deoxycytidine, in the mouse. Chemotherapy 16: 29–43
41. Blackett NM, Gordon MY (1978) Observations on the distribution of granulocytic progenitor cells (CFU-C) in human bone marrow. The importance of the manner in which the results of in vitro cultures are reported: Reply. Br J Haematol 40: 355–356
42. Blackett NM, Millard RE (1973) Differential effect of myleran on two normal haemopoietic progenitor cell populations. Nature 244: 300–301

43. Blackett NM, Millard RE (1976) Different recovery patterns of mouse hemopoietic stem cells in response to cytotoxic agents. J Cell Physiol 89: 473–480
44. Blackett NM, Millard RE, Belcher HM (1974) Thymidine suicide in vivo and in vitro of spleen colony-forming and agar colony-forming cells of mouse bone marrow. Cell Tissue Kinet 7: 309–318
45. Blackett NM, Courtenay VD, Mayer SM (1975) Differential sensitivity of colony-forming cells of hemopoietic tissue, Lewis lung carcinoma, and B16 melanoma to three nitrosoureas. Cancer Chemother Rep 59: 929–933
46. Blackett NM, Marsh JC, Gordon MY, Okell SF, Aguado M (1978) Simultaneous assay by six methods of the effect on haemopoietic precursor cells of adriamycin, methyl CCNU, ^{60}Co, γ-rays, vinblastine, and cytosine arabinoside. Exp Hematol 6: 2–8
47. Blum RH, Carter SK, Agre K (1973) A clinical review of bleomycin: A new antineoplastic agent. Cancer 31: 903–914
48. Bock HE, Allner R, Gross R (1967) Vorteile und Nachteile der hochdosierten chemotherapeutischen Stoßbehandlung von bösartigen Geschwulstbildungen. Dtsch Med Wochenschr 92: 641–646
49. Boeckl O, Heitz N, Karrer K, Mannheimer E (1964) Über die Möglichkeiten der Therapie bösartiger Tumoren mit hochdosierten Cytostatica. Arzneim Forsch 14: 797–801
50. Boggs SS, Boggs DR (1973) Cell-cycling characteristics of exogenous spleen colony-forming units. J Lab Clin Med 82: 740–753
51. Boggs DR, Athens JW, Haab OP, Cancilla PA, Raab SO, Cartwright GE, Wintrobe MM (1964) Leukokinetic studies. VII. Morphology of the bone marrow and blood of dogs given vinblastine sulfate. Blood 23: 53–67
52. Boggs DR, Athens JW, Cartwright GE, Wintrobe MM (1965) Leukokinetic studies. IX. Experimental evaluation of a model of granulopoiesis. J Clin Invest 44: 643–656
53. Boggs DR, Athens JW, Cartwright GE, Wintrobe MM (1966) The different effects of vinblastine sulfate and nitrogen mustard upon neutrophil kinetics in the dog. Proc Soc Exp Biol Med 121: 1085–1090
54. Boggs DR, Chervenick PA, Marsh JC, Cartwright GE, Wintrobe MM (1968) Neutrophil-releasing activity in plasma of normal human subjects injected with endotoxin. Proc Soc Exp Biol Med 127: 689–693
55. Boggs DR, Chervenick PA, Marsh JC, Cartwright GE, Wintrobe MM (1968) Neutrophil-releasing activity in plasma of dogs injected with endotoxin. J Lab Clin Med 72: 177–191
56. Boggs SS, Boggs DR, Neil GL, Sartiano G (1973) Cycling characteristics of endogenous spleen colony-forming cells as measured with cytosine arabinoside and methotrexate. J Lab Clin Invest 82: 727–739
57. Boggs, DR, Boggs SS, Chervenick PA, Patrene KD (1980) Murine recovery from busulfan-induced hematopoietic toxicity as assessed by three assays for colony-forming cells. Am J Hematol 8: 43–54
58. Bogliolo G, Saviane A, Massa G, Ghio R, Bianchi G, Pannacciulli I (1976) Variazioni dopo attivazione erithropoietica dell' effetto di alcuni antiblastici. Tumori 62: 445–454
59. Bohne F, Haas RJ, Fliedner TM, Fache I (1970) The role of slowly proliferating cells in rat bone marrow during regeneration following hydroxyurea. Br J Haematol 19: 533–542
60. Bollag W (1957) Tierexperimentelle Untersuchungen mit dem Cytostatikum 5-Fluorouracil. Schweiz Med Wochenschr 87: 817–820
61. Bonadonna G, Monfardini S, De Lena M, Fossati-Bellani F, Beretta G (1970) Phase I and preliminary phase II evaluation of adriamycin. Cancer Res 30: 2572–2582
62. Bonadonna G, Monfardini S, De Lena M, Fossati-Bellani F, Beretta G (1972) Clinical trials with adriamycin. Result of three-years study. In: Carter SK, Di-Marco A, Ghione M et al. (eds) International symposium on adriamycin. Springer, Berlin Heidelberg New York, pp 139–152

62a. Bonadonna G, Brusamolino E, Valagussa P, Rossi A, Brugnatelli L, Brambilla C, De Lena M, Tancini G, Bajetta E, Musumeci R, Veronesi U (1976) Combination chemotherapy as an adjuvant treatment in operable breast cancer. N Engl J Med 294: 405–410
63. Borsa J, Whitemore GF (1969) Cell killing studies on the mode of action of methotrexate on L cells in vitro. Cancer Res 29: 737–744
64. Bosch L, Harbers E, Heidelberger Ch (1958) Studies on fluorinated pyrimidines. V. Effects on nucleic acid metabolism in vitro. Cancer Res 18: 335–343
65. Botnick LE, Hannon EC, Hellman S (1976) Limited proliferation of stem cells surviving alkylating agents. Nature 262: 68–70
66. Botnick LE, Hannon EC, Hellman S (1978) Multisystem stem cell failure after apparent recovery from alkylating agents. Cancer Res 38: 1942–1947
67. Botnick LE, Hannon EC, Hellman S (1979) Nature of the hemopoietic stem cell compartment and its proliferative potential. Blood Cells 5: 195–206
68. Botnick LE, Hannon EC, Hellman S (1979) Late effects of cytotoxic agents on the normal tissue of mice. In: Vaeth JM (ed) Combined effects of chemotherapy and radiotherapy on normal tissue tolerance. Karger, Basel, pp 36–47
69. Bøyum A, Carsten AL, Laerum OD (1974) Haematopoiesis measured by spleen colony and diffusion chamber techniques in mice treated with one or two injections of cyclophosphamide. Br J Haematol 26: 605–613
70. Bradley TR, Metcalf D (1966) The growth of mouse bone marrow in vitro. Aust J Exp Biol Med Sci 44: 287–300
71. Bradley TR, Sumner MA, McInerney E (1973) Observations on enhancement of mouse marrow cell proliferation by erythrocyte extracts. In: Robinson WA (ed) Hemopoiesis in culture. DHEW Publication No. 74–205. National Institutes of Health, Bethesda, pp 77–86
72. Braunschweiger PG, Schenken LL, Schiffer LM (1980) Adriamycin-induced delayed erythropoietic injury expressed following anemia stress. Cancer Res 40: 2257–2262
73. Breivik H (1972) Response of multipotent (CFU) and granulocyte (diffusion chamber assay) progenitor cells and differentiating cells of murine hematopoietic tissues to a perturbation of the steady state. J Cell Physiol 79: 171–180
74. Brennan MJ, Vaitkevicius VK, Rebuck JW (1960) Megaloblastic anemia associated with inhibition of thymine synthesis (observations during 5-fluorouracil treatment). Blood 16: 1535–1545
75. Briganti G, Covelli V, Silini G, Srivastava PN (1970) The distribution of erythropoietic bone marrow in the mouse. Acta Haematol 44: 355–361
76. Briganti G, Galloni L, Levi G, Spaletta V, Mauro F (1975) Effects of bleomycin on mouse bone marrow stem cells. J Natl Cancer Inst 55: 53–57
77. Briganti G, Levi G, Spalletta E, Galloni L, Mauro F (1980) Effect of bleomycin on mouse haemopoietic colony-forming cells in culture (CFU-C). Cell Tissue Kinet 13: 145–151
78. Brown CH, Carbone PP (1971) Effects of chemotherapeutic agents on normal mouse bone marrow grown in vitro. Cancer Res 31: 185–190
79. Broxmeyer HE, Galbraith PR, Baker FL (1976) Relationship of colony-stimulating activity to apparent kill of human colony-forming cells by irradiation and hydroxyurea. Blood 47: 403–411
80. Bruce WR, Meeker BE (1967) Comparison of the sensitivity of haematopoietic colony-forming cells in different proliferative states to 5-Fluorouracil. J Natl Cancer Inst 38: 401–405
81. Bruce WR, Meeker BE, Valeriote FA (1966) Comparison of the sensitivity of normal hematopoietic and transplanted lymphoma colony-forming cells to chemotherapeutic agents administered in vivo. J Natl Cancer Inst 37: 233–245

82. Bruce WR, Meeker BE, Powers WE, Valeriote FA (1969) Comparison of the dose- and time-survival curves for normal hematopoietic and lymphoma colony-forming cells exposed to vinblastine, vincristine, arabinosylcytosine, and amethopterin. J Natl Cancer Inst 42:1015–1023
83. Bruce DL, Lin H-S, Bruce WR (1970) Reduction of colony-forming cell sensitivity to arabinosylcytosine by halothane anesthesia. Cancer Res 30:1803–1805
84. Buckner CD, Briggs R, Clift RA, Fefer A, Funk DD, Glucksberg H, Neiman PE, Storb R, Thomas ED (1974) Intermittent high-dose cyclophosphamide (NSC-26271) treatment of stage III ovarian carcinoma. Cancer Chemother Rep 58:697–703
85. Buckner CD, Clift RA, Fefer A, Funk DD, Glucksberg H, Neiman PE, Paulsen A, Storb R, Thomas ED (1974) High-dose cyclophosphamide (NSC-26271) for the treatment of metastatic testicular neoplasms. Cancer Chemother Rep 58:709–714
86. Buckner CD, Dillingham LA, Giddens WE, Thomas ED (1975) Toxicologic and marrow transplantation studies in Rhesus monkeys given dimethyl myleran. Exp Hematol 3:275–288
87. Buckner CD, Rudolph RH, Fefer A, Clift RA, Epstein RB, Funk DD, Neiman PE, Slichter SJ, Storb R, Thomas ED (1972) High-dose cyclophosphamide therapy for malignant disease. Toxicity, tumor response, and the effects of stored autologous marrow. Cancer 29:357–365
88. Buhles W-C, Shifrine M (1978) Increased bone marrow production of granulocytes and mononuclear phagocytes induced by mycobacterial adjuvants: Improved recovery of leukopoiesis in mice after cyclophosphamide treatment. Infect Immun 20:58–65
89. Buick RN, Messner HA, Till JE, McCulloch EA (1979) Cytotoxicity of adriamycin and daunorubicin for normal and leucemic progenitor cells of man. J Natl Cancer Inst 62:249–255
90. Burgess AW, Wilson MA, Metcalf D (1977) Stimulation by human placental conditioned medium of hemopoietic colony formation by human bone marrow cells. Blood 49:573–583
91. Burke PJ, Serpick AA, Carbone PP, Tarr N (1968) A clinical evaluation of dose and schedule of administration of cytosine arabinoside (NSC 63878). Cancer Res 28:274–279
92. Burke PJ, Owens AH, Colsky J, Shnider BI, Edmonson JH, Schilling A, Brodovsky HS, Wallace HJ, Hall TC (1970) A clinical evaluation of a prolonged schedule of cytosine arabinoside (NSC 63878). Cancer Res 30:1512–1515
93. Burke PJ, McCarthy WH, Milton GW (1971) Imidazole carboxamide therapy in advanced malignant melanoma. Cancer 27:744–750
94. Buroker TH, Padilla F, Groppe C, Guy G, Quagliana J, McCracken J, Vaitkevicius VK, Hoogstraaten B, Heilbrun L (1979) Phase II evaluation of ftorafur in previously untreated colorectal cancer. Cancer 44:48–51
95. Byron JW (1975) Cholinergic mechanisms and the hemopoietic stem cell. In: Nakao K, Fisher JW, Takaku F (eds) (1975) Erythropoiesis. Proc 4th Int. Conf. Erythropoiesis, Tokyo, 1975. University of Tokyo Press, Tokyo, pp 141–149
96. Byron JW (1972) Comparison of the action of ^{3}H-thymidine and hydroxyurea on testosterone-treated hemopoietic stem cells. Blood 40:198–203
97. Cameron GR, Courtice FC, Jones RP (1947) The effects of β,β′-dichlorodiethyl methylamine hydrochloride on the blood-forming tissues. J Pathol Biol 59:425–435
98. Camplejohn RS, Schultze B, Maurer W (1977) In vivo cell synchrony in the L 1210 mouse leukaemia studied with 5-fluorouracil or 5-fluorouracil followed by cold thymidine infusion. Br J Cancer 35:546–556
99. Carbone PP, Bono V, Frei E, Brindley CO (1963) Clinical studies with vincristine. Blood 21:640–644
100. Carter SK, Friedman MA (1972) 5-(3,3-dimethyl-1-triazeno)-imidazole-4-carboxamide (DTIC, DIC, NSC-45388). A new antitumor agent with activity against malignant melanoma. Eur J Cancer 8:85–92

101. Carter SK, DiMarco A, Ghione M, Krakoff JH, Mathé G (eds) (1972) International symposium on adriamycin. Springer, Berlin Heidelberg New York
102. Carter SK, Schabel FM, Broder LE, Johnston TP (1972) 1,3-bis(2-chloroethyl)-1-nitrosourea (BCNU) and other nitrosoureas in cancer treatment: A review. Adv Cancer Res 16: 273–332
103. Cartwright GE, Athens JW, Boggs DR, Wintrobe MM (1965) The kinetics of granulopoiesis in normal man. Ser Hematol 1: 1–12
104. Casanyi E, Elson LA (1967) Action of "mustard" and "myleran" type alkylating agents on the cellular proliferation and DNA metabolism of the haemopoietic organs of the rat. Br Empire Cancer Campaign Res 45: 32–33
105. Cavins JA, Scheer SC, Thomas ED, Ferrebee JW (1964) The recovery of lethally irradiated dogs given infusions of autologous leukocytes preserved at −80° C. Blood 23: 38–43
106. Chaffey JF, Hellman S (1971) Differing responses to radiation of murine bone marrow stem cells in relation to the cell cycle. Cancer Res 31: 1613–1615
107. Chen MG, Schooley JC (1970) Recovery of proliferative capacity of agar colony-forming cells and spleen colony-forming cells following ionizing radiation or vinblastine. J Cell Physiol 75: 89–96
108. Chervenick PA (1972) Effect of endotoxin and postendotoxin plasma on in vitro granulopoiesis. J Lab Clin Med 79: 1014–1020
109. Chervenick PA, Boggs DR (1971) Patterns of proliferation and differentiation of hematopoietic stem cells after compartment depletion. Blood 37: 568–580
110. Chervenick PA, LoBuglio AF (1972) Human blood monocytes: Stimulators of granulocyte and mononuclear colony formation in vitro. Science 178: 164–166
111. Chervenick PA, Boggs DR, Marsh JC, Cartwright GE, Wintrobe MM (1968) Quantitative studies of blood and bone marrow neutrophils in normal mice. Am J Physiol 215: 353–360
112. Chlebowski RT, Hestorff R, Sardoff L, Weiner J, Bateman JR (1978) Cyclophosphamide (NSC 26271) versus the combination of adriamycin (NSC 123127), 5-fluorouracil (NSC 19893), and cyclophosphamide in the treatment of metastatic prostatic cancer: A randomized trial. Cancer 42: 2546–2552
112a. Clement JJ, Gorman MS, Wodinsky I, Catane R, Johnson RK (1980) Enhancement of antitumor activity of alkylating agents by the radiation sensitizer misonidazole. Cancer Res 40: 4165–4172
113. Clifford P, Clift RA, Khan AG, Timmis GM (1964) Dimethyl myleran therapy combined with abdominal aortic occlusion. Br J Cancer 18: 435–448
114. Cline MJ, Golde D (1977) Mobilization of hematopoietic stem cells (CFU-C) into the peripheral blood of man by endotoxin. Exp Hematol 5: 186–190
115. Cline MJ, Rothman B, Golde D (1974) Effect of endotoxin on the production of colony-stimulating factor by human monocytes and macrophages. J Cell Physiol 84: 193–196
116. Coggins PR, Ravdin RG, Eisman SH (1960) Clinical evaluation of a new akylating agent: Cytoxan (cyclophosphamide). Cancer 13: 1254–1260
117. Cohen AM (1975) The disposition of ftorafur in rats after intravenous administration. Drug Metab Dispos 3: 303–308
118. Cohen SS, Flaks JG, Barner HD, Loeb MR, Lichtenstein J (1958) The mode of action of 5-fluorouracil and its derivatives. Proc Natl Acad Sci USA 44: 1004–1012
119. Cohen JL, Jao JY, Jusko WJ (1971) Pharmacokinetics of cyclophosphamide in man. Br J Pharmacol 43: 677–680
120. Coiffier B, Sicard B, Bryon PA, Germain D (1980) Observations on human bone marrow granulocytic progenitor cell culture: A comparison of two ways to express results. Br J Haematol 44: 335–337
121. Colvin M, Santos G (1970) High-dose cyclophosphamide administration. Proc Am Assoc Cancer Res 11: 17

122. Condit PT (1960) Studies on the folic acid vitamins. II. The acute toxicity of amethopterin in man. Cancer 13: 222–228
123. Connors TA, Roberts JJ (eds) (1974) Platinum coordination complexes in cancer chemotherapy. Springer, Berlin Heidelberg New York. Recent Results in Cancer Research, vol 48
124. Constable TB, Blackett NM (1972) Comparison of effect of four cytotoxic agents on granulocytic and erythroid repopulating ability of rat bone marrow. J Natl Cancer Inst 48: 941–948
125. Constable TB, Blackett NM (1973) Effect of cytotoxic atents on the maturing granulocytic and erythroid cells of rats. J Natl Cancer Inst 50: 515–521
126. Constable TB, Blackett NM (1974) The relationship between granulocytic and erythroid repopulating ability. Exp Hematol 2: 131–137
127. Cook PA, Page PL, Greenberg HM, Hartwell BL, Robinson SH (1977) Recovery of hemopoietic stem cells in mouse bone marrow after depletion by chemotherapy (Abstr). Blood [Suppl 1] 50: 143
128. Corder MP, Jochimsen PR, Dick FR (1979) Abnormal peripheral neutrophil and white blood cell stimulation in patients treated for regional carcinoma of the breast with adjuvant therapy (Abstr). Clin Res 37: 383
129. Costa G, Hreshchyshyn MM, Holland JF (1962) Initial clinical studies with vincristine. Cancer Chemother Rep 24: 39–44
130. Costanza ME, Nathanson L, Lenhard R, Wolter J, Colsky J, Oberfield RA, Schilling A (1972) Therapy of malignant melanoma with an imidazole carboxamide and bis-chloroethyl nitrosurea. Cancer 30: 1457–1461
131. Cowan DH, Bergsagel DE (1971) Intermittent treatment of metastatic malignant melanoma with high-dose 5-(3,3-Dimethyl-1-triazeno)imidazole-4-carboxamide (NSC-45388). Cancer Chemother Rep Part 1 55: 175–181
132. Craddock CG Jr, Perry S, Ventzke LE, Lawrence JS (1960) Evaluation of marrow granulocyte reserves in normal and disease states. Blood 15: 840–855
133. Croizat H, Frindel E, Tubiana M (1970) Proliferative activity of the stem cells in the bone marrow of mice after single and multiple irradiations (total- and partial-body exposure). Int J Radiat Biol 18: 347–358
134. Cronkite EP, Vincent PC (1969) Granulocytopoiesis. Ser Hematol II/4: 3–43
135. Cronkite EP, Bond VP, Fliedner TM, Killmann S-A (1960) The use of tritiated thymidine in the study of haemopoietic cell proliferation. In: Wolstenholme GEW, O'Connor M (eds) Ciba foundation symposium on haemopoiesis. Churchill, London, pp 70–92
136. Csany E, Elson LA (1967) Action of "mustard-" and "myleran-"type alkylating agents on the cellular proliferation and DNA metabolism of the haemopoietic organs of the rat. Br Empire Cancer Campaign Res 45: 32–33
137. Cutts JH (1968) Protective action of diethylstilbestrol on the toxicity of vinblastine in rats. J Natl Cancer Inst 41: 919–922
138. Cvitkovic E, Spaulding J, Betune V, Martin J, Whitmore WF (1977) Improvement of cis-dichlordiamine platinum (NSC-119875): Therapeutic index in an animal model. Cancer 39: 1357–1361
139. Dahlgren S, Holm G, Svanborg N, Ragnar W (1972) Clinical and morphological side-effects of busulfan (myleran) treatment. Acta Med Scand 192: 129–135
140. Dale DC, Fauci AS, Wolff SM (1973) The effect of cyclophosphamide on leukocyte kinetics and susceptibility to infection in patients with Wegener's granulomatosis. Arthritis Rheum 16: 657–664
141. Dale DC, Fauci AS, Guerry D, Wolff SM (1975) Comparison of agents producing a neutrophilic leukocytosis in man. Hydrocortisone, prednisone, endotoxin, and etiocholanolone. J Clin Invest 56: 808–813
142. Dameshek W, Weisbuse L, Stein T: Nitrogen mustard therapy in Hodgkin's disease. Blood 4: 338–379

143. Dancey JT, Deubelbeiss KA, Harker LA, Finch CA (1976) Neutrophil kinetics in man. J Clin Invest 58: 705–715
144. Deinard AS, Fortuny IE, Theologides A, Anderson GL, Boen J, Kennedy BJ (1974) Studies on the neutropenia of cancer chemotherapy. Cancer 33: 1210–1218
145. Delmonte L (1978) Effect of myleran on murine hemopoiesis. I. Granulocytic cell line specificity of action on progenitor cells. Cell Tissue Kinet 11: 347–358
146. Delmonte L (1978) Effect of myleran on murine hemopoiesis. II. Direct and host-mediated action on proliferative capacity and differentiation bias of spleen colony forming units (CFU-S). Cell Tissue Kinet 11: 359–367
147. Delmonte L, Williams N, Moore MAS (1978) Effect of myleran on murine hemopoiesis. III. Changes in the density distribution of spleen colony forming (CFU-S) and agar gel colony forming cells (CFU-C). Cell Tissue Kinet 11: 369–375
148. Denine EP, Harrison SD, Peckham JC (1977) Qualitative and quantitative toxicity of sublethal doses of methyl-CCNU in BDF_1 mice. Cancer Treat Rep 61: 409–417
149. De Palo GM, De Lena M, Di Re F, Luciani L, Valagussa P, Bonadonna G (1975) Melphalan versus adriamycin in the treatment of advanced carcinoma of the ovary. Surg Gynecol Obstet 141: 899–902
150. Deprez-deCampeneere D, Baurain R, Trouet A (1979) Pharmacokinetic, toxicologic, and chemotherapeutic properties of detrorubicin in mice: A comparative study with daunorubicin and adriamycin. Cancer Treat Rep 63: 861–867
151. Deubelbeiss KA, Dancy JT, Harker LA, Cheney B, Finch CA (1975) Marrow erythroid and neutrophil cellularity in the dog. J Clin Invest 55: 825–832
152. De Vita VT, Gold GL, Owens AH, Miller JM (1964) Preliminary studies with 1,3-bis-(2-chloroethyl)-1-nitrosourea (BCNU) (Abstr). Proc Amer Ass Cancer Res 5: 15
153. De Vita VT, Carbone PP, Owens AH, Gold GL, Krant MJ, Edmonson J (1965) Clinical trials with 1,3-bis(2-chloroethyl)-1-nitrosourea (NSC-409962). Cancer Res 25: 1876–1881
154. De Wys WJ, Mansky JM (1973) Delayed hematological recovery after cyclophosphamide treatment in the presence of an advanced tumor. Cancer Res 33: 2662–2667
155. De Wys WD, Goldin A, Mantel N (1970) Hematopietic recovery after large doses of cyclophosphamide: Correlation of proliferative state with sensitivity. Cancer Res 30: 1692–1697
156. Di Marco A (1975) Adriamycin (NSC-12327): Model and mechanisms of action. Cancer Chemother Rep 59: 91–106
157. Di Marco A, Gaetani M, Dorigotti L, Soldati M, Bellini O (1964) Daunomycin: A new antibiotic with antitumor activity. Cancer Chemother Rep 38: 31–38
158. Donaldson RC (1972) Methotrexate plus bacillus Calmette-Guérin (BCG) and isoniazid in the treatment of cancer of the head and neck. Am J Surg 124: 527–534
159. Donohue DM, Gabrio BW, Finch CA (1958) Quantitative measurement of hematopoietic cells of the marrow. J Clin Invest 37: 1564–1575
160. Donohue DM, Reiff RH, Hanson ML, Betson Y, Finch CA (1958) Quantitative measurement of the erythrocytic and granulocytic cells of the marrow and blood. J Clin Invest 37: 1571–1576
161. Douglas IDC, Price LA (1973) Bone marrow toxicity of methotrexate: A reassessment. Br J Haematol 24: 625–631
162. Dresch C, Faille A, Poirier O, Balitrand N, Najean Y (1979) Hydroxurea suicide study of the kinetic heterogeneity of colony-forming cells in human bone marrow. Exp Haematol 7: 337–344
163. Drew RM, Painter RB (1959) Action of tritiated thymidine on the clonal growth of mammalian cells. Radiat Res 11: 535–544
164. Droz JP, Mordaret N, Charbord P, Maraninchi D, Hayat M, Parmentier C (1977) Chemotherapy of differentiated thyroid carcinomas. Clinical results and effects on the granulocytic stem cell (CFU-C) compartment. Ann Radiol (Paris) 20: 814–818

165. Duménil D, Sainteny F, Frindel E (1979) Some effects of chemotherapeutic drugs on bone marrow stem cells. Cancer Chemother Pharmacol 2: 197–201
166. Dunn CDR (1972) The effect of certain nitrogen mustard derivatives on bone marrow colony-forming units and erythroid repopulating ability. I. Rats. Eur J Cancer 8: 509–516
167. Dunn CDR (1972) The effect of certain nitrogen mustard derivatives on bone marrow colony-forming units and erythroid repopulating ability. II. Mice. Eur J Cancer 8: 517–522
168. Dunn CDR (1972) Cell proliferation and drug resistance in the response of colony-forming units of rat bone marrow to repeated doses of cytotoxic agents. J Natl Cancer Inst 48: 639–649
169. Dunn CDR (1973) The proliferative capacity of haemopoietic colony forming units in the rat. Cell Tissue Kinet 6: 55–67
170. Dunn CDR (1974) Effect, with time, of melphalan on hematopoietic stem cells proliferating at different rates. J Natl Cancer Inst 52: 173–180
171. Dunn CDR (1974) The chemical and biological properties of busulphan ('Myleran'). Exp Hematol 2: 101–117
172. Dunn CDR, Constable TB (1973) A comparison of the three in vivo assays for haemopoietic stem cells. Acta Haematol 50: 9–18
173. Dunn CDR, Elson LA (1970) An apparent discrepancy between the number of colony forming units transplanted and survival of busulphan lethally treated rats. J Cell Physiol 76: 215–224
174. Dunn CDR, Elson LA (1970) The comparative effect of busulphan ('myleran') and aminochlorambucil on haemopoietic colony forming units in the rat. Cell Tissue Kinet 3: 131–141
175. Eaves AC, Bruce WR (1972) Endotoxin-induced sensitivity of hematopoietic stem cells to chemotherapeutic agents. Ser Haematol 5/2: 64–72
176. Eaves AC, Bruce WR (1974) Altered sensitivity of hematopoietic stem cells to 5-fluorouracil (NSC-19893) following endotoxin (NSC-189681), cyclophosphamide (NSC-26271), or irradiation. Cancer Chemother Rep 58: 813–820
177. Edelstein M, Vietti T, Valeriote F (1974) Schedule-dependent synergism for the combination of 1-β-D-arabinofuranosylcytosine and daunorubicin. Cancer Res 34: 293–297
178. Edelstein M, Vietti T, Valeriote F (1975) The enhanced cytotoxicity of combinations of 1-β-D-arabinofuranosylcytosine and methotrexate. Cancer Res 35: 1555–1558
179. Eliopoulos GD, André S, Anagnou NP, Fessas P (1979) Prolonged effect of Corynebacterium parvum stimulation on granulopoiesis. Scand J Haematol 23: 353–359
180. Eliopoulos G, André S, Meletis J, Tselentis J, Halpern B (1980) Effect of Corynebacterium parvum stimulation on granulopoiesis. Eur J Cancer 16: 1093–1098
181. Ellis RE (1961) Distribution of active bone marrow in the adult. Phys Med Biol 5: 255–258
182. Ellison RR, Carey RW, Holland JF (1967) Continuous infusions of arabinosyl cytosine in patients with neoplastic disease. Clin Pharmacol Ther 8: 800–809
183. Elson LA (1955) A comparison of the effects of radiation and radiomimetic chemicals on the blood. Br J Haematol 1: 104–116
184. Elson LA (1958) Hematological effects of the alkylating agents. Ann NY Acad Sci 68: 826–833
185. Elson LA, Galton DAG, Morwenna T (1958) The action of chlorambucil (CB. 1348) and busulphan (myleran) on the haemopoietic organs of the rat. Br J Haematol 4: 355–371
186. Epstein RB, Storb R, Clift RA, Thomas ED (1969) Autologous bone marrow grafts in dogs treated with lethal doses of cyclophosphamide. Cancer Res 29: 1072–1075

187. Evans R, Madison LD, Eidlen DM (1980) Cyclophosphamide-induced changes in the cellular composition of a methylcholanthrene-induced tumor and their relation to bone marrow and blood leukocyte levels. Cancer Res 40: 395–402
188. Fabricius E, Rajewsky MF (1971) Determination of hydroxyurea in mammalian tissues and blood. Rev Eur Etud Clin 16: 679–683
189. Fairman E, Corner GW (1934) The bone marrow volume of the albino rat. Anat Rec 60: 1–4
190. Fairman E, Whipple GH (1933) Bone marrow volume in adult dogs. Am J Physiol 104: 352–357
191. Falkson G, Moertel CG, Lavin P, Pretorius FJ, Carbone PP (1978) Chemotherapy studies in primary liver cancer: A prospective randomized clinical trial. Cancer 42: 2149–2156
192. Fehér J, Gidali J (1980) Protection of cycling CFU-S against hydroxyurea by low doses of actinomycin D. Cell Tissue Kinet 13: 415–424
193. Fehir KM, Rossof AH (1977) Lithium carbonate (LC) stimulation of marrow colony-forming units (CFU-c) and peripheral granulocytes (PMN) in a canine model (Abstr). Blood [Suppl 1] 50: 145
194. Ferguson FC Jr, Thiersch JB, Philips FS (1950) The action of 4-amino-N^{10}-methyl-pteroylglutamic acid in mice, rats, and dogs. J Pharmacol Exp Ther 98: 293–299
195. Ferguson RJ, Webber RH, Hayes ER (1975) Suppression and regeneration of rat bone marrow under the influence of methotrexate. Acta Anat (Basel) 92: 481–512
196. Fewer D, Wilson CB, Boldrey EB, Enot JK (1972) Phase II study of 1-(2-chloroethyl)-3-cyclohexyl-1-nitrosourea (CCNU; NSC-79037) in the treatment of brain tumors. Cancer Chemother Rep 56: 421–427
197. Finch CA, Harker LA, Cook JD (1977) Kinetics of the formed elements of human blood. Blood 50: 699–707
198. Fink ME, Calabresi P (1962) The granulocyte response to an endotoxin (Pyrexal) as a measure of functional marrow reserve in cancer chemotherapy. Ann Intern Med 57: 732–742
199. Finkelstein JZ, Hittle RE, Hammond GD (1969) Evaluation of a high-dose cyclophosphamide regimen in childhood tumors. Cancer 23: 1239–1242
200. Finley WH, Carlson WW, Frommeyer WB, Woods JW (1964) The bone marrow depressant and antitumor properties in animals of some new alkylating agents. Cancer 17: 1271–1277
201. Fisher B, Gebhardt M (1978) Comparative effects of Corynebacterium parvum, Brucella abortus extract, Bacillus Calmette-Guérin, Glucan, levamisole, and Tilorone with or without cyclophosphamide on tumor growth, macrophage production, and macrophage cytotoxicity in a murine mammary tumor model. Cancer Treat Rep 62: 1919–1930
202. Fitchen JH, Cline MJ (1980) The effect of granulopoietic stress in mice with "latent" bone marrow failure. Exp Hematol 8: 788–794
203. Fliedner TM (1974) Kinetic und Regulationsmechanismen des Granulozytenumsatzes. Schweiz Med Wochenschr 104: 98–107
203a. Floersheim GL, Elson LA (1961) Wiederherstellung der Hämatopoiese nach letaler Dosis von Dimethyl-Myleran durch isologe Knochenmarkstransplantation bei Mäusen. Versuche zur Beeinflussung der Intoleranz gegenüber homologem Knochenmark durch 6-Mercaptopurin, Aminochlorambucil und Cortison. Acta Haematol 26: 233–245
204. Foster RS (1976) The immunostimulant Corynebacterium parvum and hematopoietic toxicity of chemotherapy. Surg Forum 27: 140–142
205. Foster RS (1978) Effects of Corynebacterium parvum on granulocyte/macrophage production and toxicity of chemotherapy. Dev Biol Stand 38: 245–251
206. Foster RS (1978) Effect of Corynebacterium parvum on the proliferative rate of granulocyte-macrophage progenitor cells and the toxicity of chemotherapy. Cancer Res 38: 2666–2672

207. Foster RS (1978) Altered toxicity of 5-fluorouracil following treatment with Corynebacterium parvum. Cancer Res 38: 850–858

208. Foster RS, MacPherson BR, Browdie DA (1977) Effect of Corynebacterium parvum on colony-stimulating factor and granulocyte-macrophage colony formation. Cancer Res 37: 1349–1355

209. Fox PA, Panasci LC, Schein PS (1977) Biological and biochemical properties of 1-(2-chloroethyl)-3(β-D-glucopyranosyl)-1-nitrosourea (NSC 254157), a nitrosourea with reduced bone marrow toxicity. Cancer Res 37: 783–787

210. Fox RM, Woods RL, Tattersall MHN, Brodie GM (1979) Allopurinol modulation of high-dose fluorouracil toxicity. Lancet I: 677

211. Foyer LV, Chapman ChG, Willett FM, Adams WS (1960) Cyclophosphamide: A preliminary study of a new alkylating agent. Cancer Chemother Rep 6: 39–40

212. Fred SS, Smith WW (1968) Induced changes in transplantability of hemopoietic colony-forming cells. Proc Soc Exp Biol Med 128: 364–366

213. Frederickson T, Tambourin P, Wendling F, Jasmin C, Smajda F (1975) Target cell of the polycythemia-inducing Friend virus: Studies with myleran. J Natl Cancer Inst 55: 443–445

214. Freeman CB, Harris R, Geary CG, Leyland MJ, McIver JE, Delamore IW (1973) Active immunotherapy used alone for maintenance of patients with acute myeloid leukaemia. Br Med J 4: 571–573

215. Frei E, Franzino A, Shnider B, Costa G, Colsky J, Brindley CO, Hosley H, Holland JF, Gold GL, Jonsson U (1961) Clinical studies with vinblastine. Cancer Chemother Rep 12: 125–129

216. Frei E, Whang J, Scoggins RB, van Scott EJ, Rall DP, Ben M (1964) The stathmokinetic effect of vincristine. Cancer Res 24: 1918–1925

217. Frei E, Bickers JN, Hewlett JS, Lane M, Leary WV, Talley RW (1969) Dose schedule and antitumor studies of arabinosyl cytosine (NSC 63878). Cancer Res 29: 1325–1332

218. Fried W, Barone J (1980) Residual marrow damage following therapy with cyclophosphamide. Exp Hematol 8: 610–614

219. Fried W, Johnson C (1968) The effect of cyclophosphamide on hematopoietic stem cells. Radiat Res 36: 521–527

220. Fried W, Gregory S, Knospe WH, Trobaugh FE Jr (1970) Stimulus to proliferation of hemopoietic stem cells following injection of cyclophosphamide. Exp Hematol 20: 11–15

221. Fried W, Kedo A, Barone J (1977) Effects of cyclophosphamide and of busulfan on spleen colony-forming units and on hematopoietic stroma. Cancer Res 37: 1205–1209

222. Frindel E, Dumenil D, Sainteny F (1980) Role of pluripoietins in murine bone marrow stem cell differentiation. Leuk Res 4: 287–299

223. Fujimoto S, Inouyi T, Tsukagoshi S (1976) Effect of drug combination on antitumor activity and myelotoxicity. Gann 67: 207–211

224. Galton DAG, Morwenna T, Wiltschaw E (1958) Busulfan (1,4-dimethanesolfonyloxybutane, myleran): Summary of clinical results. Ann NY Acad Sci 68: 967–973

225. Gerner RE, Moore GE (1973) Study of 5-(3,3-Dimethyl-1-triazeno)imidazole-4-carboxamide (NSC-45388) in patients with disseminated melanoma. Cancer Chemother Rep Part 1 57: 83–84

226. Gerson SL, Page PL, Hartwell BL, Robinson SH (1977) Altered proliferative capacity of hemopoietic cells after cytotoxic perturbation (Abstr). Blood [Suppl 1] 50: 147

227. Gidáli J, Lajtha LG (1972) Regulation of haemopoietic stem cell turnover in partially irradiated mice. Cell Tissue Kinet 5: 147–157

228. Gidáli J, Fehér I, Várterész V (1969) The effect of endotoxin on the growth and differentiation of haemopoietic stem cells. Atomkernenergie 14: 235–236

229. Godwin HA, Zimmerman TS, Kimball HR, Wolff SM, Perry S (1968) Correlation of granulocyte mobilization with etiocholanolone and the subsequent development of myelosuppression in patients with acute leukemia receiving therapy. Blood 31: 580–588
230. Goldberg JH, Friedman PA (1971) Antibiotics and nucleic acids. Annu Rev Biochem 60: 775–810
231. Golde DW, Cline MJ (1975) Endotoxin-induced release of colony-stimulating activity in man. Prox Soc Exp Biol Med 194: 845–848
232. Goldie HJ, Price LA, Harrap KP (1972) Methotrexate toxicity: Correlation with duration of administration, plasma level, dose and excretion pattern. Eur J Cancer 8: 409–414
233. Goldin A, Mantel N, Greenhouse SW, Venditti JM, Humphreys SR (1953) Estimation of the antileukemia potency of antimetabolite aminopterin administered alone and in combination with citrovorum factor or folinic acid. Cancer Res 13: 843–850
234. Goldman JM, Buskard NA, Th'ng KH (1976) Bone marrow culture in acute myeloid leukaemia. Lancet 2: 260
235. Goodman JW, Hodgson GS (1962) Evidence for stem cells in the peripheral blood of mice. Blood 19: 702–714
236. Gordon MY (1977) Changes in human bone marrow colony-forming cells following chemotherapy using an agar-diffusion chamber technique. In: Baum SJ, Ledney GD (eds) Experimental hematology today. Springer, Berlin Heidelberg New York, pp 233–237
237. Gordon MY, Blackett NM (1976) The sensitivities of human and murine hemopoietic cells exposed to cytotoxic drugs in an in vivo culture system. Cancer 36: 2822–2826
238. Gordon MY, Douglas IDC (1976) Changes in proliferation rate of human bone marrow colony-forming cells measured by a cytosine arabinoside-diffusion chamber method. Eur J Cancer 12: 551–555
239. Gordon MY, Douglas IDC (1977) The effects of busulphan, hydroxyurea and cytosine arabinoside on the colony-forming cells in chronic granulocytic leukaemic and nonleukaemic marrow. Leuk Res 1: 71–73
240. Gordon MY, Douglas IDC (1977) The effect of peripheral blood contamination on colony yield from human bone marrow aspirates. Exp Hematol 5: 274–280
241. Gordon MY, Blackett NM, Douglas IDC (1975) Colony formation by human haemopoietic precursor cells cultured in semi-solid agar in diffusion chamber. Br J Haematol 31: 103–110
242. Gordon MY, Douglas IDC, Clink HM, Pickering BMJ (1976) Distribution of granulopoietic activity in the human skeleton, studied by colony growth in agar diffusion chambers. Br J Haematol 32: 537–542
243. Gottlieb JA, Drewinko B (1975) Review of the current clinical status of platinum coordination complexes in cancer chemotherapy. Cancer Chemother Rep 59: 621–628
244. Gottlieb JA, Serpick AA (1971) Clinical evaluation of 5-(3,3-dimethyl-1-triazeno)-imidazole-4-carboxamide in malignant melanoma or other neoplasms: Comparison of twice-weekly and daily administration schedules. Oncology 25: 225–233
245. Graef I, Karnofsky DA, Jager VB, Krichesky B, Smith HW (1948) The clinical and pathologic effects of the nitrogen and sulfur mustards in laboratory animals. Am J Pathol 24: 1–38
246. Graw RG Jr, Lohrmann H-P, Bull MI, Decter J, Herzig GP, Bull JM, Leventhal BG, Yankee RA, Herzig RH, Krueger GRF, Bleyer WA, Buja ML, McGinniss MH, Alter HJ, Whang-Peng J, Gralnick HR, Kirkpatrick CH, Henderson ES (1974) Bone-marrow transplantation following combination chemotherapy immunosuppression (B.A.C.T.) in patients with acute leukemia. Transplant Proc 6: 349–354

247. Greenberg PL, Van Kersen I, Mosny S (1976) Cytotoxic effects of 1-β-D-arabinofuranosylcytosine and 6-thioguanine on granulocytic progenitor cells. Cancer Res 36: 4412–4417
248. Gunz FW, Mani MK, Ravich RBM, Speden J, Vincent PC (1970) The use of etiocholanolone for the measurement of marrow granulocyte reserves. Med J Aust 1: 763–767
249. Gupta RC, Robinson WA, Kurnick JE (1976) Felty's syndrome: Effect of lithium on granulopoiesis. Ann J Med 61: 29–32
250. Gutterman JU, Cardenas JO, Blumenschein GR, Hortobagyi G, Burgess MA, Livingston RB, Mavligit GM, Gottlieb JA, Freireich EJ, Hersh EM (1976) Chemoimmunotherapy of advanced breast cancer: Prolongation of remission and survival with BCG. Br Med J 2: 1222–1225
251. Haas RJ, Fache I, Bohne F, Fliedner TM (1971) Die Wirkung von Hydroxyharnstoff auf die Hämopoiese der Ratte nach einmaliger oder fraktionierter Gabe. Arzneim Forsch 21: 974–978
252. Haas RJ, Meyer-Hamme K, Fliedner TM (1972) The role of transplanted, slowly proliferating bone marrow cells for regeneration of lethally X-irradiated rat bone marrow. Scand J Haematol 9: 121–129
253. Haas RJ, Rohruber W, Netzel B, Lau E (1979) Effects of CCNU on hematopoiesis in rats. Cancer Treat Rep 63: 377–383
254. Hall SW, Valdivieso M, Benjamin RS (1977) Intermittent high single-dose ftorafur: Phase I clinical trial with a pharmacologic-toxicity correlation. Cancer Treat Rep 61: 1495–1498
255. Halpern B, Biozzi G, Stiffel C, Mouton D (1966) Inhibition of tumour growth by administration of killed Corynebacterium parvum. Nature 212: 853–854
256. Hambsch K, Otto W (1966) Die Beeinflussung des hämopoietischen Systems der weißen Ratte durch einen N-Lost-Cyclophosphamidester (ENDOXAN-ASTA). Folia Haematol (Leipz) 86: 174–189
257. Hammond WP, Dale DC (1980) Lithium therapy of canine cyclic hematopoiesis. Blood 55: 26–28
258. Hanks GE (1964) In vivo migration of colony-forming units from shielded bone marrow in the irradiated mouse. Nature 203: 1393–1395
259. Hanks GE, Ainsworth EJ (1964) Endotoxin protection and colony-forming units. Radiat Res 32: 367–382
260. Hansen HH, Selawry OS, Holland JF, McGall CB (1971) The variability of individual tolerance to methotrexate in cancer patients. Br J Cancer 25: 298–305
261. Harbers E, Chaudhuri NK, Heidelberger C (1959) Studies on fluorinated pyrimidines. VIII. Further biochemical and metabolic investigations. J Biol Chem 234: 1255–1262
262. Harding B, MacLennan JCM (1977) Myelotoxicity of methotrexate in animals with pyogenic infection. Br J Haematol 37: 515–520
263. Harding B, Culvenor J, MacLennan ICM (1977) Effects of varying the interval between courses of methotrexate on its myelotoxic and anti-leukaemic properties. Br J Cancer 35: 40–51
264. Harker WG, Rothstein G, Clarkson D, Athens JW, Macfarlane JL (1977) Enhancement of colony-stimulating activity production by lithium. Blood 49: 263–267
265. Harriss EB, Aponte L (1968) The effect of nitrogen mustard on the hemopoietic stem cells of the bone marrow in the rat. Cell Tissue Kinet 1: 289–298
265a. Hartsock RJ, Smith EB, Petty CS (1965) Normal variations with aging of the amount of hematopoietic tissue in bone marrow from the anterior iliac crest. Am J Clin Pathol 43: 326–331
266. Haskill JS, McNeill TA, Moore MAS (1970) Density distribution analysis of in vivo and in vitro colony-forming cells in bone marrow. J Cell Physiol 75: 167–180

267. Hattori K, Ino T (1977) Several cautions on the technique of bone marrow aspiration. In: Seno S, Takaku F, Irino S (eds) Topics in hematology. Excerpta Medica, Amsterdam Oxford, pp 1061–1064
268. Hayes FD, Short RD, Gibson JE (1972) A correlation between cyclophosphamide-induced leukopenia in mice and the presence of akylating metabolites. Proc Soc Exp Biol 139: 417–421
269. Hayes DM, Cvitkovic E, Golbey RB, Schneider E, Helson E, Krakoff IH (1977) High dose cis-platinum diamine dichloride. Cancer 39: 1372–1381
270. Heal JM, Fox PA, Doukas D, Schein PS (1978) Biological and biochemical properties of the 2-hydroxyl metabolites of 1-(2-chloroethyl)-3-cyclohexyl-1-nitrosourea. Cancer Res 38: 1070–1074
271. Hedley DW, Millar JL, McElwain TJ, Gordon MY (1978) Acceleration of bone-marrow recovery by pre-treatment with cyclophosphamide in patients receiving high-dose melphalan. Lancet 2: 966–967
272. Heidelberger C (1975) Fluorinated pyrimidines and their nucleosides. In: Sartorelli AC, Johnes DG (eds) Antineoplastic and immunosuppressive agents, Part II. Springer, Berlin Heidelberg New York (Handbook of experimental Pharmacology, vol 38, part 2, pp 193–231)
273. Heidelberger Ch, Chaudhuri NK, Danneberg P, Mooren D, Griesbach L (1957) Fluorinated pyrimidines, a new class of tumor-inhibitory compounds. Nature 179: 663–666
274. Heit W, Kern P, Heimpel H, Kubanek B (1977) The role of granulocytes in colony stimulation by human white blood cells in agar cultures. Enhancement and inhibition of CSA. Scand J Haematol 18: 105–112
275. Hellman S, Botnick LE (1977) Stem cell depletion: An explanation of the late effects of cytotoxins. Int J Radiat Oncol Biol Phys 2: 181–184
276. Hellman S, Fink ME (1965) Granulocyte reserve following radiation therapy as studied by the response to a bacterial endotoxin. Blood 25: 310–324
277. Hellman S, Grate HE (1971) X-Ray and alkylating agents alter differentiation of surviving hematopoietic stem cells. Blood 38: 174–183
278. Hellman S, Grate HE (1971) Effect of cyclophosphamide on the murine hematopoietic stem cell compartment as measured by different assay techniques. Blood 38: 706–714
279. Hellman S, Hannon E (1976) Effects of adriamycin on the radiation response of murine hematopoietic stem cells. Radiat Res 67: 162–167
280. Hellman S, Grate HE, Chaffey JT, Carmel R (1970) Hematopoietic stem cell compartment: Patterns of differentiation following radiation or cyclophosphamide. In: Stolman F Jr (ed) Hemopoietic cellular proliferation. Grune & Stratton, New York, pp 49–55
281. Hellman S, Botnick LE, Hannon EC, Vigneulle RM (1978) Proliferative capacity of murine hematopoietic stem cells. Proc Natl Acad Sci USA 75: 490–494
282. Hendry JH, Lajtha LG (1972) The response of hemopoietic colony-forming units to repeated doses of X-rays. Rad Res 52: 309–315
283. Hildebrand J, Badjou R, Collard-Ronge E, Delforge A, Malarme M, Spiro T, Sztern B, Vandensteene A, Stryckmans PA (1980) Treatment of brain gliomas with high doses of CCNU and autologous bone marrow transplantation. Biomedicine 32: 71–75
284. Hill JM, Loeb E, McLellan A, Hill NO, Amanullah K, King JJ (1975) Clinical studies of platinum coordination compounds in the treatment of various malignant diseases. Cancer Chemother Rep 59: 647–659
285. Hillcoat BL, Banerjee M, McCulloch PB, Williams CKO (1977) Prediction of marrow toxicity in patients treated by intravenous infusion of 5-fluorouracil. Eur J Cancer 13: 81–87
286. Hodgson G, Blackett N (1977) In vivo synchronisation of haemopoietic stem cells with hydroxyurea. Exp Hematol 5: 423–426

287. Hodgson GS, Bradley TR (1979) Properties of haematopoietic stem cells surviving 5-fluorouracil treatment: Evidence for a pre-CFU-S cell? Nature 281: 381–382
288. Hodgson GS, Bradley TR, Martin RF, Sumner M, Fry P (1975) Recovery of proliferating haemopoietic progenitor cells after killing by hydroxyurea. Cell Tissue Kinet 8: 51–60
289. Hopkins HA, Kovacs CJ, Looney WB, Wakefield JA (1976) Differential recovery of intestine, bone marrow, and thymus of rats with solid tumors following 5-fluorouracil administration. Cancer Biochem Biophys 1: 303–312
290. Hopkins HA, Looney WB, Wakefield JA, Morris HP, MacLeod MS (1978) The kinetics of host and experimental solid tumor responses after adriamycin. Br J Cancer 37: 1006–1014
291. Høst H (1966) Regeneration of bone marrow cells in rats following cyclophosphamide or total body irradiation. Acta Radiol Ther Phys Biol 4: 337–352
292. Høst H (1966) Comparative effects of cyclophosphamide, nitrogen mustard, and total-body irradiation on survival and on white blood cells in rats. Radiat Res 27: 638–651
293. Høst H (1966) Effect of intermittent hypoxia on regeneration of haematopoiesis in rats treated with cyclophosphamide or total body irradiation. Scand J Haematol 3: 193–204
294. Hrsak J, Pavicic S (1974) Comparison of the effects of 5-fluorouracil and ftorafur on the haematopoiesis in mice. Biomedicine 21: 164–167
295. Hryniuk WM (1972) Purineless death as a link between growth rate and cytotoxicity by methotrexate. Cancer Res 32: 1506–1511
296. Humphrey EW, Hymes AC, Ansman RK, Ferguson DJ (1961) An evaluation of actinomycin D and mitomycin C in patients with advanced cancer. Surgery 50: 881–885
297. Huybrechts M, Symann M, Trouet A (1979) Effects of daunorubicin and doxorubicin free and associated with DNA, on hemopoietic stem cells. Cancer Res 39: 3738–3743
298. Iscove NN, Till JE, McCulloch EA (1970) The proliferative states of mouse granulopoietic progenitor cells. Proc Soc Exp Biol Med 134: 33–36
299. Israels LG, Sinclair C, Graf J, Zipursky A (1962) Comparative effects of nitrogen mustard (HN_2), chlorambucil (CB 1348), and busulfan (myleran) on the peripheral blood and the ferrokinetic patterns in dogs. Can J Biochem Physiol 40: 667–677
300. Itoga T, Laszlo J (1962) Döhle bodies and other granulocytic alterations during chemotherapy with cyclophosphamide. Blood 20: 668–674
301. Jacobson LO, Spurr CL, Barron ES, Smith T, Lushbaugh C, Dick GF (1946) Nitrogen mustard therapy. Studies on the effect of metyhl-bis-(β-chloroethyl)amine hydrochloride on neoplastic diseases and allied disorders of the hemopoietic system. J Am Med Ass 132: 263–271
302. Jacobson LO, Marks EK, Gaston E, Block MH (1949) The effects of nitrogen mustard on induced erythroblastic hyperplasia in rabbits. J Lab Clin Med 34: 902–924
303. Janssen PAJ (1976) The levamisole story. In: Jucker E (ed) Progress in research 20. Birkhäuser, Basel Stuttgart, p 347
304. Jenkins VK, Costanzi JJ, Ellis HN (1976) Effects of single and combined chemotherapeutic agents on hemopoietic stem cells in mice. Am J Hematol 1: 79–88
305. Jensen RH, Sharp JG, Zajic GH, Anderson RW (1977) Inverse relationship between splenomegaly and stem cell compartment size in mice treated with nitrogen mustard. Scand J Haematol 18: 309–316
306. Johnson RK, Garbjanian BT, Houchens DP, Kline J, Gaston MR, Syrkin AB, Goldin A (1976) Comparison of 5-fluorouracil and ftorafur. I. Quantitative and qualitative differences in toxicity to mice. Cancer Treat Rep 60: 1335–1345
306a. Jones BC, Radley JM, Bradley TR, Hodgson GS (1980) Enhanced megakaryocyte repopulating ability of stem cells surviving 5-fluorouracil treatment. Exp Hematol 8: 61–64

307. Jones SE, Salmon SE (1979) Adjuvant therapy of cancer II. Grune & Stratton, New York
308. Josvasen N, Bøyum A (1973) Haematopoiesis in busulphan-treated mice. A comparison between two different stem cell assays. Scand J Haematol 11: 78–86
309. Joyce RA, Chervenick PA (1977) Corticosteroid effect on granulopoiesis in mice after cyclophosphamide. J Clin Invest 60: 277–283
310. Joyce RA, Chervenick PA (1979) Lithium effect on granulopoiesis following vinblastine (Abstr). Clin Res 27: 388A
311. Joyce RA, Hartmann O, Chervenick PA (1979) Splenic granulopoiesis in mice following administration of cyclophosphamide. Cancer Res 39: 215–218
312. Kaboth W, Trepel F, Schick P, Wernekke G, Begemann H (1968) Morphologische und funktionelle Veränderungen im Blutzellsystem des Meerschweinchens nach Behandlung mit cytostatischen Substanzen und Prednisolon. Z Gesamte Exp Med 148: 306–336
313. Karev NI, Blokkina NG, Vozny EK, Pershin MP (1972) Experience with ftorafur treatment in breast cancer. Neoplasma 19: 347–350
314. Kaul M, Hudson G (1969) Recovery of haemopoiesis after cyclophosphamide. Acta Haematol 41: 170–179
315. Kennedy BJ, Theologides A (1961) The role of 5-fluorouracil in malignant disease. Ann Intern Med 55: 719–730
316. Kern P, Heimpel H, Heit W, Kubanek B (1977) Granulocytic progenitor cells in aplastic anemia. Br J Haematol 35: 613–623
317. Killman S-A, Cronkite EP, Fliedner TM, Bond VP (1962) Mitotic indices of human bone marrow cells. I. Number and cytologic distribution of mitoses. Blood 19: 743–750
318. Kindred JE (1949) The blood cells and the hemopoietic and other organs of dogs given intravenous injections of 2-chloroethyl vesicants. Arch Pathol 47: 378–398
319. Kirkwood JM, Frei E III (1978) 5-Fluorouracil (FU) with thymidine (TdR): A phase I study. Proc Amer Ass Cancer Res 19: 159
320. Kociba RJ, Sleight SD (1971) Acute toxicologic and pathologic effects of cis-diamine dichloroplatinum (NSC-119875) in male rats. Cancer Chemother Rep 55: 1–8
321. Koizumi S, Yamagami M, Veno Y, Miura M, Taniguchi N (1980) Resistance of human bone marrow CFU-C to high-dose methotrexate cytotoxicity. Exp Hematol 8: 635–640
322. Kolb HJ, Storb R, Weiden PL, Ochs HD, Kolb H, Graham TC, Floersheim GL, Thomas ED (1974) Immunologic, toxicologic and marrow transplantation studies in dogs given dimethyl myleran. Biomedicine 20: 341–352
323. Korn AP, Henkelman RM, Ottensmeyer FP, Till JE (1973) Investigations of a stochastic model of haemopoiesis. Exp Hematol 1: 362–375
324. Korte W, Bredebach H (1967) Operation and hochdosierte zytostatische Behandlung (1,5 g bis 5,0 g pro Stoß) beim Ovarialkarzinom. Fortschr Med 85: 299–304
325. Kovach JS, Moertel CG, Schutt AJ, Reitemeier RG, Hahn RG (1973) Phase II study of cis-diaminedichloroplatinum (NSC-119875) in advanced carcinoma of the large bowel. Cancer Chemother Rep 57: 357–359
326. Krakoff IH, Lippman AJ (1974) Clinical trials of cis-platinum (II) diaminedichloride (PDD) in patients with advanced cancer. In: Connors TA, Roberts JJ (eds) Platinum coordination complexes in cancer chemotherapy. Springer, Berlin Heidelberg New York Recent Results in Cancer Research, vol 48, pp 183–190
327. Kubanek B, Bock E, Bock O, Heit W (1975) Growth patterns of foetal hemopoiesis after injury. In: Nakao K, Fisher JW, Takaku F (eds) Erythropoiesis. Proceedings of the Fourth International Conference on Erythropoiesis. University of Tokyo Press, Tokyo, pp 371–379
328. Kubanek B, Bock O, Heit W, Bock E, Harriss EB (1973) Size and proliferation of stem cell compartments in mice after depression of erythropoiesis. In: Wolstenholme GEW,

O'Connors M (eds) Hemopoietic stem cells, Ciby Foundation Symposium 13. Amsterdam, Associated Scientific Publishers, p. 243–262
329. Kühböck J, Pietschmann H, Rothenbuchner G (1967) Untersuchungen des menschlichen Knochenmarkes unter Vinblastinsulfatwirkung. Folia Haematol (Leipz) 87: 220–229
330. Kühböck J, Peitschmann H, Rothenbuchner G (1971) Klinische Erfahrungen mit Vinblastinsulfat. Wien Klin Wochenschr 83: 185–188
331. Kurland J, Moore MAS (1977) Modulation of hemopoiesis by prostaglandins. Exp Hematol 5: 357–373
332. Kurland JI, Bockman RS, Broxmeyer HE, Moore MAS (1978) Limitation of excessive myelopoiesis by the intrinsic modulation of macrophage-derived prostaglandin E. Science 199: 552–555
333. Ladisch SL, Poplack DG, Bull JM (1978) Acceleration of myeloid recovery from cyclophosphamide-induced leukopenia by pretreatment with bacillus Calmette-Guérin. Cancer Res 38: 1049–1051
334. Ladisch SL, Reaman GH, Poplack DG (1979) Bacillus Calmette-Guérin enhancement of colony stimulating activity and myeloid colony formation following administration of cyclophosphamide. Cancer Res 39: 2544–2546
335. Lahiri SK (1976) Kinetics of haemopoietic recovery in endotoxin-treated mice. Cell Tissue Kinet 9: 31–39
336. Lajtha LG (1970) Stem cell kinetics. In: Gordon AS (ed) Regulation of hematopoiesis; vol 1: Red cell production. Appleton Century Crofts, New York, pp 111–131
337. Lajtha LG, Schofield R (1974) On the problem of differentiation in haemopoiesis. Differentiation 2: 313–320
338. Lampert F (1967) Morphologische und quantitativ-cytochemische Veränderungen der normalen menschlichen Knochenmarkszellen durch Cytostatika. Z Gesamte Exp Med 111: 189–202
339. Lee Ch, Castles TR, Kinter LD (1973) Single-dose toxicity of cyclophosphamide (NSC-26271) in dogs and monkeys. Cancer Chemother Rep 4: 51–71
340. Lee M, Durch S, Dale D, Finch C (1979) Kinetics of tumor-induced murine neutrophilia. Blood 53: 619–632
341. Lee MY, Sperlin A, Dale DC (1980) Distribution of granulocytopoietic committed stem cells in mice with tumor-induced neutrophilia. Exp Hematol 8: 249–255
342. Lempert N, Leather RP, Scharfman WB (1963) Methods of altering nitrogen mustard toxicity in dogs. I. Spleen and mesenteric artery exclusion. Blood 21: 213–220
343. Levitt LJ, Questenberry PJ (1980) Effect of lithium on murine hematopoiesis in a liquid culture system. New Engl J Med 302: 713–719
344. Levitt M, Mosher MS, DeConti RC (1973) Improved therapeutic index of methotrexate. Cancer Res 33: 1729–1834
345. Lichtman MA, Weed RI (1972) Alteration of the cell periphery during granulocyte maturation: Relationship to cell function. Blood 39: 301–316
346. Liss RH, Chadwick M (1974) Correlation of 5-fluorouracil (NSC-19893) distribution in rodents with toxicity and chemotherapy in man. Cancer Chemother Rep 58: 777–786
347. LoBue J (1973) Stem cell and neutrophilic granulocyte kinetics. Med Clin North Am 57: 265–287
348. Lohrmann H-P (1978) Thymidine-suicide of human granulocytic progenitor cells (CFU-C). Biomedicine 28: 319–323
349. Lohrmann H-P (1979) Das Reaktionsmuster der normalen menschlichen Granulopoiese auf zytostatische Chemotherapie. Habilitationsschrift, Universität Ulm
349a. Lohrmann H-P (1979) Tolerance of hemopoiesis for repeated cytotoxic drug therapy. Blut 39: 237–244
350. Lohrmann H-P, Schreml W (1979) Sensitivity of human granulopoiesis in vitro to adriamycin before and after exposure in vivo. Cancer Res 39: 527–530

351. Lohrmann H-P, Schreml W, Fliedner TM, Heimpel H (1977) Studies on blood granulocytic precursor cells (CFU-C) following high-dose chemotherapy in man. Exp Hematol [Suppl 2] 5: 95
352. Lohrmann H-P, Hansi W, Heimpel H (1978) Human placenta-conditioned medium for stimulation of human granulopoietic precursor cell (CFU-C) colony growth in vitro. Blut 36: 81–88
353. Lohrmann H-P, Schreml W, Lang M, Betzler M, Fliedner TM, Heimpel H (1978) Changes of granulopoiesis during and after adjuvant chemotherapy of breast cancer. Br J Haematol 40: 369–381
354. Lohrmann H-P, Schreml W, Fliedner TM, Heimpel H (1979) Reaction of human granulopoiesis to high-dose cyclophosphamide therapy. Blut 8: 9–16
355. Looney WB, Macleod MS, Hopkins HA (1978) Solid tumor models for the assessment of different treatment modalities. VII. Single vs fractionated doses of 5-fluorouracil on two solid tumours and their hosts. Br J Cancer 37: 841–848
355a. Looney WB, Hopkins HA, Macleod MS (1979) Solid tumor models for the assessment of different treatment modalities. VIII. The scheduling of treatment for a chemotherapeutically resistant experimental solid tumor. Cancer 43: 1201–1210
356. Lord BI (1975) Cell proliferation changes in hemopoietic tissue as a result of irradiation or drug administration: The control of cell proliferation in hemopoietic tissue. In: Nygaard OF, Adler HI, Sinclair WU (eds) Radiation research: Biomedical, chemical and physical perspectives. Academic Press, New York, pp 826–833
357. Lord BI (1976) Stem cell reserve and its control. In: Cairnie AB, Lala PK, Osmond DG (eds) Stem cells of renewing cell populations. Academic Press, New York, pp 165–179
358. Lord BI, Lajtha LG, Gidali J (1974) Measurement of the kinetic status of bone marrow precursor cells. Three cautionary tales. Cell Tissue Kinet 7: 507–515
359. Lord BI, Mori KJ, Wright EG (1977) A stimulator of stem cell proliferation in regenerating bone marrow. Biomedicine 27: 223–226
360. Lord BI, Mori KJ, Wright EG, Lajtha LG (1976) An inhibitor of stem cell proliferation in normal bone marrow. Br J Haematol 34: 441–445
361. Luce JK, Ihurman WG, Isaacs BL, Talley RW (1970) Clinical trials with the antitumor agent 5-(3,3-dimethyl-1-triazeno)-imidazole-4-carboxamide (NSC-45388). Cancer Chemother Rep 54: 119–124
362. Lyman G, Williams CC, Preston D (1980) The use of lithium carbonate to reduce infection and leukopenia during systemic chemotherapy. N Engl J Med 302: 257–260
363. MacVittie TJ (1979) Alterations induced in murine hemopoietic stem cells following a single injection of Corynebacterium parvum. In: Baum SJ, Ledney GD (eds) Experimental Hematology Today. Springer, New York Heidelberg Berlin, p 3
364. MacVittie TJ, Walker RI (1978) Endotoxin-induced alterations in canine granulopoiesis: Colony-stimulating activity, colony-forming cells in culture, and growth of cells in diffusion chambers. Exp Hematol 6: 613–618
365. MacVittie TJ, Walker RI (1980) Hematologic responses induced by endotoxin in normal and endotoxin tolerant dogs. Exp Hematol 8: 599–609
366. Maloney MA, Dorie MJ, Lamela RA, Roliers ZR, Patt HM (1978) Hematopoietic stem cell regulatory volumes as revealed in studies of the bg^J/bg^J: W/W^v chimera. J Exp Med 147: 1189–1197
367. Marsh JC (1976) The effects of cancer chemotherapeutic agents on normal hematopoietic precursor cells: A review. Cancer Res 36: 1853–1882
368. Marsh JC (1979) Comparison of the sensitivities of human, canine, and murine hematopoietic procursor cells to adriamycin and N-trifluoro-acetyladriamycin-14-valerate. Cancer Res 39: 360–364
369. Martini H, Scheef W, Knecht W (1967) Verträglichkeit und Wirkung sehr hoch dosierter Endoxanstöße in der Tumortherapie. Med Welt 18: 1573–1578

370. Massa G, Saviane A, Bogliolo G, Mitra G, Pannacciulli I (1977) Effetti des salasso sulla suscettibilita delle CFU-S di topi C57Bl/C3H a vari antiblastici. Boll Soc Ital Biol Sper 53: 1252–1256
371. Massa G, Saviane A, Bogliolo G, Pannacciulli I (1976) Confronti die effetti di alchilanti, di antimetaboliti, e di antiblastici di altro tipo sulle CFU emopoietiche del topo. Boll Soc Ital Biol Sper 52: 460–464
372. Mathé G, Amiel JL, Schwarzenberg L, Schneider L, Cattan A, Schlumberger JR, Hazart M, De Vassal F (1969) Active immunotherapy for acute lymphoblastic leukaemia. Lancet I: 697–699
373. Mathé G, Pouillart P, Lapeyraque F (1969) Active immunotherapy in L1210 leukaemia applied after the graft of tumour cells. Br J Cancer 23: 814–824
374. Mauro F, Briganti G, Elli R, Schiaffini G, Zupi G (1976) Plateau phase cultures as a system for studying the effects of bleomycin in view of its utilization in vivo. Prog Bichem Pharmacol 11: 93–106
375. McCulloch EA, Thompson NM, Siminovitch L, Till JE (1970) Effects of bacterial endotoxin on hemopoietic colony-forming cells in the spleens of normal mice and mice of genotype Sl/Sl^d. Cell Tissue Kinet 3: 47–54
376. McElwain TJ, Hedley DW, Gordon MY, Jarman M, Millar JL, Pritchard J (1979) High dose melphalan and non-cryopreserved autologous bone marrow treatment of malignant melanoma and neuroblastoma. Exp Hematol [Suppl 5] 7: 360–371
377. McNeill TA (1970) Antigenic stimulation of bone marrow colony-forming cells. III. Effect in vivo. Immunology 18: 61–72
378. Metcalf D (1972) Effect of thymidine siuciding on colony formation in vitro by mouse hematopoietic cells. Proc Soc Exp Biol Med 139: 511–514
379. Metcalf D (1977) Hemopoietic colonies. Springer, Berlin Heidelberg New York (Recent Results in Cancer Research, vol 61)
380. Metcalf D, Wilson JW (1976) Endotoxin-induced size change in bone marrow progenitors of granulocytes and macrophages. J Cell Physiol 89: 381–392
381. Meyer LM, Fliedner TM, Cronkite EP (1964) Autologous bone-marrow transfusion following chemotherapy. Ann NY Acad Sci 114: 499–508
382. Michaillow W, Mitrov GG, Zographov DG (1972) Über den Einfluß der Kombination von ionisierenden Strahlen und Cyclophosphamid auf die koloniebildenden hämopoietischen Stammzellen. Strahlentherapie 144: 87–95
383. Micklem HS, Ogden DA (1976) Ageing of haematopoietic stem cell populations in the mouse. In: Cairnie AB, Lala PK, Osmond DG (eds) Stem cells of renewing cell populations. Academic Press, New York, pp 331–341
384. Micklem HS, Anderson N, Ross E (1975) Limited potential of circulating hemopoietic stem cells. Nature 256: 41–43
385. Middleman E, Luce J, Frei E III (1971) Clinical trials with adriamycin. Cancer 28: 844–850
386. Milenkovic P, Pavlovic-Kentera V (1980) Regeneration of erythroid committed precursor cells in polycythemic mice treated with cyclophosphamide. Exp Hematol 8: 44–51
387. Millar JL, McElwain TJ (1978) Combinations of cytotoxic agents that have less than expected toxicity on normal tissues in mice. Antibiot Chemother 23: 271–282
388. Millar JL, Hudspith BN, McElwain TJ, Phelps TA (1978) Effect of high-dose melphalan on marrow and intestinal epithelium in mice pretreated with cyclophosphamide. Br J Cancer 38: 137–142
389. Millard RE, Blackett NM (1974) The recovery of haemopoietic progenitor cells in the mouse following cytotoxic agents. Br J Haematol 27: 361–362
390. Millard RE, Okell SF (1975) The effect of cytosine arabinoside in vitro on agar colony-forming cells and spleen colony-forming cells of C57Bl mouse bone marrow. Cell Tissue Kinet 8: 33–40

391. Millard RE, Blackett NM, Okell SF (1973) A comparison of the effect of cytotoxic agents on agar colony-forming cells, spleen colony-forming cells, and the erythrocytic repopulating ability of mouse bone marrow. J Cell Physiol 82: 309–317
392. Miller RC, Hill RB, Nichols WW, Meadows AT (1978) Acute and long-term cytogenetic effects of childhood cancer chemotherapy and radiotherapy. Cancer Res 38: 3241–3246
393. Moertel CG, Reitemeier RJ, Hahn RG (1968) Therapy of advanced gastrointestinal cancer with 1-3-bis-(2-chloroethyl)-1-nitrosourea (BCNU). Clin Pharmacol Ther 9: 652–656
394. Moertel CG, Reitemeier RJ, Hahn RG, Schutt AJ (1970) Study of 5-(3.3-Dimethyl-1-triazeno)imidazole-4-carboxamide (NSC-45388) in patients with gastrointestinal carcinoma. Cancer Chemother Rep Part 1 54: 471–473
395. Momparler RL, Karon M, Siegel SE, Avila F (1976) Effect of adriamycin on DNA, RNA, and protein synthesis in cell-free systems and intact cells. Cancer Res 36: 2891–2895
396. Monette FC, Gilio MJ, Chalifaux P (1974) Separation of proliferating CFU from G_0 cells of murine bone marrow. Cell Tissue Kinet 7: 443–450
397. Moore GE, Bross ID, Ausman R,Nadler S (1968) Effects of 5-fluorouracil (NSC-19893) in 389 patients with cancer. Cancer Chemother Rep 52: 641–653
398. Moore GE, DiPaolo J, Kondo T (1958) The chemotherapeutic effects and complications of actinomycin D in patients with advanced cancer. Cancer 11: 1204–1214
399. Moore MAS, Williams N, Metcalf D (1973) In vitro colony formation by normal and leukemic human hematopoietic cells. Interaction between colony-forming and colony-stimulating cells. J Natl Cancer Inst 50: 591–602
400. Morardet N, Parmentier C (1977) Description of a suicide technique in vitro for granulocytic stem cells (CFU) by hydroxyurea on normal human bone marrow. Biomedicine 27: 349–353
401. Morley A, Blake J (1974) An animal model of chronic aplastic marrow failure. I. Late marrow failure after busulfan. Blood 44: 49–56
402. Morley A, Blake J (1974) Haemopoietic precursor cells in experimental hypoplastic marrow failure. Aust J Exp Biol Med Sci 52: 909–914
403. Morley A, Stohlman F Jr (1970) Cyclophosphamide-induced cyclical neutropenia. N Engl J Med 282: 643–646
404. Morley A, Trainor K, Blake J (1975) A primary stem cell lesion in experimental chronic hypoplastic marrow failure. Blood 45: 681–688
405. Morley A, Trainor K, Remes J (1976) Residual marrow damage: Possible explanation for idiosyncrasy to chloramphenicol. Br J Haematol 32: 525–531
406. Morley AA, Trainor KJ, Seshadri RS (1978) Chronic hypoplastic marrow failure and residual injury. Blood Cells 4: 253–266
407. Morse BS, Stohlman F Jr (1966) Regulation of erythropoiesis. XVIII. The effect of vincristine and erythropoietin on bone marrow. J Clin Invest 45: 1241–1250
408. Morse BS, Rencricca NJ, Stohlman F Jr (1969) The effect of hydroxyurea on differentiated marrow erythroid precursors. Proc Soc Exp Biol Med 130: 986–989
409. Morse BS, Rencricca NJ, Stohlman F Jr (1970) Relationship of erythropoietin effectiveness to the generative cycle of erythroid precursor cells. Blood 35: 761–774
410. Morton DL, Eilber FR, Holmes EC, Hunt JS, Ketcham AS, Silverstein MJ, Sparks FS (1974) BCG-immunotherapy of malignant melanoma: Summary of a seven-year experience. Ann Surg 180: 635–643
411. Müller-Nübling J, Fliedner TM (1979) Präklinische Untersuchungen über die Reaktion der Blut-CFU-C-Konzentration auf eine einmalige Applikation von Cyclophosphamid. Blut 38: 175–179
412. Mullins GM, Colvin M (1975) Intensive cyclophosphamide (NSC-26271) therapy for solid tumors. Cancer Chemother Rep 59: 411–419

413. Murphy DL, Goodwin FK (1971) Leukocytosis during lithium treatment. J Psychiatry 127:1559–1561
414. Myers CE, McGuire WP, Liss RH, Ifrim I, Grotzinger K, Young RC (1977) Adriamycin: The role of lipid peroxidation in cardiac toxicity and tumor response. Science 197:165–167
415. Nagourney RA, Fox P, Schein PS (1978) A comparison of the biological and biochemical properties of 1-(4-amino-2-methylpyrimidin-5-yl)methyl-3-(2-chloroethyl)-3-nitrosourea and 2-[3-(2-chloroethyl)-3-nitrosoureido]-D-glucopyranose. Cancer Res 38:65–68
416. Nakayama M, Schuster J, Schoyerer W (1967) Klinische und tierexperimentelle Erfahrungen mit der Endoxan-Stoßtherapie. Dtsch Med Wochenschr 92:1915–1919
417. Nakeff A, McLellan WL, Bryan J, Valeriote FA (1979) Response of megakaryocyte, erythroid, and granulocyte-macrophage progenitor cells in mouse bone marrow to gamma-irradiation and cyclophosphamide. In: Baum SJ, Ledney GD (eds) Experimental Hematology Today 1979. Springer, New York Heidelberg Berlin, pp 99–104
418. Nasrallah AG, McGarry MP (1976) In vivo distinction between a target cell for Friend virus (FVP) and murine hematopoietic stem cells. J Natl Cancer Inst 57:443–445
419. Necas E, Neuwirt J (1976) Control of haemopoietic stem cell proliferation by cells in DNA synthesis. Br J Haematol 33:395–400
420. Necas E, Neuwirt J (1976) Proliferation rate of haemopoietic stem cells after damage by several cytostatic agents. Cell Tissue Kinet 9:479–487
421. Necas E, Neuwirt J (1977) Effect of hydroxyurea and vinblastine on the proliferation of the pluripotent stem cells. Neoplasma 24:29–40
422. Necas E, Ponka P, Neuwirt J (1978) Changes in stem cell compartments in mice after hydroxyurea. Cell Tissue Kinet 11:119–127
423. Necas E, Ponka P, Neuwirt J (1978) Disappearance of haemopoietic stem cells from blood after hydroxyurea. Folia Biol (Praha) 24:78–90
424. Nesbit ME, Lowman JT (1969) Hematopoiesis and serum iron changes following vincristine sulfate. Blood 34:633–644
425. Niho Y, Till JE, McCulloch EA (1976) Effect of arabinosyl cytosine on granulopoietic colony formation by marrow cells from leukemic and non-leukemic patients. Exp Hematol 4:63–69
426. Ninkov V, Piletic O (1974) Hematopoietic response after treatment with cyclophosphamide and autotransplantation of non-damaged bone marrow cells. Acta Biol Med Ger 33:35–41
427. Niskanen E (1967) Bone marrow cell proliferation after busulphan treatment and its relation to humoral control mechanisms. Acta Pathol Microbiol Scand [Suppl 190] 70
428. Niskanen E, Rytömaa T, Kivilaakso E (1971) Reversion of the inhibitory effect of busulphan on bone marrow cell proliferation, by chlorambucil. Acta Pathol Microbiol Scand [A] 79:102–108
429. Nissen-Meyer R, Host H (1960) A comparison between the haematological side effects of cyclophosphamide and nitrogen mustard. Cancer Chemother Rep 9:51–55
430. Northup JD, Bull JM, Carbone PP (1972) Proliferative activity of human granulocytes, as estimated quantitatively by in vitro colony formation. J Natl Cancer Inst 48:629–637
430a. Nowrousian MR, Schaefer UW, Oehl S, Boecker WR, Schmidt CG (1980) Effekte der zytostatischen Langzeitchemotherapie mit Bleomycin auf die Hämatopoese (Abstr). Blut 41:320
431. Nye RN (1931) Bone marrow volume in rabbits. Proc Soc Exp Biol Med 29:34–37
432. O'Connell RA (1970) Leukocytosis during lithium carbonate treatment. Int J Pharmacopsychiatry 4:30–34
433. O'Donnell JF, McKoy WS, Makuch RW, Bull JM (1979) Increased in vitro toxicity to mouse bone marrow with 1,3-(2-chloroethyl)-1-nitrosourea and hyperthermia. Cancer Res 39:2547–2549

434. Ogawa M, Bergsagel DE, McCulloch EA (1971) Differential effects of melphalan on mouse myeloma (adj. PC-5) and hemopoietic stem cells. Cancer Res 31: 2116–2119
435. Ogawa M, Bergsagel DE, McCulloch EA (1973) Chemotherapy of mouse myeloma: Quantitative cell cultures predictive of response in vivo. Blood 41: 7–15
436. Ogawa M, Bergsagel DE, McCulloch EA (1973) Sensitivity of human and murine hemopoietic precursor cells to chemotherapeutic agents assessed in cell culture. Blood 42: 851–856
437. Ogawa M, Gale GR, Keirn SS (1975) Effect of cis-diamminedichloroplatinum (NSC 119875) on murine and human hemopoietic precursor cells. Cancer Res 35: 1398–1401
438. Old LJ, Clarke DA, Benacerraf B (1959) Effect of bacillus Calmette-Guérin (BCG) infection on transplanted tumours in the mouse. Nature 184: 291–292
439. Oliverio VT (1976) Pharmacology of the nitrosoureas: An overview. Cancer Treat Rep 60: 703–707
440. Osband M, Cohen H, Cassady JR, Faffe N (1977) Severe and protracted bone marrow dysfunction following long-term therapy with methyl-CCNU. Proc Am Ass Cancer Res 18: 303
441. Page PL, Cook PA, Greenberg HM, Hartwell BL, Robinson SH (1978) Cytotoxic reduction of murine marrow stem cells and subsequent recovery (Abstr.) Exp Hematol [Suppl 3] 6: 68
441a. Page PL, Gerson SL, Hartwell BL, Robinson SH (1978) Chemotherapy-induced alterations in proliferative capacity of marrow stem cells (Abstr.) Clin Res 26: 537A
442. Panasci LC, Fox PA, Schein PS (1977) Structure-activity studies of methylnitrosourea antitumor agents with reduced bone marrow toxicity. Cancer Res 37: 3321–3328
443. Panasci LC, Green D, Schein PS (1979) Chlorozotocin. Mechanism of reduced bone marrow toxicity in mice. J Clin Invest 64: 1103–1111
444. Pannacciulli I, Bogliolo G, Massa G, Ronco D, Fresco G, Saviane A, Dolocino G, Celle G (1975) Ricerca sperimentale sui rapporti tra attivazione eritropoietica ed emotossicità di alcuni antiblastici. Tumori 61: 179–198
445. Pannacciulli I, Ghio R, Bigliolo G, Massa G, Saviane A, Bianchi G (1976) Cellule staminali emopoietiche ed antiblastici. 1. Variazioni delle cellule formatrici die colonie in vivo e in vitro dopo somministrazione in dose singola di ciclofosfamide, vinblastina e azatioprina. Haematologica 61: 433–448
446. Pannacciulli IM, Massa G, Saviane AG, Bianchi G, Bogliolo GV, Ghio R (1977) The effects of chronic administration of cyclophosphamide on haemopoietic stem cells. Scand J Haematol 19: 217–223
447. Papac RJ (1968) Clinical and hematologic studies with 1-β-D-arabinosylcytosine. J Natl Cancer Inst 40: 997–1002
448. Parker LM, Hirst M, Israel M (1978) N-Trifluoroacetyladriamycin-14-valerate. Additional mouse antitumor and toxicity studies. Cancer Treat Rep 62: 119–127
449. Parmentier C, Droz JP, Tubiana M (1978) Ways of expressing results of human bone marrow progenitor cell culture. Br J Haematol 40: 105–109
450. Parmentier C, Maraninchi D, Morardet N, Droz JP (1978) Observations on the distribution of granulocytic progenitor cells (CFU-C) in human bone marrow: The importance of the manner in which the results of in vitro cultures are reported. Br J Haematol 40: 353–354
451. Patt HM (1957) A consideration of myeloid-erythroid balance in man. Blood 12: 777–787
452. Patt HM, Maloney MA (1972) Relationship of bone marrow cellularity and proliferative activity: A local regulatory mechanism. Cell Tissue Kinet 5: 303–309
453. Pegg DE (1963) The hematological side effects of cyclophosphamide and a discussion of autologous bone marrow grafting after cancer chemotherapy. Cancer Chemother Rep 27: 39–44

454. Perez C, Sutow WW, Wang YM, Herson J (1979) Evaluation of overall toxicity of high-dosage methotrexate regimens. Med Pediatr Oncol 6: 219–228
455. Philips FS, Sternberg SS, Schwartz HS, Cronin AP, Sodergren JE, Vidal PM (1967) Hydroxyurea. I. Acute cell death in proliferating tissues in rats. Cancer Res 27: 61–74
456. Pike BL, Robinson WA (1970) Human bone marrow colony growth in agar gel. J Cell Physiol 76: 77–84
457. Pinedo HM, Zaharko DS, Bull J, Chabner BA (1977) The relative contribution of drug concentration and duration of exposure to mouse bone marrow toxicity during continuous methotrexate infusion. Cancer Res 37: 445–450
458. Pinedo HM, Zaharko DS, Bull JM, Chabner BA (1976) The reversal of methotrexate cytotoxicity to mouse bone marrow cells by leucovorin and nucleosides. Cancer Res 36: 4418–4428
459. Pinedo HM, Zaharko DS, Chabner BA, Bull J (1976) Evidence for early recruitment of granulocyte precursors during high-dose methotrexate infusion in mice. Blood 48: 301–307
460. Pliess G, Fassbender D (1961) Die Wirkung subletaler Dosen Endoxan auf die Hämopoese der Ratte. Arzneim Forschung 11: 179–188
461. Pluznik DH, Sachs L (1965) The cloning of normal mast cells in tissue culture. J Cell Comp Physiol 66: 319–324
462. Porteous DD, Lajtha LG (1966) On stem-cell recovery after irradiation. Br J Haematol 12: 177–188
463. Pouillart P, Palangie T, Schwarzenberg L, Brugerie H, Lhéritier J, Mathé G (1976) Effect of BCG on hematopoietic stem cells: Experimental and clinical study. Cancer Immunol Immunother 1: 163–169
464. Powles RL (1976) Immunotherapy in the management of acute leukaemia. Br J Haematol 32: 145–149
465. Preisler HD, Henderson ES (1972) Effect of suppression of erythropoiesis on hematopoietic stem cells in the mouse. J Cell Physiol 79: 103–110
466. Preisler HD, Henderson ES (1971) Effect of cytosine arabinoside and 1,3-bis(2-chloroethyl)-1-nitrosourea on hematopoietic precursors in the mouse. J Natl Cancer Inst 47: 971–977
467. Quesenberry PJ, Morley A, Miller M, Rickard K, Howard D, Stohlman F Jr (1973) Effect of endotoxin on granulopoiesis and the in vitro colony-forming cell. Blood 41: 391–398
468. Quesenberry PJ, Morley A, Ryan M, Howard D, Stohlman F Jr (1973) The effect of endotoxin on murine stem cells. J Cell Physiol 82: 239–244
469. Quesenberry P, Morley A, Stohlman F Jr, Rickard K, Howard D, Smith M (1972) Effect of endotoxin on granulopoiesis and colony-stimulating factor. N Engl J Med 286: 227–232
470. Quesenberry P, Zuckerman K, Ryan M, Stohlman F Jr (1977) A dichotomy between the release of bone marrow granulocytes and stem cells. Proc Soc Exp Biol Med 154: 53–56
471. Radley JM, Scurfield G (1979) Effects of 5-fluorouracil on mouse bone marrow. Br J Haematol 43: 341–351
472. Ragab AH, Gilkerson E, Myers M (1974) The effect of 6-mercaptopurine and allopurinol on granulopoiesis. Cancer Res 34: 2246–2249
473. Ragab AH, Gilkerson E, Myers M, Choi SC (1974) The culture of colony-forming units from the peripheral blood and bone marrow of children with acute lymphocytic leukemia. Cancer 34: 663–669
474. Randolph VL, Wittes RE (1978) Weekly administration of cis-diamminedichloroplatinum (II) without hydration or osmotic diuresis. Eur J Cancer 14: 753–756

475. Razek A, Valeriote F, Vietti T (1972) Survival of hemopoietic and leukemic colony-forming cells in vivo following the administration of daunorubicin or adriamycin. Cancer Res 32: 1496–1500
476. Reimer RR, Hoover R, Fraumeni JF, Young RC (1977) Acute leukemia after alkylating-agent therapy of ovarian cancer. N Engl J Med 297: 177–180
477. Reissmann K, Ito K (1966) Selective eradication of erythropoiesis by actinomycin D as a result of interference with hormonally controlled effector pathway of cell differentiation. Blood 28: 201–212
478. Reissmann K, Samorapoompichit S (1969) Effect of erythropoietin on regeneration of hematopoietic stem cell after 5-fluorouracil administration. J Lab Clin Med 73: 544–550
479. Reissmann KR, Samorapoompichit S (1970) Effect of erythropoietin on proliferation of erythroid stem cells in the absence of transplantable colony-forming units. Blood 36: 287–296
480. Reissmann KR, Udupa KB (1972) Effect of erythropoietin on proliferation of erythropoietin-responsive cells. Cell Tissue Kinet 5: 481–489
481. Reissmann KR, Udupa KB, Kawada K (1974) Effects of erythropoietin and androgens on erythroid stem cells after their selective suppression by BCNU. Blood 44: 649–657
482. Reissmann K, Udupa KB, Okamura H (1970) Effect of endotoxin on normal and 5-fluorouracil-suppressed hemopoietic stem cells. J Lab Clin Med 76: 652–658
483. Rich IN, Heit W, Kubanek B (1980) The effect of actinomycin D on hemopoiesis. I. Short-term effects. Blut 41: 29–40
484. Richman CM, Weiner RS, Yankee RA (1976) Increase in circulating stem cells following chemotherapy in man. Blood 47: 1031–1039
485. Rickard KA, Morley A, Howard D, Stohlman F Jr (1971) The in vitro colony-forming cell and the response to neutropenia. Blood 37: 6–22
486. Rickard KA, Shadduck RK, Howard DE, Stohlman F Jr (1970) A differential effect of hydroxyurea on hemopoietic stem cell colonies in vitro and in vivo. Proc Soc Exp Biol Med 134: 152–156
487. Rizzoli V, Jacobs S, Butturini U (1978) Selectivity in rescue of high-dose methotrexate. In: Periti P (ed) High-dose methotrexate: Pharmacology, toxicology, and chemotherapy. Editrice Giuntina, Florence (Chemioterapia Oncologica, Supplemento dicembre) pp 71–84
488. Robinson WA, Mangalik A (1975) The kinetics and regulation of granulopoiesis. Semin Hematol 12: 7–25
489. Rojas AF, Mickiewicz E, Feierstein JN, Glait H, Olivari AJ (1976) Levamisole in advanced human breast cancer. Lancet 1: 211–215
490. Rosenberg B, Van Camp L, Krigas T (1965) Inhibition of cell division in Escherichia coli by electrolysis products from a platinum electrode. Nature 205: 698–699
491. Rosenblum ML, Reynolds AF, Smith KA, Rumack BH, Walker MD (1973) Chloroethyl-cyclohexyl-nitrosourea (CCNU) in the treatment of malignant brain tumors. J Neurosurg 39: 306–314
492. Rosendaal M, Hodgson GS, Bradley TR (1979) Organisation of haemopoietic stem cells: The generation-age hypothesis. Cell Tissue Kinet 12: 17–29
493. Rosenoff SH, Bull JM, Young RC (1975) The effect of chemotherapy on the kinetics and proliferative capacity of normal and tumorous tissues in vivo. Blood 45: 107–118
494. Rosenhoff SH, Bostick F, Young RC (1975) Recovery of normal hematopoietic tissue and tumor following chemotherapeutic injury from cyclophosphamide (CTX): Comparative analysis of biochemical and clinical techniques. Blood 45: 465–475
495. Rossof AH, Slayton RE, Perlia CP (1972) Preliminary clinical experience with cis-diamminodichloroplatinum (II) Cancer 30: 1451–1456
496. Rothstein G, Clarkson DR, Larsen W, Grosser BI, Athens JW (1978) Effect of lithium on neutrophil mass and production. N Engl J Med 298: 178–180

497. Salasoo S, Freedman A (1978) Prevention of methotrexate toxicity: Effect of infusion rate on clearance. In: Periti (ed) High-dose methotrexate: Pharmacology, toxicology, and chemotherapy. Editrice Giuntina, Firenze (Chemoterapia oncologica Supplemento dicembre) 1978, pp 163–172
498. Santelli G (1977) Potentiation of 5-fluorouracil cytotoxicity by thymidine against leukemia cells. Proc Am Assoc Cancer Res and Amer Soc Clin Oncol 18: 148
499. Santelli G, Valeriote F (1978) In vivo enhancement of 5-fluorouracil cytotoxicity to AKR leukemia cells by thymidine in mice. J Natl Cancer Inst 61: 843–847
500. Santos GW, Tutschka PJ (1974) Marrow transplantation in the busulfan-treated rat: Preclinical model of aplastic anemia. J Natl Cancer Inst 53: 1781–1785
501. Saviane A, Massa G, Bogliolo G, Pannacciulli I (1976) L'azione die antiblastia ciclo-spezifici e non ciclo spezifici scelle CFU emopoietiche del topo depo salasso. Boll Soc Ital Biol Sper 52: 465–468
502. Scaro JL, Alvarez Prado de Tombolesi AR, Guidi EE (1970) Effect of actinomycin D on the erythropoietic restoring capacity of mouse bone marrow cells. Acta physiol Lat Am 20: 265–270
503. Scaro JL, Rendo MEB, De Tombolesi ARAP (1972) Hematopoietic recovery after a single high dose of cyclophosphamide in the mouse. Acta physiol Lat Am 22: 258–265
504. Scaro JL, Rendo ME, Buys MC, Zenteno A (1973) Studies on hemopoietic stem cell kinetics after a single high dose of actinomycin D (AM), cyclophosphamide (CY) and busulphan (BU) in the mouse. Acta physiol Lat Am 23: 548–550
505. Schaefer UW, Nowrousian MR, Öhl S, Boecker WR, Scheulen ME, Schilcher B, Schmidt CG (1980) Autologous bone marrow transplantation. The influence of prolonged cytotoxic chemotherapy. In: Thierfelder S, Rodt H, Kolb HJ (eds) Immunobiology of bone marrow transplantation. Springer, Berlin Heidelberg New York, pp 275–283
506. Schaeppi U, Heyman IA, Fleischman RW, Rosenkrantz H, Ilievski V, Phelan R, Cooney DA, Davis RD (1973) cis-Dichlorammineplatinum (II) (NSC-119875): Preclinical toxicologic evaluation of intravenous injection in dogs, monkeys, and mice. Toxicol Appl Pharmacol 25: 230–241
507. Schein PS, Winokur SH (1975) Immunosuppressive and cytotoxic chemotherapy: Long-term complications. Ann Intern Med 82: 84–95
508. Schein PS, Bull JM, Doukas D, Hoth D (1978) Sensitivity of human and murine hematopoietic precursor cells to 2-[3-(2-chloroethyl)-3-nitrosoureido]-D-glucopyranose and 1,3-bis(2-chloroethyl)-1-nitrosourea. Cancer Res 38: 257–260
509. Schick P, Trepel F, Begemann H (1968) Morphologische und funktionelle Veränderungen im Blutzellsystem des Meerschweinchens nach Behandlung mit cytostatischen Substanzen, Prednisolon und Phenylbutazon. Z Gesamte Exp Med 148: 275–305
510. Schneider R (1962) Vergleichende Untersuchungen über die Wirksamkeit einiger Zytostatika und der Röntgenbestrahlung. Strahlentherapie 119: 104–110
511. Schneider R (1965) Beitrag zur Wirkungsweise einiger Zytostatika und ionisierender Strahlen. 1. Teil: Morphologische und funktionelle Untersuchungen von Knochenmark und Milz normaler Inzuchtratten ohne Impftumoren. Strahlentherapie 126: 213–235
512. Schofield R (1978) The relationship between the spleen colony-forming cell and the haemopoietic stem cell. A hypothesis. Blood Cells 4: 7–25
513. Schreml W, Betzler M, Lang M, Lohrmann H-P, Kubitza P, Schlag P, Flad H-D, Herfarth Ch, Heimpel H (1980) Adjuvant intermittent chemo-immuno-therapy of breast cancer. In: Mouridsen HT, Palshof T (eds) Breast cancer, experimental and clinical aspects. Pergamon Press, Oxford New York, pp 165–168
514. Schreml W, Bock O, Bock E, Heit W, Kubanek B (1974) Different action of suicidal doses of tritiated thymidine and hydroxyurea on murine haemopoietic cells. Cell Tissue Kinet 7: 517–527
515. Schreml W, Lohrmann H-P (1979) No effects of levamisole on cytotoxic drug-induced changes of human granulopoiesis. Blut 38: 331–336

516. Schreml W, Lohrmann H-P (1979) Effect of high-dose methotrexate with citrovorum factor on human granulopoiesis. Cancer Res 39: 4195–4199
517. Schreml W, Lohrmann H-P (1979) Hematotoxicity of adjuvant therapy. In: Jones SE, Salmon SE (eds) Adjuvant therapy of cancer II. Grune & Stratton, New York, pp 63–70
517a. Schreml W, Lohrmann H-P (1981) Effect of two nitrosoureas (methyl-CCNU, BCNU) with 5-fluorouracil upon the human granulopoietic system. In: Serrou B, Schein PS, Imbach J-L (eds) Nitrosoureas in Cancer Treatment. Elsevier/North Holland, Amsterdam, p 207–213
518. Schubert JCF, Fischer M, Hilbert L (1969) Erfahrungen mit „ultrahohen" Cyclophosphamid-Dosen an 42 Kranken mit soliden und lymphoretikulären Tumoren. Dtsch Med Wochenschr 94: 2583–2592
519. Schutt AJ, Hahn RG, Reitemeier RJ, Moertel CG (1973) A phase 2 study of intermittent high-dose cyclophosphamide therapy of advanced gastrointestinal cancer. Cancer Res 33: 2218–2220
520. Schwartz PM, Dunigan JM, Marsh JC, Handschumacher RE (1980) Allopurinol modification of the toxicity and antitumor activity of 5-fluorouracil. Cancer Res 40: 1885–1889
521. Scott MT (1974) Corynebacterium parvum as an immunotherapeutic anti-cancer agent. Semin Oncol 1: 367–378
522. Seidel HJ (1977) Hematologic effects of a single dose of methylnitrosourea. Exp Hematol 5: 19–26
523. Seidel HJ, Kreja L (1980) Erythroid stem cell regeneration in normal and plethoric mice treated by cytosinarabinoside. Exp Hematol 8: 541–548
524. Seidel H-J, Opitz U (1979) Effect of actinomycin D and busulphan on stem cells in normal and Friend virus-infected mice. Blut 38: 349–360
525. Seidel H-J, Opitz U (1979) Hematopoietic stem cells in Friend murine leukemia virus-infected mice undergoing chemotherapy: Remission and relapse of erythropoietin-indepedent erythropoiesis induced by hydroxyurea. J Natl Cancer Inst 62: 531–536
526. Seidel H-J, Opitz U (1979) Erythroid stem cell regeneration in normal and plethoric mice treated with hydroxyurea. Exp Hematol 7: 500–508
527. Seifert P, Baker LH, Reed ML, Vaitkevicius VK (1975) Comparison of continuously infused 5-fluorouracil with bolus injection in treatment of patients with colorectal adenocarcinoma. Cancer 36: 123–128
528. Senn JS, McCulloch EA (1970) Kinetics of regeneration after cyclophosphamide in human marrow assessed by a cell culture method (Abstr). Exp Hematol 20: 8–9
529. Sensenbrenner LL, Owens AH (1967) The effects of mechlorethamine on bone marrow function and iron metabolism in man. Hopkins Med J 121: 162–174
530. Sensenbrenner LL, Owens AH Jr, Zawatzsky LS, Elfenbein G (1972) The comparative effects of selected cytotoxic agents on transplanted hematopoietic cells. Transplantation 14: 347–351
531. Sensenbrenner LL, Owens AH, Heiby JR, Jeejeebhoy HF (1973) Comparative effects of cytotoxic agents on transplanted hematopoietic and antibody-producing cells. J Natl Cancer Inst 50: 1027–1033
532. Sensenbrenner LL, Marini JJ, Colvin M (1979) Comparative effects of cyclophosphamide, isophosphamide, 4-methylcyclophosphamide, and phosphoramide mustard on murine hematopoietic and immunocompetent cells. J Natl Cancer Inst 62: 975–981
533. Sharp JG, Thomas DB (1971) The effects of mustine hydrochloride on the colony-forming units of murine bone marrow. Acta Haematol 46: 271–274
534. Sharp JG, Thomas DB, Briscoe CV (1973) Effects of mustine hydrochloride on mouse haematopoietic and lymphoid tissues. Chemotherapy 18: 304–313

535. Sharp JG, Thomas DB, Briscoe CV, Littlewood V (1975) Prolonged effects of nitrogen mustard on mouse haemotopoietic and lymphoid tissues. Scand J Haematol 14: 313–319
536. Shnider BI, Gold GL, Hall T, Dederick M, Nevinny HB, Potee KG, Lasagna L, Owens AH, Hreschyshyn M, Selawry O, Holland JF, Jones R, Colsky J, Franzino A, Zubrod GG, Frei E, Brindley C (1960) Preliminary studies with cyclophosphamide. Cancer Chemother Rep 8: 102–111
537. Shopsin B, Friedmann R, Gershon S (1971) Lithium and leukocytosis. Clin Pharmacol Ther 12: 923–928
538. Sieber SM, Adamson RH (1975) Toxicity of antineoplastic agents in man: Chromosomal aberrations, antifertility effects, congenital malformations, and carcinogenic potential. Adv Cancer Res 22: 57–155
539. Silini G, Elli R, Siracusa G, Pozzi LV (1968) Repopulation of the bone-marrow stem-cell compartment after irradiation. Cell Tissue Kinet 1: 111–122
540. Simpson HW, Stoney PJ (1977) A circadian variation of melphalan (L-phenylalanine nitrogen mustard) toxicity to murine bone marrow: Relevance to cancer treatment protocols. Br J Haematol 35: 459–464
540a. Sinclair WK (1965) Hydroxyurea: Differential lethal effects on cultured mammalian cells during the cell cycle. Science 150: 1729–1731
541. Sladek NE (1973) Bioassay and relative cytotoxic potency of cyclophosphamide metabolites generated in vitro and in vivo. Cancer Res 33: 1150–1158
542. Smart CR, Townsend LB, Rusho WJ, Eyre HJ, Quagliana JM, Wilson ML, Edwards CB, Mannings SJ (1975) Phase I study of ftorafur, an analog of 5-fluorouracil. Cancer 36: 103–106
543. Smith LH, Clayton ML (1970) Distribution of injected ^{59}Fe in mice. Exp Hematol 20: 82–86
544. Smith WW, Wilson SM (1967) Effects of vinblastine and vincristine on survival and hemopoiesis in irradiated mice. J Natl Cancer Inst 39: 1055–1066
545. Smith WW, Wilson SM (1970) Persistence of radiation damage: Hemopoietic effects in irradiated mice treated with actinomycin D. In: Stohlman F Jr (ed) Hemopoietic cellular proliferation. Grune & Stratton, New York, p 49–55
546. Smith WW, Alderman IM, Cornfield J (1961) Granulocyte release by endotoxin in normal and irradiated mice. Am J Physiol 201: 396–402
547. Smith WW, Brecher G, Fred S, Budd RA (1966) Effect of endotoxin on the kinetics of hemopoietic colony-forming cells in irradiated mice. Radiat Res 27: 710–717
548. Smith WW, Wilson SM, Fred SS (1968) Kinetics of stem cell depletion and proliferation: Effects of vinblastine and vincristine in normal and irradiated mice. J Natl Cancer Inst 40: 847–854
549. Smith JP, Rutledge FN, Delclos L (1975) Postoperative treatment of early cancer of the ovary: A random trial between postoperative irradiation and chemotherapy. Natl Cancer Inst Monogr 42: 149–153
549a. Spiro TE, Mattelaer M-A, Efira A, Stryckmans P (1981) Sensitivity of myeloid progenitor cells in healthy subjects and patients with chronic myeloid leukemia to chemotherapeutic agents. J Natl Cancer Inst 66: 1053–1059
550. Spitz S (1948) The histological changes of nitrogen mustards on human tumors and tissues. Cancer 1: 383–398
551. Spitzer G, Verma DS, Barlogie B, Beran MA, Dicke KA (1979) Possible mechanisms of action of lithium on augmentation of in vitro spontaneous myeloid colony formation. Cancer Res 39: 3215–3219
552. Spurr CL, Jacobson LO, Smith TR, Guzman Barron ES (1943) The clinical application of a nitrogen mustard compound methyl-bis-(β-chloroethyl)-amine to the treatment of neoplastic disorders of the hemopoietic system. Cancer Res 7: 51–52
553. Squires DJP, Lamerton LF (1975) The effect of various cytotoxic agents on bone marrow progenitor cells as measured by diffusion chamber assays. Br J Haematol 29: 31–42

554. Stalzer RC, Kiely JM, Pease GL, Brown AL Jr (1965) Effect of 5-fluorouracil on human hematopoiesis. Cancer 18: 1071–1078
555. Standen G, Philip MA, Fletcher J (1980) The proliferative state of granulocytic progenitor cells in human blood and marrow. Cell Tissue Kinet 13: 105–113
556. Stein RS, Beaman C, Ali MY, Hansen R, Jenkins DD, Jume'an HG (1977) Lithium carbonate attenuation of chemotherapy-induced neutropenia. N Engl J Med 297: 430–431
557. Stein RS, Hanson G, Koethe S, Hansen R (1977) An in vivo evaluation of lithium-induced granulocytosis. Blood [Suppl 1] 50: 161
558. Stein RS, Hanson G, Koethe S, Hansen R (1978) Lithium-induced granulocytosis. Ann Intern Med 88: 809–810
559. Stein RS, Flexner JM, Graber SE (1979) Lithium and granulocytopenia during induction therapy of acute myelogenous leukemia. Blood 54: 636–641
560. Steinbach KH, Schick P, Trepel F, Raffler H, Döhrmann J, Heilgeist G, Heltzel W, Li K, Past W, van der Woerd-de-Lange JA, Theml H, Fliedner TM, Begemann H (1979) Estimation of kinetic parameters of neutrophilic, eosinophilic, and basophilic granulocytes in human blood. Blut 39: 27–38
560a. Steinbach KH, Raffler H, Pabst G, Fliedner TM (1980) A mathematical model of canine granulocytopoiesis. J Math Biol 10: 1–12
561. Stevens EE, Dicke KA (1976) Bone marrow transfusion in mice treated with BCNU. Proc Am Assoc Cancer Res 17: 57
562. Stohlman F Jr, Quesenberry P, Niskanen E, Morley A, Tyler W, Rickard K, Symann M, Monette F, Howard D (1973) Control of granulopoiesis. In: Haemopoietic stem cells (Ciba Foundation Symposium 13). Elsevier Excerpta Medica/North Holland, Amsterdam London New York, pp 205–219
563. Stohlman F Jr, Quesenberry PJ, Tyler WS (1973) The regulation of myelopoiesis as approached with in vivo and in vitro techniques. Prog Hematol 8: 259–297
564. Stolinsky DC, Pugh RP, Bateman JR (1975) 5-Fluorouracil therapy for pancreatic carcinoma: Comparison of oral and intravenous route. Cancer Chemother Rep 59: 1031–1033
565. Stoller RG, Kenneth RH, Jacobs SA, Rosenberg SA, Chabner BA (1977) Use of plasma pharmacokinetics to predict and prevent methotrexate toxicity. N Engl J Med 297: 630–634
566. Stoller RG, Kaplan HG, Cummings FJ, Calabresi P (1979) A clinical and pharmacological study of high-dose methotrexate with minimal leucovorin rescue. Cancer Res 39: 908–912
567. Storb R, Buckner CD, Dillingham LA, Thomas ED (1970) Cyclophosphamide regimens in rhesus monkeys with and without marrow infusion. Cancer Res 30: 2195–2203
568. Straw JA, Talbot DC, Tailor GA, Harrap KR (1977) Some observations on the reversibility of methotrexate toxicity in normal proliferative tissue. J Natl Cancer Inst 58: 91–97
569. Suit HD (1957) A technique for estimating the bone marrow cellularity in vivo using ^{59}Fe. J Clin Pathol 10: 267–269
570. Svoboda V (1974) Distribution of colony-forming cells in mouse bone marrow. Acta Haematol 51: 113–120
571. Symoens J (1977) Levamisole, an antianergic chemotherapeutic agent: An overview. In: Chirigos M (ed) Control of neoplasia by modulation of the immune system. Raven, New York
572. Symoens J, Veys E, Mielants M, Pinals R (1978) Adverse reactions to levamisole. Cancer Treat Rep 62: 1721–1730
573. Szmigielski S, Jeljaszewicz J (1976) Inhibition of normal granulopoiesis by cytostatic agents. Folia Haematol (Leipz) 103: 678–685
574. Taketa ST, Carsten AL, Cohn SH, Atkins HL, Bond VP (1970) Active bone marrow distribution in the monkey. Life Sci 9: 169–174

575. Talbot TR, Elson LA (1958) Protection of august rats against lethal doses of a dimethyl homologue of myleran by isologous bone marrow. Nature 181: 684–686
576. Talley RW, Vaitkevicius VK (1963) Megaloblastosis produced by a cytosine antagonist, 1-β-D-arabinofuranosylcytosine. Blood 21: 352–362
577. Talley RW, O'Bryan RM, Tucker WG, Loo RV (1967) Clinical pharmacology and human antitumor activity of cytosine arabinoside. Cancer 20: 809–816
578. Talley RW, O'Bryan RM, Gutterman JU, Brownlee RW, McCredie KB (1973) Clinical evaluation of cis-diamminedichloroplatinum (NSC-119875): Phase I clinical study. Cancer Chemother Rep 57: 465–471
579. Tanaka T, Craig AW, Lajtha LG (1970) A kinetic study on murine myeloid leukaemia. Br J Cancer 24: 138–148
580. Terasima T, Takabe Y, Katsumata T, Watanabe M, Umezawa H (1972) Effect of bleomycin on mammalian cell survival. J Natl Cancer Inst 49: 1093–1100
581. Terry WD (1978) Concluding remarks. In: Terry WD, Windhorst D (eds) Immunotherapy of cancer: Present states of trials in man. Raven, New York, pp 669–671
582. Thiersch JB (1949) Bone marrow changes in man after treatment with aminopterin, amethopterin, and aminoanfol. Cancer 2: 877–883
583. Thomas DB, Briscoe CV (1973) The effects of intravenous injections of endotoxin on the distribution of cells between murine blood and bone marrow. J Anat 114: 407–419
584. Thomas ED, Fliedner TM, Thomas D, Cronkite EP (1965) The problem of the stem cell: Observations in dogs following nitrogen mustard. J Lab Clin Med 65: 794–803
585. Thompson HS, Gale GR (1971) cis-Dichlordiammineplatinum (II): Hematopoietic effects in rats. Toxicol Appl Pharmacol 19: 602–609
586. Till JE (1976) Regulation of hemopoietic stem cells. In: Cairnie AB, Lala PK, Osmond DG (eds) Stem cells of renewing cell populations. Academic Press, New York, pp 143–155
587. Till JE, McCulloch EA (1961) A direct measurement of the radiation sensitivity of normal mouse bone marrow cells. Radiat Res 14: 213–222
588. Tisman G, Herbert V, Rosenblatt S (1973) Evidence that lithium induces human granulocyte proliferation: Elevated serum vitamin B_{12} binding capacity in vivo and granulocyte colony proliferation in vitro. Br J Haematol 24: 767–771
589. Torelli U (1977) An overlooked aspect of the mechanism of action of most antineoplastic drugs: The inhibition of macromolecular RNA metabolism. Eur J Cancer 13: 1363–1368
590. Trainor KJ, Morley AA (1976) Screening of cytotoxic drugs for residual bone marrow damage. J Natl Cancer Inst 57: 1237–1239
591. Trainor KJ, Seshadri RS, Morley AA (1979) Residual marrow injury following cytotoxic drugs. Leuk Res 3: 205–210
592. Trainor KJ, Morley AA, Seshardi RS (1980) A proliferative defect of marrow cells in experimental chronic hypoplastic marrow failure (aplastic anaemia). Exp Hematol 8: 674–682
593. Trouet A, Deperez-De Champeneere D, de Duve C (1972) Chemotherapy through lysosomes with a DNA-daunomycin complex. Nature (New Biol) 239: 110–112
594. Trouet A, Deperez-De Champeneere D, de Smedt-Malengreaux M, Atassi G (1974) Experimental leukemia chemotherapy with a "lysosomotropic" adriamycin-DNA complex. Eur J Cancer 10: 405–411
595. Twentyman PR (1972) Leucocyte response to bacterial endotoxin in mice pre-treated with cytotoxic agents. Br J Haematol 23: 69–78
596. Twentyman PR, Bleehen NM (1973) The sensitivity to bleomycin of spleen colony-forming units in the mouse. Br J Cancer 28: 66–70
597. Udupa KB, Reissmann KR (1974) Acceleration of granulopoietic recovery by androgenic steroids in mice made neutropenic by cytotoxic drugs. Cancer Res 34: 2517–2520

598. Udupa KB, Reissmann KR (1979) In vivo erythropoietin requirements of regenerating erythroid progenitors (BFU-e, CFU-e) in bone marrow of mice. Blood 53: 1164–1171
599. Udupa KB, Okamura H, Reissmann KR (1972) Granulopoiesis during myleran-induced suppression of transplantable hematopoietic stem cells. Blood 39: 317–325
600. Ujj G, Kovács P, Hernádi F (1979) In vitro estimation of the proliferative state of murine bone marrow colony forming units in culture (CFU-C) with hydroxyurea (HU). Biomedicine 31: 61–62
601. Urabe A, Asano S, Sato N, Chiba S, Kosaka K, Chiyoda S, Mizoguchi H, Miura Y, Takaku F (1976) Recovery of bone marrow precursor cells after administration of cytosine arabinoside in mice. 16th Congr Int Soc Hematol, Kyoto 1976 (Abstr 0–14)
602. Uyeki EM, Pazdernik TL, El Askar A (1976) Toxicity of antitumor agents on hemopoietic colony-forming cells. J Pharmacol Exp Ther 198: 246–253
603. Vaitkevicius VK, Talley RW, Tucker JL, Brennan MJ (1962) Cytological and clinical observations during Vincaleukoblastine therapy of disseminated cancer. Cancer 15: 294–306
604. Valdivieso M, Bodey GP, Gottlieb JA, Freireich EJ (1976) Clinical evaluation of ftorafur (pyrimidine-deoxyribose-N_1-2-furanidyl-5-fluorouracil). Cancer Res 36: 1821–1824
605. Valeriote FA, Bruce WR (1967) Comparison of the sensitivity of hematopoietic colony-forming cells in different proliferative states to vinblastine. J Natl Cancer Inst 38: 393–399
606. Valeriote FA, Tolen SJ (1972) Survival of hematopoietic and lymphoma colony-forming cells in vivo following the administration of a variety of alkylating agents. Cancer Res 32: 470–476
607. Valeriote FA, Van Putten L (1975) Proliferation-dependent cytotoxicity of anticancer agents: A review. Cancer Res 35: 2619–2630
608. Valeriote FA, Bruce WR, Meeker BE (1966) Comparison of the sensitivity of normal hematopoietic and transplanted lymphoma colony-forming cells of mice to vinblastine administered in vivo. J Natl Cancer Inst 36: 21–27
609. Valeriote FA, Collins DC, Bruce WR (1968) Hematological recovery in the mouse following single doses of gamma-radiation and cyclophosphamide. Radiat Res 33: 501–511
610. Valeriote F, Vietti T, Tolen S (1973) Kinetics of the lethal effect of actinomycin D on normal and leukemic cells. Cancer Res 33: 2658–2661
611. Valeriote F, Vietti T, Edelstein M (1976) Combined effect of cytosine arabinoside and thiopurines. Cancer Treat Rep 60: 1925–1934
612. Valeriote FA, Vietti T, Coulter D (1980), Cytotoxicity of adriamycin combined with methotrexate against L1210 leukemia in mice. J Natl Cancer Inst 64: 801–805
613. Van Putten LM (1974) Are cell kinetic data relevant for the design of tumor chemotherapy schedules? Cell Tissue Kinet 7: 493–504
614. Van Putten LM, Lelieveld P (1970) Factors determining cell killing by chemotherapeutic agents in vivo. I. Cyclophosphamide. Eur J Cancer 6: 313–321
615. Van Putten LM, Lelieveld P (1971) Factors determining cell killing by chemotherapeutic agents in vivo. II. Melphalan, chlorambucil and nitrogen mustard. Eur J Cancer 7: 11–16
616. Van Putten LM, Lelieveld P, Kram-Idsenga LKJ (1972) Cell-cycle specificity and therapeutic effectiveness of cytostatic agents. Cancer Chemother Rep, Part 1 56: 691–700
617. Van Putten LM, Lelieveld P, Kram-Idsenga LKJ (1973) Abhängigkeit der Wirksamkeit phasenspezifischer Zytostatika vom Zellzyklus: Interpretation von Dosis-Wirkungskurven. In: Wüst G (ed) Aktuelle Probleme der Therapie maligner Tumoren. Thieme, Stuttgart, pp 197–208

618. Van Putten LM, Kram-Idsenga LKJ, Pijpers-de-Bruin M (1974) A comparison of the cell killing in the mouse after exposure to ftorafur and to 5-fluorouracil. Br J Cancer 30: 179–180
619. Vassort F, Frindel E, Tubiana M (1971) Effects of hydroxyurea on the kinetics of colony-forming units of bone marrow in the mouse. Cell Tissue Kinet 4: 423–431
620. Vassort F, Winterholer M, Frindel E, Tubiana M (1973) Kinetic parameters of bone marrow stem cells using in vivo suicide by tritiated thymidine or by hydroxyurea. Blood 41: 789–796
621. Vecchi A, Fioretti M, Mantovani A, Barzi A, Spreafico F (1976) The immunosuppressive and hematotoxic activity of imidazole-4-carboxamide, 5-(3,3-dimethyl-1-triazeno) in mice. Transplantation 22: 619–624
622. Vodopick H, Hamilton HE, Jackson HL, Peng CT, Sheets RF (1969) Metabolic fate of tritiated busulfan in man. J Lab Clin Med 73: 266–276
623. Vogel CL, Lipscomb DL, Silverman DA, Kerns AL, Mansell PW, Sugarbaker EU (1976) Levamisole granulocytopenia in patients receiving an adjuvant chemoimmunotherapy program after surgery for breast carcinoma with axillary lymph node involvement. Cancer Treat Rep 62: 1587–1589
624. Vogel JM, Kimball HR, Wolff SM, Perry S (1967) Etiocholanolone in the evaluation of marrow reserves in patients receiving cytotoxic agents. Ann Intern Med 67: 1226–1238
625. Vogel SJ, Presant CA, Ratkin GA, Klahr C (1979) Phase I study of thymidine plus 5-fluorouracil infusions in advanced colorectal carcinoma. Cancer Treat Rep 63: 1–5
626. Vogler WR, Mingioli ES, Garwood FA (1973) The effect of methotrexate on granulocytic stem cells and granulopoiesis. Cancer Res 33: 1628–1633
627. Vogler WR, Mingioli ES, Garwood FA (1972) Granulopoietic stem cell regulators in murine urine: Alterations in activity after methotrexate. J Lab Clin Med 79: 379–387
628. Vos O (1972) Multiplication of haemopoietic colony-forming units (CFU) in mice after X-irradiation and bone marrow transplantation. Cell Tissue Kinet 5: 341–350
629. Vos O, Buurman WA, Ploemacher RE (1972) Mobilization of haemopoietic stem cells (CFU) into the peripheral blood of the mouse: Effects of endotoxin and other compounds. Cell Tissue Kinet 5: 467–479
629a. Wagemaker G, Visser TP (1980) Erythropoietin-independent regeneration of erythroid progenitor cells following multiple injections of hydroxyurea. Cell Tissue Kinet 13: 505–517
629b. Wagemaker G, Peters MF, Bol SJL (1979) Induction of erythropoietin responsiveness in vitro by a distinct population of bone marrow cells. Cell Tissue Kinet 12: 521–537
630. Wagner DE, Ramirez G, Weiss AJ, Hill G Jr (1971) Combination phase I–II study of imidazole carboxamide (NCS 45388). Oncology 26: 310–316
631. Walker RI, Herion JC, Palmer JG (1962) Leukocyte kinetics studied by nitrogen mustard-induced alterations in DNA phosphorus labeling. Blood 20: 72–76
632. Wallace HJ Jr, Higby DJ (1974) Phase I evaluation of cis-platinum(II)diamminedichloride (PDD) and a combination of PDD plus adriamycin. In: Connors TA, Roberts JJ (eds) Platinum coordination complexes in cancer chemotherapy. Springer, Berlin Heidelberg New York. Recent Results in Cancer Research, vol 48, pp 167–177
633. Ward HWC (1978) Central nervous system tumors of childhood treated with CCNU, vincristine, and radiation. Med Pediatr Oncol 4: 315–320
634. Weiner RS, Richman CM, Yankee RA, Parker L (1979) Clinical results of autotransplantation after nitrosourea therapy. Exp Hematol [Suppl 5] 7: 384–388
635. Wendling F, Tambourin P, Moreau-Gachelin F (1978) Incapacity of hematopoietic stem cell-deprived mice to produce tumor colonies induced by Friend virus-infected cells. Exp Hematol 6: 777–784

636. Werner W, Haller M, Höpfner V, Küchler J, Ziervogel J (1971) Verlauf der hämatotoxischen Cyclophosphamidwirkung bei der Ratte. Exp Pathol (Jena) 5: 123–127
637. Wheeler AG, Dansby D, Hawkins HC, Payne HG, Weikel JH (1962) A toxicologic and hematologic evaluation of cyclophosphamide (cytoxan) in experimental animals. Toxicol Appl Pharmacol 4: 324–343
638. White FR (1959) New agent data summaries: Cytoxan. Cancer Chemother Rep 2: 21–25
639. Wodinsky I, Swiniarski J, Kensler CJ (1967) Spleen colony studies of leukemia L1210. II. Differential sensitivities of normal and leukemic bone marrow colony-forming cells to single- and divided-dose therapy with cytosine arabinoside (NSC-63878). Cancer Chemother Rep 51: 423–429
640. Wolmark N, Fisher B (1974) The effect of a single and repeated administration of Corynebacterium parvum on bone marrow macrophage colony production in syngeneic tumor-bearing mice. Cancer Res 34: 2869–2872
641. Worton RG, McCulloch EA, Till JE (1969) Physical separation of hemopoietic stem cells from cells forming colonies in culture. J Cell Physiol 74: 171–182
642. Wu C-T, Lajtha LG (1975) Hemopoietic stem cell kinetics during continuous radiation. Int J Radiat Biol 27: 41–50
643. Yagoda A, Watson RC, Gonzalez-Vitale JC, Grabstald H, Whitmore WF (1976) cis-Dichlordiammineplatinum (II) in advanced bladder cancer. Cancer Treat Rep 60: 917–923
644. Yoffey JM (1973) Stem cell role of the lymphocyte-transitional cell (LT) compartment. In: Haemopoietic stem cells. Elsevier/Excerpta Medica/North Holland, Amsterdam London New York (CIBA Foundation Symposium 13, pp 5–39)
645. Young RC, deVita VT (1970) The effect of chemotherapy on the growth characteristics and cellular kinetics of leukemia L1210. Cancer Res 30: 1789–1794
646. Young RG, Walker MD, Canellos GP, Schein PS, Chabner BA, deVita VT (1973) Initial clinical trials with methyl-CCNU, 1-(2-chloroethyl)-3-(4-methylcyclohexyl)-1-nitrosourea (MeCCNU). Cancer 31: 1164–1169
647. Zuckerman KS, Sullivan R, Quesenberry PJ (1978) Effects of actinomycin D in vivo on murine erythroid stem cells. Blood 51: 957–969

Subject Index

Recent Results in Cancer Research

Sponsored by the Swiss League against Cancer. Editor in Chief: P. Rentchnick, Genève

For information about Vols. 1–9, please contact your bookseller of Springer-Verlag

10 NELSON, R. S.: Radioactive Phosphorus in the Diagnosis of Gastrointestinal Cancer.
11 FREEMAN, R. G. and J. M. KNOX: Treatment of Skin Cancer.
12 LYNCH, H. T.: Hereditary Factors in Carcinoma.
13 Tumours in Children, 2nd Edition. Edited by H. B. MARSDEN and J. K. STEWARD.
14 ODARTCHENKO, N.: Production Cellulaire Erythropoïétique.
15 SOKOLOFF, B.: Carcinoid and Serotonin.
16 JACOBS, M. L.: Malignant Lymphomas and Their Management.
17 Normal and Malignant Cell Growth. Edited by R. J. M. FRY, M. L. GRIEM, and W. H. KIRSTEN (Symposium).
18 ANGLESIO, E.: The Treatment of Hodgkin's Disease.
19 BANNASCH, P.: The Cytoplasm of Hepatocytes during Carcinogenesis. Electron- and Lightmicroscopical Investigations of the Nitrosomorpholineintoxicated Rat Liver.
20 Rubidomycin. A new Agent against Cancer. Edited by J. BERNARD, R. PAUL, M. BOIRON, C. JACQUILLAT, and R. MARAL.
21 Scientific Basis of Cancer Chemotherapy. Edited by G. MATHÉ (Symposium).
22 KOLDOVSKÝ, P.: Tumor Specific Transplantation Antigen.
23 FUCHS, W. A., J. W. DAVIDSON, and H. W. FISCHER: Lymphography in Cancer. With contributions by G. JANTET AND H. RÖSLER.
24 HAYWARD, J.: Hormones und Human Breast Cancer. An Account of 15 Years Study.
25 ROY-BURMAN, P.: Analogues of Nucleic Acid Components. Mechanisms of Action.
26 Tumors of the Liver. Edited by G. T. PACK and A. H. ISLAMI.
27 SZYMENDERA, J.: Bone Mineral Metabolism in Cancer.
28 MEEK, E. S.: Antitumour and Antiviral Substances of Natural Origin.
29 Aseptic Environments and Cancer Treatment. Edited by G. MATHÉ (Symposium).
30 Advances in the Treatment of Acute (Blastic) Leukemias. Edited by G. MATHÉ (Symposium).
31 DENOIX, P.: Treatment of Malignant Breast Tumors. Indications and Results.
32 NELSON, R. S.: Endoscopy in Gastric Cancer.
33 Experimental and Clinical Effects of L-Asparaginase. Edited by E. GRUNDMANN and H. F. OETTGEN (Symposium).
34 Chemistry and Biological Actions of 4-Nitroquinolin 1-Oxide. Edited by H. ENDO, T. ONO, and T. SUGIMURA.
35 PENN, I.: Malignant Tumors in Organ Transplant Recipients.
36 Current Concepts in the Management of Lymphoma and Leukemia. Edited by J. E. ULTMANN, M. L. GRIEM, W. H. KIRSTEN, and R. W. WISSLER (Symposium).
37 CHIAPPA, S., R. MUSUMECI, and C. USLENGHI: Endolymphatic Radiotherapy in Malignant Lymphomas. With contributions by G. BONADONNA, B. DAMASCELLI, G. FAVA, F. PIZZETTI, U. VERONESI.
38 KOLLER, P. C.: The Role of Chromosomes in Cancer Biology.
39 Current Problems in the Epidemiology of Cancer and Lymphomas. Edited by E. GRUNDMANN and H. TULINIUS (Symposium).
40 LANGLEY, F. A. and A. C. CROMPTON: Epithelial Abnormalities of the Cervix Uteri.
41 Tumours in a Tropical Country. A Survey of Uganda (1964–1968). Edited by A. C. TEMPLETON.
42 Breast Cancer: A Challenging Problem. Edited by M. L. GRIEM, E. V. JENSEN, J. E. ULTMANN, and R. W. WISSLER (Symposium).
43 Nomenclature, Methodology and Results of Clinical Trials in Acute Leukemias. Edited by G. MATHÉ, P. POUILLART, L. SCHWARZENBERG (Symposium).
44 Special Topics in Carcinogenesis. Edited by E. GRUNDMANN (Symposium).
45 KOLDOVSKÝ, P.: Carcinoembryonic Antigens.
46 Diagnosis and Therapy of Malignant Lymphoma. Edited by K. MUSSHOFF (Symposium).
47 Investigation and Stimulation of Immunity in Cancer Patients. Edited by G. MATHÉ and R. WEINER (Symposium).
48 Platinum Coordination Complexes in Cancer Chemotherapy. Edited by T. A. CONNORS and J. J. ROBERTS (Symposium).
49 Complications of Cancer Chemotherapy. Edited by G. MATHÉ and R. K. OLDHAM (Symposium).
50 Cancer Registry, Edited by E. GRUNDMANN and E. PEDERSEN (Symposium).
51 Gliomas. Current Concepts in Biology, Diagnosis and Therapy. Edited by J. HEKMATPANAH (Symposium).

52 The Ambivalence of Cytostatic Therapy. Edited by E. GRUNDMANN and R. GROSS (Symposium).

53 A. CLARYSSE, Y. KENIS, and G. MATHÉ: Cancer Chemotherapy.

54 Malignant Bone Tumors. Edited by E. GRUNDMANN.

55 MATHÉ, G.: Cancer Active Immunotherapy, Immunoprophylaxis, and Immunorestoration.

56 Lymphocytes, Macrophages, and Cancer. Edited by G. MATHÉ, I. FLORENTIN, and M.-C. SIMMLER (Symposium).

57 Breast Cancer: A Multidisciplinary Approach. Edited by G. ST. ARNEAULT, P. BAND, and L. ISRAËL (Symposium).

58 B. S. SCHOENBERG: Multiple Primary Malignant Neoplasms.

59 Selective Heat Sensitivity of Cancer Cells. Edited by A. ROSSI-FANELLI, R. CAVALIERE, B. MONDOVI, and G. MORICCA.

60 Tumors of the Male Genital System. Edited by E. GRUNDMANN and W. VAHLENSIECK (Symposium).

61 D. METCALF: Hemopoietic Colonies.

62 Tactics and Strategy in Cancer Treatment. Edited by G. MATHÉ (Symposium).

63 Antitumor Antibiotics. Edited by S. K. CARTER, H. UMEZAWA, J. DOUROS, and Y. SAKURAI (Symposium).

64 Lymphoid Neoplasias I: Classification, Categorization, Natural History.

65 Lymphoid Neoplasias II: Clinical and Therapeutic Aspects.
Lymphoid Neoplasias I & II. Proceedings of the 1977 CNRS-EORTC International Colloquium. Editors: G. MATHÉ, M. SELIGMANN, M. TUBIANA. Devided into two volumes.

66 Carcinogenic Hormones. Edited by C. H. LINGEMAN.

67/68 Adjuvant Therapies and Markers of Post-Surgical Minimal Residual Disease I & II. Proceedings of the 1978 Annual Plenary Meeting of the EORTC. Editors: G. BONADONNA, G. MATHÉ, S. E. SALMON. Divided into two volumes.

67 Markers and General Problems of Cancer Adjuvant Therapies.

68 Adjuvant Therapies of the Various Primary Tumors.

69 Strategies in Clinical Hematology. Edited by R. GROSS and K.-P. HELLRIEGEL.

70 New Anticancer Drugs. Edited by S. K. CARTER

71 Endocrine Treatment of Breast Cancer. Edited by B. HENNINGSEN, F. LINDER, C. STREICHELE.

72 CAWLEY, J. C., BURNS, G. F., HAYHOE, F. G. J.: Hairy-Cell Leukaemia.

73 Thyroid Cancer. Edited by W. DUNCAN.

74 Cancer Chemo- and Immunopharmacology. 1. Chemopharmacology. Edited by G. MATHÉ and F. M. MUGGIA.

75 Cancer Chemo- and Immunopharmacology. 2. Immunopharmacology, Relations and General Problems. Edited by G. MATHÉ and F. M. MUGGIA.

76 New Drugs in Cancer Chemotherapy. Edited by S. K. CARTER, Y. SAKURAI, H. UMEZAWA

77 K. STANLEY, J. STJERNSWÄRD, M. ISLEY: The Conduct of a Cooperative Clinical Trial.

78 Prostate Cancer. Edited by W. DUNCAN.

79 Chemotherapy and Radiotherapy of Gastrointestinal Tumors. Edited by H. O. KLEIN.

80 Adjuvant Therapies of Cancer. Edited by G. MATHÉ, G. BONADONNA, S. SALMON.

81 H. P. LOHRMANN and W. SCHREML: Cytotoxic Drugs and the Granulopoietic System.

MIX
Papier aus verantwortungsvollen Quellen
Paper from responsible sources
FSC® C105338

If you have any concerns about our products,
you can contact us on
ProductSafety@springernature.com

In case Publisher is established outside the EU,
the EU authorized representative is:
Springer Nature Customer Service Center GmbH
Europaplatz 3, 69115 Heidelberg, Germany

Printed by Libri Plureos GmbH
in Hamburg, Germany